Assessing
Clinical Competence

Victor R. Neufeld, M.D., FRCP(C)
Geoffrey R. Norman, Ph.D.
Editors

Foreword by William B. Spaulding,
M.D., FRCP(C), FACP

SPRINGER PUBLISHING COMPANY
New York

Springer Publishing Co.
536 Broadway
New York, N.Y. 10012

88 89 / 10 9 8 7 6 5 4 3

Library of Congress Cataloging in Publication Data

Main entry under title:
Assessing clinical competence.
    (Springer series on medical education ; v. 7)
    Includes bibliographies and index.
    1. Medicine—Ability testing. 2. Medicine, Clinical—Ability testing.
I. Neufeld, Vic. II. Norman, Geoffrey R. III. Series: Springer series on medical education ; 7. [DNLM: 1. Clinical Competence. 2. Educational Measurement—methods.
W1 SP685SE v. 7 / W 18 A834]
R837.A2A86 1984   610'.76   84-10555
ISBN 0-8261-3330-4

Printed in the United States of America

To John C. Sibley, M.D. (1923-1981)

Jack Sibley was a consultant internist who practiced in the Hamilton community for 30 years. In 1968, he joined the Faculty of Health Sciences at McMaster University where he was an insightful and effective clinical teacher; his strongest educational technique was the quality of his own clinical practice. His research contribution was in the assessment of the quality of patient care. He was preparing a chapter on this subject when he died unexpectedly on August 4, 1981.

We dedicate this book to the memory of Jack Sibley—friend, researcher, educator, and competent clinician.

Contents

Foreword   xi
> *William B. Spaulding*

Contributors   xiii

Acknowledgments   xvii

Part I: Introduction and Definitions of Competence   1

1.   Historical Perspectives on Clinical Competence   3
> *Victor R. Neufeld*

2.   Defining Competence: A Methodological Review   15
> *Geoffrey R. Norman*

Part II: Methods   37

3.   An Introduction to Measurement Properties   39
> *Victor R. Neufeld*

4.   Direct Observation   51
> *Jacqueline Wakefield*

5.   Oral Examinations   71
> *Linda J. Muzzin and Lawrence Hart*

6. Written Examinations   94
   Victor R. Neufeld

7. Global Rating Scales   119
   David L. Streiner

8. Medical Record Review   142
   Peter Tugwell and Caroline Dok

9. Patient Management Problems   183
   John W. Feightner

10. Computer Simulations   201
    Geoffrey R. Norman and Catherine Painvin

11. Simulated Patients   219
    Geoffrey R. Norman, Howard S. Barrows,
    Gayle Gliva, and Christel Woodward

Part III: Applications   231

12. Evaluation of the Doctor-Patient Relationship   233
    Christel Woodward and Brian Gerrard

13. Assessment of Technical Skills   259
    John Watts and William B. Feldman

14. Assessment of the Use of Diagnostic Tests   275
    R. Brian Haynes, David L. Sackett, and Peter Tugwell

Part IV: Implications   295

15. Implications for Education   297
    Victor R. Neufeld

16. Implications for Licensure and Certification   311
    C. Barber Mueller

17. Implications for Research   330
    Geoffrey R. Norman

18. Implications for Health Care   342
    J. Fraser Mustard

Index   353

Foreword

Every medical school strives to select the good student and reject the bad, amplify the goodness, and graduate individuals who will be competent doctors. Some people, including even a few medical educators, think that judging accurately a doctor's performance presents no problems. Ask patients whether they have a good doctor and the answer is likely to be prompt and clear-cut. They respond as if they know. But get behind the general concept, try to analyze, define, measure, and compare—then the difficulties arise. In less sophisticated days, medical educators believed they knew what they were talking about. Assumptions were more often accepted than questioned. If an able student (i.e., with good marks) from a respectable family applied to medical school, the Dean was pleased to approve admission with the hope that the student would pass the medical school and the licensing examinations, thereby providing society with another good doctor. If this graduate avoided being found guilty of malpractice, then no questions were asked about clinical competence, indeed the phrase rarely cropped up. Nowadays the term, with its solid, satisfying ring, is heard frequently whenever medical educators or members of certifying boards get together. Employed uncritically the words may create the illusion that medical educators know what they mean by clinical competence, are able to recognize competence when they see it, can measure it, grade it, and take appropriate steps to ensure that competent clinicians stay that way. But of course the truth is very different.

As this book convincingly demonstrates, the way toward understanding and evaluating clinical competence is beset with more traps and pitfalls than the uninitiated would ever imagine. All along the path lie semantic snares and methodological delusions, so well hidden that before you know it, national medical organizations have approved mandatory recertification oblivious of the fact that the full spectrum of clinical competence still needs to be defined in detail, proven measurable, and then shown to have a positive relationship to the well-being of patients. For the interested amateur, which includes most physicians and health educators, this book should provide an effective, sobering, and educational antidote to naive enthusiasms.

Sir Peter Medawar in his discussion of scientific discovery entitled "The Art of the Soluble"[1] emphasized that the scientific method can be applied successfully only to problems for which scientists have already mastered the necessary concepts and investigative techniques. Questions posed too soon elude answers which may be revealed to investigators of a later time. Have we reached the time for fruitful research into clinical competence? Many fervently hope so because it makes such good sense to ensure that doctors begin their careers clinically competent and remain so. Even if the key concepts and research approaches are at hand, this book shows how much shrewdly planned and sheer hard work lies ahead before the profession can confidently assure the public that all practitioners are clinically competent.

Each essayist who is included in this volume has contributed personally to the understanding and measurement of clinical competence by reviewing and critically analyzing the literature. The varied approaches and viewpoints help to provide a clearer comprehension of this complex topic, which must continue to be addressed in efforts to improve medical care.

William B. Spaulding, M.D., FRCP(C), FACP
Professor of Medicine
Faculty of Health Sciences
McMaster University

[1]P. B. Medawar. *The Art of the Soluble.* Methuen & Co. Ltd., London, 1967.

Contributors

Howard S. Barrows is a neurologist and innovator in education. From 1971 to 1981 he held a number of leadership positions in medical education at McMaster. He is presently Dean, Education Affairs, at Southern Illinois University School of Medicine, Springfield, Illinois.

Caroline Dok received her M.Sc. in Epidemiology and Health from McGill University. She has been a research associate in the Department of Clinical Epidemiology and Biostatistics at McMaster since 1979. As a result of belonging to a research group in continuing medical education, she has developed an interest in assessing the efficacy of various educational interventions. Methodological issues involved in the assessment of quality of care constitute another of her prime interests.

John W. Feightner is a family physician at McMaster. He completed a residency in Family Medicine at McMaster in 1972 and joined the faculty in the same year. He has maintained a major interest in clinical evaluation and research in clinical problem-solving in addition to continuing teaching responsibilities at the undergraduate and postgraduate level. He is presently completing a degree in Design, Measurement, and Evaluation at McMaster.

William B. Feldman is a pediatrician and educator. He was professor of pediatrics at McMaster from 1970 to 1981. During these years he was responsible for the residency program in pediatrics and was chief examiner for the Royal College. He has also conducted a number of epidemiological studies of children and recently took up a position as professor of pediatrics and community medicine and epidemiology at the University of Ottawa.

Brian Gerrard holds doctoral degrees in both psychology and evaluation. For several years he was the director of a major research project at McMaster in the area of continuing education. He has a major interest in communications between patients and health professionals and has studied and written on this topic. He is currently on the faculty at the University of Guelph, Ontario.

Gayle Gliva is a research assistant in the Program for Educational Development at McMaster. She has herself been a simulated patient and is the coordinator of the Simulated Patient Program in the Faculty of Health Sciences.

R. Brian Haynes is an internist, epidemiologist, and educator. He recently became Director of the Program for Educational Development at McMaster. Prior to assuming this responsibility he chaired the Masters Program in Design, Measurement, and Evaluation. In addition to his educational interests, he has had continuing research interests in patient compliance, use of laboratory tests, and dissemination and use of available knowledge by health professionals.

Lawrence Hart is a senior resident in internal medicine and rheumatology as well as a graduate student in research methodology. As a medical student in South Africa, he became interested in new methods of medical education, an interest that brought him to Hamilton, Ontario, Canada. His research interests include the measurement of clinical competence and the assessment of observer variation in the clinical examination.

C. Barber Mueller is a surgeon and educator. He was one of the original faculty at McMaster. In addition to his teaching and clinical activities, he has been an active consultant to licensing and certification bodies in both Canada and the United States for many years.

J. Fraser Mustard was until recently the Vice-President of McMaster's Faculty of Health Sciences. He is widely known for his biomedical research in the area of thromboembolism and arteriosclerosis. He has been increasingly involved in considerations of health and health care both regionally and nationally.

Linda J. Muzzin is currently a research associate in the Program for Educational Development and a graduate student in the Department of Sociology at McMaster. She received her M.A. in Experimental Psychology in 1972 and has held various research positions in psychiatry, sociology, and administration since that time.

Catherine Painvin is a physician and epidemiologist. Trained in France, she spent several years in the Office of Medical Education at Laval University before coming to McMaster in 1978. She is presently continuing her career in medical education at the University of Western Ontario, London.

David L. Sackett is an epidemiologist and internist. Internationally known for his research in clinical epidemiology, he has also made major contributions to McMaster's education and research programs. He was the founding chairman of the Department of Clinical Epidemiology and Biostatistics and is currently the chairman of the clinical clerkship year in the Undergraduate M.D. Program.

William B. Spaulding is a general internist and a founder of the McMaster medical school. In addition to his major contribution to the medical school, he has been active in many medical organizations at the local, national, and international levels. He has recently been the Vice-President of the American College of Physicians.

David L. Streiner is a clinical psychologist and professor in the Department of Psychiatry and in Clinical Epidemiology and Biostatistics at McMaster. In addition to his clinical activities, he has conducted extensive research in psychiatry and has pursued applications of computers and statistics to medicine.

Peter Tugwell is Professor and Chairman of the Department of Clinical Epidemiology and Biostatistics at McMaster. He is a rheumatologist and epidemiologist by training, but has had a continuing major interest in medical education, particularly in the use of the medical record to assess clinical skills and quality of care.

Jacqueline Wakefield is a professor in the Department of Family Medicine at McMaster. She is the Director of the Family Medicine Residency Program. She has had a long-standing research interest in the evaluation of the physician-patient encounter by direct observation.

John Watts is a pediatrician originally from Britain, who is now the Director of a busy neonatal intensive care unit. He has been involved in various educational activities at McMaster, including the development of learning resources.

Christel Woodward is a psychologist and a member of the Department of Clinical Epidemiology and Biostatistics and the Department of Psychiatry at McMaster. She has also had a major role in the Program for Educational Development with responsibility for follow-up studies of McMaster graduates. Her interests include assessment of the quality of the doctor-patient relationship and health services research.

Acknowledgments

When we began this book, it seemed like a straight-forward task. However, true to tradition, our naive estimates of the amount of time and energy required to complete the task at hand were well off the mark. Now that the book is complete, we must acknowledge a tremendous debt to the contributors, who individually invested many hours of research and writing time to complete this useful and critical review of the topic.

In addition, there are many unsung heroes who assisted us in editing, typing, and correcting the numerous drafts. These include Linda Muzzin, who provided major editorial help in addition to contributing a chapter; Morag Horsman, who had major responsibility for typing the texts; Lee Fielding, who mastered some complex computer programs in order to enter and revise the extensive bibliography; and Liza Thong, who spent endless hours ensuring that the figures and tables were accurate and understandable. Finally, we thank the Program for Educational Development at McMaster for providing financial support, and the staff of the Computation Services Unit for assisting with word processing and providing free computer services when the funds ran low.

To all involved, a sincere thanks.

PART I

Introduction and Definitions of Competence

This section introduces the reader to the reasons for writing this book. The first chapter traces three historical perspectives that have been concerned with clinical competence. These are the influence of the profession, the perspective of society, and the impact of research and development. These three "force fields" converge to raise important questions about our current understanding of clinical competence, how we measure it, and how we apply our understanding. The chapter closes with a brief description of the scope and style of the book.

In Chapter 2, we review various approaches that have been used to come to an understanding of what is meant by clinical competence. Several distinct perspectives are presented. These include the "armchair" approaches, task analysis and other formalized methods used by specialty boards and licensing examinations, and the indirect viewpoint on competence provided by a variety of research methods—epidemiological, psychological, and quality of care.

CHAPTER 1

Historical Perspectives on Clinical Competence

VICTOR R. NEUFELD

Clinical competence is a battered child: a child because it is a relatively new area of interest, with most of the research and development having been done in the past 10 to 15 years; battered because it has been mistreated by researchers, who cannot agree on what it is and how to measure it. Consider these examples of confusion about clinical competence:

Ask any number of clinical educators or professional groups to define the term *clinical competence* and somewhat different responses will be obtained from each of them. Until recently, there has been little attempt to study what a clinician actually does, and it is even rarer to find performance assessment procedures which are systematically based on new insights into clinical methods.

Measures of clinical competence have been described in the literature which appear to have been adopted prematurely, without the benefit of step-by-step methodological development. In some cases, the measures are in the early "pilot project" stage or are simply untested ideas.

Systems and institutions have arisen outside of the medical profession, each of which are concerned with some aspect of clinical competence. These responsibilities may include the selection of applicants to a particular training program, the program itself, and the licensing, certification, or recertification of individual physicians. Frequently, the boundaries of responsibility are unclear. More importantly, it is unusual for questions such as these to be asked: Is the system working? What is the evidence that an intended result is being achieved? Given a particular approach, how does it compare with a more standard or alternate regimen?

This book aims to clarify some of these issues. Primarily, it is written for clinical educators—the people in academic institutions and other professional organizations who are the *users* of the research on clinical competence. The book should also be useful to methodologists who are *doing* the research in this area.

Historical Perspectives

For many decades, the medical profession has struggled with the question of competence. The motivation to do so has come from a variety of sources. Three of the most important are the influence of the profession itself; the influence of society; and the influence of research and development. These three are interrelated and overlap to some extent. We shall first look at them separately, and then examine the combined effects of these "force fields" on the profession at the present time.

The Influence of the Profession

The medical profession, through its various institutions, has used a number of different strategies to assure the competence of clinicians. A recent book (Samph and Templeton, 1979) reviews the role of various American professional and government institutions in assuring competence. While this panorama of involved groups is perhaps more complicated in the United States than in other countries, a similar pattern could be described in Canada, Great Britain, and other countries of the world. Some of these patterns will be described later in the book.

In general terms, the profession has used three strategies to produce competent clinicians: the accreditation process, the licensing and certification process, and specific training programs.

The Accreditation Process. The earliest approach used in North America, accreditation was based on the assumption that if the setting in which physicians are trained met acceptable standards, then the performance of the individual professionals should be acceptable. The American Medical Association as early as 1905 devised a rating system consisting of a number of categories for assessing medical schools. Since those early days, the accreditation process has become vastly more complex and has spread along the "continuum of medical education" to include post-graduate (residency training) programs, then lately extending into programs in continuing medical education.

Paralleling the accreditation of training programs has been the accreditation of health care institutions, particularly hospitals, but also ambulatory care settings. Now called "quality assurance," this activity, particularly in the United States, has swollen into a large and complicated bureaucracy, stimulated by the legislation which gave rise to the Professional Standards Review Organizations (PSRO), and is having a significant impact on the struggle to understand clinical competence.

From a methodological point of view, the question could be asked: What is the evidence that the accreditation process, in its various forms, assures the competence of *individual* clinicians; and does it have any significant effect on health outcomes? The evidence to date is not particularly encouraging.

Licensing and Certification. The second strategy used by the profession to assure clinical competence is that of licensing and certification, focusing on the performance of the individual practitioner in contrast to that of an institution. The history of the process in the United States is well described by Derbyshire (in Samph and Templeton, 1979). It is a fascinating story. There has been much change from the time, a number of decades ago, when senior retired clinicians on state medical boards grilled candidates with archaic questions ("describe mercury inunction"), to the current use of computer-marked comprehensive multiple-choice examinations.

The certification story is similar. From virtually no standards other than some sort of acceptable apprenticeship, there has been a steady evolution to prescribed training programs and structured certification examinations. This trend is influenced by the phenomenon of increasing subspecialization. The American Board of Medical Specialties, for example, now consists of 23 separate boards, each with its own approach to certification. The Royal College of Physicians and Surgeons of Canada has 36 individually recognized medical and surgical specialties. Over the years, each specialty group has come to define the required training, usually stated in terms of a prescribed number of years and rotations, but rarely in terms of performance objectives.

There is a wide range in the format of certification examinations. Some are simple, using only multiple-choice examinations. Some are complex; an example is the certification examination of the Canadian College of Family Physicians, which includes written examinations, simulated patients, and simulated "office orals" in which the examiner is himself a patient, married to an equally complicated scoring system. An additional recent development in Canada is the use of institutional reports from residency program directors to contribute directly to the certification decision (Valberg and Firstbrook, 1977).

Finally, there is the phenomenon of relicensure and recertification. Virtually every group within the profession of medicine has in the last few years wrestled with the issue of assuring continuing competence of individual practitioners. The strategies employed range from encouragement to attend continuing education events through to mandatory recertification and relicensure. The methods proposed for the latter again are wide ranging, from self-assessed office medical records to computer-based patient management problems.

Again questions need to be asked from the methodological perspective: Which competencies are being tested in today's examination for licensure and certification? Is it generally agreed that they are the most important? How good are the measures employed? Is there any evidence that the increasingly complex machinery for relicensure and recertification has any actual influence on the continuing competence of a physician? Do our current certification procedures discriminate accurately—that is, do they pass the sufficiently competent, but hold back those that are not ready for independent practice?

Training Programs. The third strategy employed by the profession to assure competence is the structured educational process itself. We have already referred to the accreditation of institutions, which attempts to ensure a basic level of quality in a training program. Several components of an education program can affect the development of competence in individual trainees, including the selection system, the curriculum itself, and the evaluation system.

Medical schools in North America (and, to some extent, residency programs) are in a luxury situation. There are many more candidates than places, currently about three candidates per place. Many of the unsuccessful applicants are probably quite acceptable and may eventually become adequate physicians. It has been observed that important qualities required for successful completion of a training program and for professional practice are already present in applicants to medical school. Given this situation, an opportunity exists for devising selection methods and procedures which will most optimally match an applicant's ability and interest with the style and objective of a particular training program and eventually with the demands and opportunities of a professional practice. In the interests of educating future physicians well, there should be an optimal match between candidates and programs.

A curriculum is designed to prepare a certain kind of "product." The term *curriculum* usually encompasses the formal or structured learning experiences of students—the lectures, laboratories, clinical tutorials and seminars, elective experiences, and direct participation in patient care under supervision. There is also considerable evidence that the "informal curriculum" is important in shaping future professionals. These informal factors include interaction with peers, unplanned and often unrecognized "role modeling" of supervising residents and attending physicians, unobtrusive influences of the medical school as a social entity, the personal and family demands on an individual, and the general social climate of the time (Funkenstein, 1977).

Of the many components of a training program, perhaps none is quite as influential as the manner in which student performance is assessed. Generations of medical students have discovered that the "bottom line" of getting through medical school involves understanding the evaluation system and complying with the behavior pattern that it demands. It is in the evaluation system that the "real" objectives of any program are displayed, and the truly important values become apparent.

These considerations again suggest a number of questions: To what extent does a training program in fact influence the eventual performance of a clinician? Which component is the most important: the selection system, the structure of the curriculum, the "informal" learning environment, or the evaluation system? To what extent does each of these components relate to educational objectives, explicit or implicit? And do the objectives of a training program reflect the range of competencies required in actual professional life?

The Influence of Society

Modern society exerts an influence on its professions through formal mechanisms and through informal influences, such as the general climate in which potential physicians grow up, including the level of public awareness about health and disease. Examples of formal mechanisms are specific laws and policies governing professional behavior and the legal arrangements reflected in malpractice suits.

Formal Mechanisms. The legal statements which define the limits of professional responsibility tend to be "responsive"; that is, they formalize a system which is already in place. It is unlikely that they have a direct influence on the performance of individual practitioners.

Perhaps more influential are government policies that relate to "cost containment" and to "quality assurance." A current example is the PSRO legislation in the United States where a large and complicated bureaucracy has been constructed, aimed at controlling hospital costs through the application of guidelines on duration of hospital stay. A recent Canadian example involves the government of Ontario. In an attempt to control costs, the Ministry of Health has declared maximum hospital bed ratios per given population and is actually involved in closing down some smaller hospitals. In many countries, the government participates directly in medical insurance, resulting in a direct influence on physician fee structures and salary levels. This level of participation in the health system has a direct effect on what individual physicians and groups of physicians actually do in professional practice.

Another formal mechanism that influences physican performance is the malpractice phenomenon, prominent in the United States, where the legal tradition differs somewhat from that of Canada and Western Europe. Large sums of money are paid by American physicians for malpractice insurance, and the clinical behavior of physicians is directly influenced by the spectre of malpractice. This is evident in the practice of "protective medicine"—for example, the excessive ordering of laboratory and radiological investigations in an emergency room.

Informal Mechanisms. Related to the malpractice situation is the widely accepted observation that the public is more interested in and knowledgeable about health and disease. Patients, quite appropriately, demand explanations about an illness, its prognosis, investigation, and treatment. Further, we wish to participate in our own health management—a concept that expresses itself in various ways: self-health manuals, participation by partners in childbirth, holistic health clinics, consumer participation in health councils, and the proclamation of statements of patient rights. For the individual practitioner, this means spending more time on patient education and involving the patient and his family more in direct health care activities.

The recently published studies of Funkenstein and his colleagues (1977) report on the perception and career choices of Harvard medical students over a 20-year period, incorporating five social eras, and show that the values and to some extent the career choices of the graduates were influenced by the prevailing social environment.

These formal and informal influences that affect the practice situation and individual professional activity present for methodologists a number of challenges. For example, can reliable and valid methods be developed to select students who represent the social spectrum of society? To what extent do the factors influence physician performance? Can some of them be measured, and can physician behavior be altered in a way that makes health care less costly but still effective?

The Influence of Research and Development

A third stream of influence on the performance of clinicians is research and technological development, as seen in the availability of sophisticated technology to practicing physicians and in the rise of new fields of research which relate to clinical competence. Some of its facets will be described briefly.

Virtually every physician is affected by the availability of increasingly sophisticated technology. Through automated blood testing systems, laboratory results which were not ordered are frequently brought to the physician's attention. They are answers to unasked questions, which, in turn, lead to new questions; and these new questions frequently are unrelated to the patient's initial illness. Another example of rapidly advancing technology is represented in diagnostic imaging. Consider the available tests in a large hospital for investigating a suspected pancreatic mass.

Which devices should be used and in what sequence—a barium meal, angiography, or whole-body computerized tomography? The answers are by no means clear to practicing physicians.

A different example is the use of the computer in testing. Computers have been used for storing and retrieving multiple-choice questions (the so-called item bank); computers are also used increasingly as a basis for simulating clinical thinking. Probably the very availability of the technology was the main reason for developing the simulations, rather than any compelling logic to use a computer for purposes such as this.

There has been an increased interest in research in medical education. In the United States, this interest dates back approximately 20 years, when educational researchers joined faculties of medicine and other medical professional organizations. Stimulated by the desire to enhance teaching and evaluation, specific methodological techniques were applied to the area of clinical competence. There was also an increased awareness of concepts of educational measurement such as validity (in its various forms), reliability, and objectivity, which were used to examine existing methods of assessing competence and to design new assessment tools.

A related research area might be called "health care research," a broad and heterogeneous area of investigation which includes the work of clinical epidemiologists, operations researchers, health economists, and biostatisticians. Much of this work is focused on the problem of developing health outcome measures and applying these measures to the pursuit of specific health care questions. The progress that has occurred in the "quality assurance" movement is attributable mainly to the work of this group of researchers. Both health care research and educational research have had a profound influence on definition and measurement of competence. These areas form the basis for the remainder of this book.

A Convergence of Forces

In this review of three "force fields" influencing clinical competence over the past two decades, we have discussed the activities of the profession itself, the less direct influence of society, and the influence of research and technological development. All have their effect on the clinical activity of an individual practitioner. These three developments appear now to be converging, producing much of the urgency and some of the confusion about our current understanding of clinical competence. Here are some examples:

In its concern for demonstrating to the public that physicians are competent, the profession has started down the path of recertification and relicensure. In some jurisdictions, these concepts have been taken to the stage of government mandate. But from a methodological point of view, this trend would appear to be premature. The same types of instruments used for initial certification are now being used (in the absence of anything better) for recertification. The irony is that these tools have not yet been demonstrated to possess adequate validity for certification. Quite apart from the whole question of whether recertification is an appropriate idea philosophically, it is highly doubtful from a methodological point of view whether we are ready for it.

The computer-marked multiple-choice examination is now the most widely used evaluation instrument; it is also a favorite format in certification. This approach seems to have been accepted as an adequate tool for these critical decision points in the career of an individual physician. It is generally agreed that the tool is useful for sampling the knowledge base of an individual, but not much more than this. This overreliance on one instrument has occurred despite repeated pleas from thoughtful clinician-educators that many other attributes should be included in a definition of competence. The same plea is heard from the public. A survey sponsored by the Ontario Medical Association, but conducted independently under the direction of Mr. Edward Pickering, reported, for example, that patients identified the main deficit in the medical profession in the areas of "human relations" and access to care (Pickering, 1973). This imbalance is particularly troublesome in the absence of any convincing evidence of a correlation between the demonstration of an adequate medical knowledge base and the actual performance of a physician (Wingard and Williamson, 1973).

From the health care research literature has emerged the sobering evidence that many health outcomes are not directly attributable to what physicians do (McKeown, 1976). Through the use of such design strategies as the randomized clinical trial, many of the treatments we once thought to be beneficial turn out, in fact, not to be, and some result in more harm than good (Haynes et al., 1978). Observations such as those should significantly influence the means by which the competence of physicians, both individually and as a group, are assessed. And yet it is extremely difficult to change behavior once a certain trend is established. As an example, consider the probably excessive use of coronary artery bypass surgery. Governments and private institutions are evidently prepared to fund cardiovascular surgery units—sometimes several in the same city. Patients ask for the procedure. And the profession, armed with the technical know-how, proceeds with this therapeutic strategy, in advance of convincing evidence of its specific effectiveness for certain conditions.

These situations demand clear and critical thought. Our hope is that this book will help the clinician-educator sort out some of the "fallout" from the convergence of these developments of recent history.

Scope and Style

For the most part, this book is limited to a discussion of the clinical competence of physicians since most of the available research has used physicians or student-physicians as subjects. Comprehensive reviews of clinical competence of other health professionals are available (Morgan and Irby, 1978). We think, however, that much of what we will be saying will also be useful to other health professionals.

A methodological perspective pervades this review. We are primarily concerned with the empirical basis for our understanding of clinical competence, the methods used to assess it, and the systems which assure its development or continuance. It follows that this book is not primarily a "how to do it" cookbook, or a sales pitch for a particular approach or device. Rather, it attempts to look as objectively as possible at the available evidence, with comments based on specific predetermined criteria.

There is a special emphasis on education and on research studies which were conducted in a learning environment. In contrast to such areas as general health care research and the rapidly growing field of "quality assurance," there is a paucity of methodological reviews where clinical education is the primary focus. The contributors to this book are deeply involved in education and are seeking to apply critical thought to the learning setting and to their behavior as educators. Learning is fundamentally related to competence. We view educational measurement and evaluation as part of the learning process. And competence, both initial and continuing, is the end product of effective learning.

The contributors are all from the Faculty of Health Sciences at McMaster University, where for the past ten years or so some new ideas in medical education have been explored, and a number of the methods and approaches which will be described have been tested. It was thought that the flow of ideas in the book would be facilitated by collegial discussion and feedback; this is obviously easier when all the contributors work in the same place.

Part I includes this general introduction and a chapter in which we review various approaches that have been used to come to an understanding of what is meant by clinical competence. Several distinct perspectives are presented: the "armchair" approaches to definition of competence illustrated by textbooks on clinical diagnosis, task analysis, and other formalized methods used by specialty boards and licensing examinations, and the indirect viewpoint on competence provided by a variety of research methods—epidemiology, psychology, and quality of care research.

Part II, Methods, identifies and describes criteria to be applied to any method with purports to measure clinical competence. Each chapter then focuses on one instrument (or class of instrument). Included is a synthesis of the strengths and weaknesses of the tool under discussion and suggestions for further research.

The review of individual measures is followed in Part III, Applications, by consideration of how the measures can be used. Three chapters are devoted to looking at the application of tools to special components of professional performance where it is likely that more than a single method is appropriate. These are the use of diagnostic tests, the assessment of technical proficiency, and the measurement of physician-patient interaction.

The final section, Part IV, Implications, takes the form of a synthesis, under four headings: education, research, certification, and health care. Each chapter attempts to provide a "where do we go from here" statement, based on the perspectives presented in the earlier sections of the book.

References

Derbyshire, R. C.: State and local agencies. In Samph, T., Templeton, B. (Eds.) Evaluation in medical education: past, present and future. Cambridge, Mass: Ballinger (1979).

Funkenstein, D.: Medical students, medical schools and society during five eras. Cambridge, Mass.: Ballinger (1977).

Haynes, R. B., et al.: Increased absenteeism from work after detection and labeling of hypertensive patients. N Engl J Med 199, 741-744 (1978).

McKeown, T.: The role of medicine: dream, mirage or nemesis. London, England: The Nuffield Provincial Hospitals Trust (1976).

Morgan, M, Irby, D.: Evaluating clinical competence in the health professions. St. Louis. Mo.: CV Mosby (1978).

Pickering, E. A.: Report of the special study regarding the medical profession in Ontario. Toronto, Ontario Medical Association (1973).

Samph, T., Templeton, B.: Evaluation in medical education: past, present, future. Cambridge, Mass.: Ballinger (1979).

Valberg, L. S., Firstbrook, J. B.: A project to improve the measurement of professional competence for specialty certification in internal medicine. Ann R Coll Phys Surg Can 10, 278-282 (1977).

Wingard, J. R., Williamson, J. W.: Grades as predictors of physicians' career performance: an evaluative literature review. J Med Educ, 48, 311-322 (1973).

CHAPTER 2

Defining Competence: A Methodological Review

GEOFFREY R. NORMAN

What is clinical competence? The present chapter reviews the various methods used to define competence and points out the strengths and limitations of each. The focus is the clinical encounter—the activities of the physician in diagnosing and managing a patient's problems. Although other aspects of physician activity such as attitudes or relationships with colleagues and other health professionals, participation in professional associations, and scholarly or research activities may be important components of professional activity, they are excluded from the present discussion.

The Dimensions of Competence

Senior (1976) has made a distinction between "competence" and "performance," the former meaning what a physician is capable of doing, and the latter meaning what a physician actually does in his day-to-day practice. The distinction parallels the separation between the efficacy and effectiveness of a drug—the former is an indicator of the performance of a drug under ideal circumstances, with carefully chosen patients and near-perfect compliance, and the latter refers to the performance of the drug under actual conditions, with less than perfect compliance and a more heterogeneous patient population.

Competence in a specialty can be defined along a number of dimensions. For example, the American Board of Internal Medicine (1979) outlines four dimensions which must be considered in defining competence: (1) the relevant abilities of the physician—knowledge, technical skills, and interpersonal skills, (2) problem-solving tasks—data gathering, diagnosis, continuing care, etc., (3) the nature of the medical illness—the problems encountered by the physician, and (4) the social and psychological aspects of the patient's problem, especially those which relate to diagnosis and management.

Other specialties and certifying bodies have used variations on a matrix approach to the definition of competence (Burg et al., 1976; McDermott et al., 1977). The American Board of Medical Specialties (1979) suggests a conceptual framework with three principal dimensions: (1) the tasks of the physician (history taking, use of tests, etc.), (2) the clinical situations or subject matter of the discipline, and (3) prerequisite abilities (knowledge, problem-solving ability, attitudes, etc.). Although these schema suggest that several dimensions must be considered in a definition of competence, many approaches to a detailed specification of competence in a speciality deal only with one or two dimensions.

Methods of Defining Physician Activity: An Overview

There are two main sources used in defining the activity of the effective clinician—the writings of individual experts, which commonly appear in the introductory chapters of textbooks on clinical diagnosis, and the consensus of groups of experts (American Board of Medical Specialties, 1979) which have been compiled as detailed and structured taxonomies and published by specialty boards. There is also, however, an extensive research literature in disciplines ranging from psychology to epidemiology relevant to the definition of competence. The primary goal of this research may not have been to define competence, but some of it has a direct bearing on describing relevant dimensions of competence: the thinking processes of clinicians, the manifestations of these processes in observed behaviors, the nature of problems confronting the clinician, and the nature of the interaction between the physician's activities and the patient's problem resulting in a change in health status.

A further breakdown of these methods is defined below. In the remainder of the chapter we shall review each method in greater detail.

1. *Reflective/philosophical.* Historically the earliest definition of the profession, this "method" involves consideration of the qualities deemed important by a single recognized authority, and generally appears in the context of philosophical writings or textbooks on clinical diagnosis.

2. *Task analysis.* Andrew (1976) has defined task analysis as "a process whereby the activities that physicians engage in . . . are documented and described in such a way as to make explicit the purposes of the activity, the procedures that the physician utilizes in performing the activity, and the outcomes or expected products of the activity." She identifies three streams in task analysis: the consensus of expert opinions; the critical incident approach; and the use of activity logs.

3. *Descriptive studies.* Observational and epidemiological studies in primary care and some specialties focus on the type of problems seen by the physician. This method is fundamental in defining the subject matter or clinical problems seen by the physician.

4. *Studies of diagnostic thinking.* Medical diagnosis has been studied by psychologists as an example of "problem-solving" activity. Several research paradigms have been used in investigating clinical reasoning, including information-processing studies, in which physicians are observed and questioned in the course of solving a clinical problem; clinical judgment studies, in which physician judgments are described by mathematical models; and decision analysis, using Bayes' theorem in conjunction with the probability of various outcomes and their expected value in developing an optimal approach to diagnosis or management of a particular problem.

5. *Consumer opinion.* These studies of patient attitudes and expectations lead to a definition of competence from the client's perspective.

6. *Epidemiologic and quality of care.* With these approaches competence is defined from a health care perspective,

ideally in terms of those aspects of performance which can be shown to result in improvement or deterioration of health status.

A detailed review of each approach follows.

Reflective/Philosophical Statements

From the time of the Greek philosophers, the leading physicians of the day have put forth personal statements bearing on the principles and practice of medicine. Plato states, "Now the most skillful physicians are those who, from their youth upwards, have combined with a knowledge of their art, the greatest experience of disease; they had better not be of robust health and should have had all manner of disease in their own person." Hippocrates is cited as saying that the physician should have a good working knowledge of astrology! Osler, in an address to the graduating class at the University of Pennsylvania in 1889, defines three primary qualities of the clinician: the "Art of Detachment," which refers not to scientific objectivity, but to personal detachment from the pursuits and pleasure of youth; "The Virtue of Method," scientific method and practice management; and the "Quality of Thoroughness," not in history-taking and physical examination, but in scientific knowledge. More recent treatises on the practice of medicine cannot claim the literacy or ascetism of Osler's admonitions but are otherwise similar. For example, Tyrer and Eadie (1976) have described one aspect of clinical reasoning in the following manner:

> As more and more evidence of various sorts is accumulated, the physician, by reasoning in relation to his knowledge, is able to formulate possible diagnoses in his mind and then narrow down the list of suspect diseases until a definite diagnosis can be made. Should insufficient or invalid evidence of facts be obtained ... a correct diagnosis is unlikely.... Should the knowledge of the clinician be defective ... it would be difficult for him to reach a correct diagnosis ... or should his reasoning be defective he may be unable to isolate the correct diagnosis from the forest of alternatives presented to him. ...

Tumulty (1973) defines the skills of the clinician in the following manner:

> An effective clinician must have a number of skills. He must be a scientist. He must be knowledgeable about the natural course of com-

mon and uncommon clinical disease. He must be able to harvest clinical evidence from all available sources. He must be a keen analyst of these gathered facts. . . . The clinician must have the facility to communicate with [the patient] and his family members.

These descriptions of the effective clinician are not confined to textbooks on clinical medicine; similar statements can be found in medical journals (Dudley, 1970; King, 1967; McWhinney, 1972). Some of these writings have had a major impact on medical education and clinical practice and, although philosophical and possibly idiosyncratic, cannot be lightly dismissed.

Critique. Reconciling these definitions with the more systematic descriptions derived from the formal or research approaches is difficult. These writings have some bearing on both prerequisite abilities and problem-solving activities. Yet each treatise, considered alone, would be a poor prototype on which to develop an evaluation method. Although common threads can be developed, the writings are a reflection of the viewpoint of a single individual. There may be agreement among practitioners that the writings are a reasonable representation of clinical practice, and presumably the extent to which an individual author can capture the attitudes of his peers is related to the popularity of his writings. But each description is, of itself, incomplete and lacking in content validity and often presents a utopian view of how medicine should be practiced.

Task Analysis Approaches

In contrast to the philosophical stance of the reflective approaches, task analysis is rooted in a much more pragmatic base. The three streams identified by Andrew (1976) vary in the extent to which they use actual incidents of behavior or subjective judgments but the goal is the same—to describe the components of competence required by an adequate but not necessarily exemplary practitioner of the specialty. The description is deliberately comprehensive, and it attempts to deal with all four dimensions of competence—abilities, processes, problems, and interactions with the patient.

The Consensus of Experts. Experts in a field are frequently used in defining the content of a discipline. They may do so explicitly as members of a committee whose goals are to formulate educational objectives and define the components of competence of a specialty, or implicitly as members of test committees designing examinations for licensure or certification. Explicit competency statements have been developed for a number of specialities, such as the American Board of Pediatrics (1974), The American Board of Internal Medicine (1979), and the College of Family Physicians of Canada (1973). The process used by these various specialty boards is similar. Initially, a committee of acknowledged experts in the field is designated; the group may vary in size from fewer than 10 to 50 or more members. The committee or subcommittees then develop detailed specifications of competence along predetermined dimensions (for example, subject matter, abilities, tasks). These statements are then collated, reviewed, and discussed until a consensus is reached.

Andrew (1976) has documented a number of potential biases in this approach. The first problem is one of sampling: If the group of experts is too small, or if they do not represent a sufficiently broad perspective, consensus may be difficult to achieve and may have little relationship to the actual practice of the specialty. A second bias is that competency statements should derive from the independent judgments of the experts, in order to capitalize on the diversity of interests represented in the committee. After initial generation of competency statements, however, dominant members of the committee may alter the final consensus. Another problem is simply a reflection of the magnitude of the task. It is a mammoth undertaking, requiring hundreds of hours of professional time, and may deter many specialties from developing such statements. A last problem is that the definition which emerges is a statement of the ideal. The extent to which the statement of competence reflects how the specialty should be practiced, rather than the actual practice of the specialty, is unknown.

Critical Incident Approaches. The "critical incident" approach (Flanagan, 1954) overcomes some of the defects present in the previous method. A large number of practitioners are asked to identify, from their own experience, incidents which appear to have either a positive or a negative effect on the quality of care delivered to the patient. The method was used by the National Board of Medical Examiners (Flanagan, 1960) to define clinical competence for their examination. The study involved 600 practitioners and a total of 3,300 critical incidents, described as "clinical situations in which they had personally observed interns doing something that impressed them as examples of conspicuously good or poor clinical practice." These incidents were then grouped and classified into nine major categories.

The technique was also employed to develop a certification examination for the American Board of Orthopedic Surgery (Miller, 1968), this time involving 1,700 critical incidents contributed by 1,100 specialists, and grouped into 94 subcategories. Sanazaro and Williamson (1970) used the technique to study a number of primary care specialties involving a total of 2,000 physicians and 12,000 incidents. Cowles (1965), in a variation of the method, classified a total of 2,300 critical comments retrospectively derived from written evaluations of clinical clerks and scored each comment in an attempt to develop an objective means of evaluating verbal statements.

These studies and the resulting examinations have had a major impact on the development of clinical evaluation methods. The National Board study continues to be used as a guideline for developing new evaluation methods, and the orthopedic examination format has been copied, with modifications, by other specialties, notably the College of Family Physicians of Canada (Lamont, 1972). The method overcomes many of the problems of the expert committee approach. The criterion group is very large and is deliberately chosen to be representative. Incidents are not deleted in the final summary, but are simply categorized, removing personal biases from this stage of the process.

What problems exist with the method? The first is inherent in the method: By definition, there is no attempt to determine what constitutes adequate practice, only very good and very poor practice. As a result, a standard of acceptable performance cannot be interpolated easily and one is left with judgments about how many good incidents are good enough and how many poor incidents are too many. The second problem is one of validity. Although, at first glance, one might dismiss the possibility of bias because of the large samples involved, the potential for bias still exists. The method is based on actual performance, but the performance is judged through the eyes of the criterion physician. As one example, thoroughness emerges as a principal feature of good intern performance in the National Board study, yet thoroughness on history and physical has been shown to be unrelated to diagnosis and management, and thoroughness of laboratory workup at hospital admission has been shown to be inversely related to quality of care (Barrows et al., 1978; Sackett, 1978).

This method, then, has played a historically significant role in defining clinical competence and has several methodological advantages. Nevertheless, a potential for different types of bias remains.

Procedural Logs. To avoid the biases inherent in the previous methods, a more direct definition of competence must derive from the actual activities of competent physicians. One approach has been to gather data on day-to-day performance through the use of activity logs, in which physicians maintain a detailed record of their daily activities over a period of time. One difficulty with this method is a logistical one of ensuring accurate recording by physicians as the events occur, rather than retrospectively. Problems also exist in developing an adequate and representative sample, and avoiding volunteer bias. Finally, in contrast to the critical incident method, there is no way of determining from the log which activities constitute good or competent behavior, which are poor, and which activities fall in the mid-range.

Critique. To the extent that there is a conventional approach to the definition of competence, the three methods summarized in this section epitomize this approach. Most discussions about defining competence focus on these methods. We have described the strengths and weaknesses of each method in the preceding discussion, but there are inherent problems common to all three methods. One methodological problem is sampling. The sampling must meet two possibly conflicting criteria; on the one hand, it is necessary to sample at random a large number of practitioners to ensure that the resulting definition is representative; by contrast, the individuals whose opinions are to culminate in the definition of competence must be accepted exemplars in the field and therefore not randomly chosen. The second criticism of these methods is that, like the philosophical statements, they are derived, not from actual samples of clinical practice, but from aspects of practice which are, in one way or another, perceived as important by the practitioners. The extent to which the competencies described in the final document are a reflection of practice is contingent on the judgment of the practitioners, and such judgments are liable to a number of biases which may affect the validity of these products. Finally, as Lloyd (1979) has indicated, the most serious limitation of such approaches is that they have a tendency to become ends in themselves, rather than means to ends.

Descriptive Studies:
Observational and Epidemiological

All of the task analysis approaches in the previous section have the explicit goal of a comprehensive definition of competence. In contrast to this formalized process, there is an extensive literature, primarily in family medicine and general practice, which takes a more pragmatic view of clinical competence, defining the entity in terms of the daily activities of competent practitioners. These studies have three main foci: (1) detailed observation of a small sample of physicians over an interval of several days, (2) epidemiological studies of the types of problems seen by physicians, classified by complaint and/or diagnosis, and (3) studies of defined activities, such as history taking and physical examination.

Observational Studies. Two intensive studies using similar methodology have been conducted in this area, by Peterson et al. (1956) in North Carolina and by Clute (1963) in Canada. Both studies used ethnographic methods, in which the investigators visited physicians in their practices, held discussions with them, and observed their activities over a period of several days.

The studies presented a wealth of data describing many aspects of general practice, ranging from the use of cytologic smears and tuberculin tests to the occupation of the physician's father. The studies can be criticized as objective descriptions of clinical competence in general practice, however, since performance in history, clinical examination, and use of investigations was judged against an external criterion. For example, Peterson states, "Almost no good histories dealing with anemia or hypertension were observed," suggesting that the histories were being judged against criteria which may have been inappropriate for family practice. Peterson and colleagues had accepted that "most, if not all, physicians performed complete physical examinations on all new patients. . . . That such was not the case soon became evident." In light of what we now know about the limited value of screening tests, the general practitioners may have been practicing more rational medicine that was credited to them.

Clute's study involved 44 general practitioners in Ontario and 42 in Nova Scotia. Again, the data gathered from the study was comprehensive and included previous education, office facilities, work load, membership in professional societies, income, and social activities, in addition to a detailed breakdown of the kinds of problems seen and quality of care delivered. Once again, however, a large portion of the book is devoted to assessing the quality of care delivered, and although the authors devote considerable space to a rationale for their scoring methods, they might still be interpreted as arbitrary.

Price et al. (1971) conducted a series of studies of physicians in Utah over two decades. A 1964 study involved the assessment of 80 criterion measures on each of 800 physicians ranging from grade point average in the first two years of medical school to the dollar value of office equipment. The 80 variables were then used to provide some empirical basis for defining the domains of competence. The investigators developed a variety of methods to combine and weight these variables into an overall measure of competence. Of particular interest to the present chapter, those variables which were judged most important to competence had no direct relationship to patient care but were based on peer judgments—for example, the number of times a physician was nominated as an outstanding contributor by colleagues. These investigators went a step further in defining competence in a second study. Critical comments about physician behavior were obtained from 100 physicians used in the first study. These were then rated by ten different consumer and professional groups, ranging from nurses and medical students to hippies. Although these comments do not provide a detailed specification of competence on which an examination could be structured, they do provide insight into domains considered important by providers and consumers.

Studies of Patient Problems. A ubiquitous feature of general practice research is a preoccupation with defining the types of problems seen by the practitioners. Limited studies have been conducted in Canada (McFarlane, Norman, and Spitzer, 1971; McFarlane, O'Connell, and Hay, 1971) and Britain (Fry, 1966; Hodgkin, 1973) and two major studies have been done in the United States (National Center for Health Statistics, 1978; Marsland et al., 1976). More similarities than differences have emerged from these studies, conducted in widely different geographic locations. The most common problems dealt with by general practitioners are acute upper respiratory infections, followed by cardiovascular disease and emotional problems. The prevalence of emotional problems shows greatest variation from study to study, presumably more as a function of the physicians involved than their patients.

The implication of these studies for educational programs directed at training primary care physicians is significant. The family physician is competent to the extent that he can manage the problems he is likely to encounter: management of emotional problems, the problems of detection and compliance in the 10 percent of his adult practice who are hypertensive, and so forth. The futility of attempting to train such a physician in the academic medical center is elegantly demonstrated by White (1961).

Studies of Practice Activities. Other studies in general practice have focused on other aspects of the patient encounter—for example, the proportion of patients with new or old conditions who received only history, history and limited physical examination, investigations, and so on (Hull, 1972; Morrell, 1972). A complete, or even extensive physical examination is a relative rarity in general practice, occurring in less than 10 percent of visits.

Critique. The three classes of research we have reviewed in this section do not, of themselves, define clinical competence. They do, however, yield insights into the performance of physicians. As more studies are initiated in a variety of domains, it is increasingly evident that physicians frequently do not practice medicine in the manner they have been taught in medical school, and their actual performance may not bear a very close resemblance to how they believe they practice, or think they ought to practice. Thus, there may be considerable distortion when competence is defined "from the armchair" using the methods described previously.

The study of presenting problems is perhaps the best approach to a definition of the clinical situations encountered by the physician, which in turn defines the relevant subject matter. However, the transfer from a description of practice activity to a definition of competence is not completely straightforward. The criteria imposed on practitioners by Clute and Peterson comprised a definition of competence which in retrospect appears to have been arbitrarily high. Yet the actual performance of physicians cannot be presumed to define the lower limits of competence in the absence of some external criteria. In addition, although prevalence studies of presenting complaints and diagnoses assess one dimension of the subject matter of a discipline, they do not directly translate to a definition of the appropriate content areas. The physician must be competent to deal with rare but potentially serious conditions and make the appropriate decisions to treat, consult, or refer. These situations are not adequately addressed by simple considerations of disease prevalence.

Studies of Diagnostic Thinking

Medical diagnosis has been of interest to psychologists for some time as an example of human problem-solving activity. Clinicians have been studied using a variety of experimental paradigms, and, in turn, this research has affected our view of the nature of clinical reasoning, eliminating some of the mystique, but frequently substituting a plethora of simple models lacking in credibility and seemingly unrelated to each other.

The studies reviewed in this section do not presume to describe all aspects of clinical competence; their focus is on the mental strategies used by clinicians to seek out information, generate diagnostic hypotheses, weigh the information against these hypotheses to arrive at a conclusion, and develop a management plan with due consideration of the costs and benefits associated with alternative therapies. Excluded from the discussion are the domains of technical skills, interpersonal skills, and prerequisite knowledge. Instead, the focus is on understanding what many would view as the essential feature of clinical competence—the mental problem-solving strategies involved in using the available data to arrive at a diagnosis and management plan.

The studies fall into three general classes (Elstein and Bordage, 1979) characterized by the goal of the research and the experimental methods employed. We shall focus on two in this review.

1. *Information-processing approaches.* The goal of this research is to understand how humans solve problems. The method involves detailed observation of human behavior and of verbalized thought processes, while the subjects approach diagnostic problems. The goal is a theory which describes both the process of problem solving and the relationship between process and outcome.
2. *Decision analysis and Bayesian approaches.* This research approach is further removed from the study of human thought. The goal is to seek an optimal means of combining the data to arrive at a correct or best outcome using information about the probability and utility of various possible end states.

Information Processing Approaches. Studies of clinicians using this paradigm have "the goal . . . to define precisely the processes and states that a particular subject is using to solve a particular problem, and to be able to list—for example, in the form of a computer program—the exact sequence of operations used" (Kleinmuntz, 1968). Several studies have been conducted in medicine, and all use similar experimental techniques. The subject physician is presented with a clinical problem, either as a simulated patient or orally by the investigator, and is asked to approach the problem in his usual style. His thought processes are captured, either by thinking aloud as he works through the problem, or by reviewing a videotape subsequently. Subjects have included neurologists (Kleinmuntz, 1968), criterion internists (Elstein et al., 1978), neurology residents (Barrows and Bennett, 1972), family physicians (Barrows et al., 1978; Feightner et al., 1977), medical students (Neufeld et al., 1981), and residents in family and internal medicine (Scherger, 1980).

A common finding of these studies is the formation of multiple diagnostic hypotheses very early in the encounter, frequently within a few seconds of obtaining the chief complaint. These hypotheses serve an essential role in determining both the process and the outcome of the encounter. Elstein et al. (1978) and Barrows et al. (1978) found that the hypotheses strongly dictated the subsequent search for information. Most of the data were gathered to confirm one hypothesis or another. Furthermore, using a simple three-point weighting of each finding against each hypothesis, the investigators in both studies were able to accurately predict the clinician's ultimate choice of diagnosis, suggesting that the clinical reasoning involved in arriving at a diagnosis may not be as complex as we had supposed. Barrows et al. (1978) found that the number of hypotheses and many other measures of the process, in particular the amount of significant data gathered, were unrelated to diagnosis and management. What was important in diagnosis was whether the clinician had entertained the correct diagnosis as an hypothesis during the encounter. These investigators also examined differences by specialty type (family medicine or internal medicine) and educational level, from entry into medical school to graduation. With the exception of the content of the hypotheses, most features of the encounter, such as number of hypotheses or amount of data, were essentially the same for all subgroups. These results suggest that the process of problem solving may be a general feature, and the important consequence of education and/or experience is the acquisition of content.

Although the studies can be faulted on methodological grounds, since they frequently involve a small sample of subjects, and only a few clinical problems, they are based on actual performance. Furthermore, they have begun to explore the mental problem-solving strategies of clinicians, an area of competence which formerly could only be inferred from the introspective, and frequently erroneous, accounts of experienced clinicians.

What are the implications of these studies for a definition of competence? The findings may be viewed by some as disquieting. The notion of the clinician as the passive and objective observer of illness finds little confirmation in these studies. Similarly, the artful balancing of positive and negative information to arrive at a diagnosis appears much simpler than has been formerly construed.

Bayesian Diagnosis and Decision Analysis. The methods discussed above have an obvious role to play in defining the nature of clinical reasoning and clinical competence as actually practiced by clinicians. But also relevant is an extensive literature based on the manipulations by computers of disease probabilities, conditional probabilities of various signs and symptoms, and the value of various treatment outcomes. The literature has roots in business and psychology and uses various labels—computer-aided diagnosis, Bayesian diagnosis, and decision analysis (McNeil, 1975). It is not intended to understand the clinician's thinking processes. Rather, the method uses, as input, information derived from actual disease probabilities, and its goal is to determine an optimal diagnosis or management decision based on the available data (optimal in the sense of maximizing the probability of particular diagnostic end states, or the utility, to patient or physician, of particular treatment outcomes).

This literature is viewed with suspicion by many clinicians for a number of reasons (Elstein, 1976; Feinstein, 1979); it is highly mathematical and not readily understandable, and the computer models attempt to treat all patients with a given condition by a single model, the antithesis of individualized clinical care.

Although how these methods can be applied to a definition of clinical competence is unclear, the findings of a number of studies in the area are a disquieting reminder of human fallibility in clinical reasoning. Computer diagnosis has been shown to be, at worst, as accurate as physician diagnosis, and at best, when actual probability data are available, considerably better than human diagnosis (Beach, 1975; Leaper et al., 1972). Further, as the literature on decision analysis grows, the method is evolving as an ideal criterion against which actual physician performance can be judged.

Critique. Will the application of these methods lead to the replacement of the clinician's reasoning with the numerical manipulations of a computer? Despite the fallibility of human judgment, we feel such an outcome is unlikely. Methods such as decision analysis may, however, have an educational role to play in improving clinical judgments through explicating the range of available alternatives and the value of possible end points (Elstein, 1976). The apparently contradictory conclusions of different clinicians in the same situation may then be shown to have a rational basis in differing subjective probabilties or different values placed on a range of possible outcomes.

Similar comments might be made about the clinical judgment and information-processing approach, which will not, of itself, lead to a definition of competence. What it has accomplished is the illumination of a central area of competence—problem solving or clinical reasoning—which was previously considered unobservable and which lay primarily in the realm of the art of medicine. Although specific measures of these areas of competence do not exist in any practical form as yet, the insights provided by the research could potentially result in the development of such measures in the near future.

Patient and Consumer Opinion

It is the nature of professional practice that the client is not in a position to judge the competence of the individual practitioner, and decisions about competence are made by legislative bodies such as state boards and medical associations. The patient indeed has no valid means at his disposal to determine the technical skills of a surgeon or the diagnostic acumen of an internist. Yet there is one area in which the patient is informed and is the best judge of competence—the domain of doctor-patient relationship and interpersonal skills.

Korsch and co-workers (1968) studied the relationship between the physician's interviewing techniques and patient satisfaction using 800 tape-recorded encounters with pediatric patients and follow-up interviews in an emergency room setting. Significant relationships were found between satisfaction and (1) the friendliness and sympathy of the physician; (2) the physician's communication skills; (3) physician explanations of the nature and cause of the illness; and (4) his or her dealing directly with the patient's concerns and anxieties. Dissatisfaction was related to unfulfilled patient expectations for lab tests, X-rays, physical examinations, or drugs.

Hulka (1971, 1975) has developed a methodology to directly assess physician awareness of patient concerns using a problem-specific scale completed by both physician and patient. Physician awareness has been related to a number of physician and practice characteristics, such as specialty certification and residency training; however, the relationships are complex and not consistent, nor is there a consistent relationship between physician awareness and health outcomes.

Critique. Like the research on problem solving, these studies do not provide a comprehensive framework for a definition of competence; rather, they serve to elucidate one area which previously resided in the domain of the "art" of medicine. At the present time, it is unclear precisely how patient satisfaction is influenced by the expectations of the patient or other patient variables, and how the dimensions of physician performance related to patient satisfaction can be characterized. Nevertheless, it is apparent with the rise of consumer advocacy in North America that increasing attention must be paid to this domain of competence.

Epidemiologic and Quality-of-Care Approaches

Although the research approaches we have reviewed in this chapter are focused on the performance dimension, these approaches tend to be of a descriptive nature. By contrast, research on quality of care attempts to measure physician performance on specific conditions against an absolute standard of acceptable care. This literature has been reviewed by Williamson (1976) and others.

A feature of all research conducted in this tradition is a focus on actual performance—the actual quality of care delivered to a series of patients with one or more conditions in a hospital or clinic setting. Quality of care may be measured against standards set by some external body, similar to the criteria used in the Clute (1963) and Peterson (1956) studies cited earlier, so-called process measures, or may be based on measures of patient morbidity or mortality resulting from the care received—referred to as "outcome measures." These outcomes are related to various measures of process in the health care system to indicate which features of the process of health care are significantly related to improved outcomes.

Some examples will illustrate these distinctions. A study by Moses and Mosteller (1968) examined the postoperative death rates from cholecystectomy and gastric resection in various hospitals. After correcting for a variety of patient variables, the death rate in teaching hospitals was three to five times lower than in nonteaching hospitals. Similar results were found by Lipworth, Lee, and Morris (1963) in an examination of case fatality rate for a variety of conditions in teaching and nonteaching hospitals. Morbidity associated with appendicitis (peritonitis or abscess) was used in a study of Goran and Gonnella (1975) of various sources of health payments.

Process and outcome measures were both used in a study by Brook and Appel (1973) of 296 patients in a single hospital. They also used implicit judgments by faculty of quality of care in comparison with explicit criteria developed by the same panel. In terms of assessment of clinical competence, a major concern emerging from these studies is that frequently very little relationship was found between performance and such conventional measures of clinical competence as board certification or years in practice. Furthermore, the study of Goran et al. (1973) directly compared performance on management of urinary tract infection with an evaluation of competence using patient management problems and found that clinic teams did very well on the written examinations and very poorly on the actual clinic management of similar problems.

Critique. Studies of actual performance have a clear role to play in defining clinical competence, if for no other reason than that the great discrepancy between these measures and conventional evaluation methods strongly suggests that they assess a different, and undoubtedly important, domain of competence. Nevertheless, these methods have certain disadvantages: They are extremely expensive, and they are usually constrained to examination of a particular problem area. As such, they cannot be used to contribute to a broad definition of competence.

Summary and Conclusions

No single method can adequately define the prerequisite knowledge, skills, and attitudes required of a competent physician in a particular specialty. Each method has certain limitations. These may derive from biases inherent in the method, such as the critical incident studies or consensual approach, or may be a result of the limited focus of the method, such as the information-processing studies.

Regardless of the method chosen, the goal is the detailed specification of the necessary knowledge or skills of the competent practitioner. These individual components are usually arranged or sorted into domains of competence, such as knowledge, technical skills, or interpersonal skills. The detailed specification of the individual elements within each domain is beyond the scope of this book and is a task we leave to the members of objectives committees and specialty boards. The domains of competence are of immediate concern, however, since each evaluation method to be considered in subsequent chapters may be useful for assessing only some of the dimensions of competence. We must begin by outlining these areas in order to critically examine the appropriate role of each evaluation method.

The scheme we will use for the purposes of organizing this book is shown in the Table 2.1. It is no more or less optimal than

TABLE 2.1
A Categorization of Clinical Competence

The following abilities are required in encounters between a physician and individual patients:

1. Clinical Skills

   The ability to acquire clinical information by talking with and examining patients, and interpreting the significance of the information obtained.

2. Knowledge and Understanding

   The ability to remember relevant knowledge about clinical conditions in order to provide effective and efficient care for patients.

3. Interpersonal Attributes

   The expression of those aspects of a physician's personal and professional character that are observable in interactions with patients.

4. Problem Solving and Clinical Judgment

   The application of relevant knowledge, clinical skills, and interpersonal attributes to the diagnosis, investigation and management of the clinical problems of a given patient.

5. Technical Skills

   The ability to use special procedures and techniques in the investigation and management of patients.

any other categorization reviewed in this chapter and serves, not to define competence, but to provide a reference point for the discussions of specific methods which follow. The scheme will be introduced again in the discussion of educational implications in Chapter 15, at which time we shall suggest the potential role of each of the evaluation methods we have reviewed in assessing competence.

REFERENCES

American Board of Internal Medicine: Clinical competence in internal medicine. Ann Intern Med 90, 402-411 (1979).

American Board of Medical Specialties: Definitions of competence in specialties of medicine. Chicago: Author (1979).

American Board of Pediatrics: Foundations for evaluating the competency of pediatricians. Chapel Hill (1974).

Andrew, B. J.: Validation by task analysis. In Extending the validity of certification. Chicago: American Board of Medical Specialties (1976).

Barrows, H. S., Bennett, K.: Experimental studies of the diagnostic (problem-solving) skill of the neurologist. Arch Neurol 26, 273-277 (1972).

Barrows, H. S., Neufeld, V. R., Feightner, J. W., Norman, G. R.: An analysis of the clinical methods of medical students and physicians. Final report to Ontario Ministry of Health, Toronto (1978).

Beach, B. H.: Expert judgment about uncertainty: Bayesian decision making in realistic settings. Organizational Behavior and Human Performance 14, 10-59 (1975).

Brook, R. H., Appel, F. A.: Choosing a method for peer review. N Engl J Med 288, 1323-1332 (1973).

Burg, F. D., et al.: A method for defining competency in pediatrics. J Med Educ 51, 824-828 (1976).

Clute, K. F.: The general practitioner. Toronto: University of Toronto Press (1963).

College of Family Physicians of Canada: Educational objectives for certification in family medicine. Toronto (1973).

Cowles, J. T.: A critical comments approach to the rating of medical students' clinical performance. J Med Educ 40, 188-198 (1965).

Dudley, H. A. F.: The clinical task. Lancet ii, 1352-1354 (1970).

Elstein, A. S.: Clinical judgment: psychological research and medical practice. Science 194, 696-700 (1976).

Elstein, A. S., Shulman, L. S., Sprafka, S. A.: Medical problem solving: An analysis of clinical reasoning. Cambridge: Harvard University Press (1978).

Elstein, A. S., Bordage, G.: Psychology of clinical reasoning. In G. Stone, F. Cohen, and N. Adler (eds.): Health psychology: a handbook. San Francisco: Jossey-Bass (1979).

Feightner, J. W., et al.: Solving problems—how does the family physician do it? Can Fam Physician 23, 67-71 (1977).

Feinstein, A. R.: The haze of Bayes, the aerial places of decision-analysis, and the computerized ouija board. Clin Pharmacol Ther 21, 482-496 (1979).

Flanagan, W., et al.: The definition of clinical competence in medicine: Performance dimensions and rationales for clinical skill areas. Palo Alto: American Institutes for Research in the Behavioral Sciences (1960).

Flanagan, W. The critical incident technique. Psychol Bull 51, 327-358 (1954).

Fry, J.: Profiles of disease. London: E&S Livingston (1966).

Goran, M. J., Williamson, J. W., Gonnella, J. S.: The validity of patient management problems. J Med Educ 48, 171-177 (1973).

Goran, M. J., Gonnella, J. S.: Quality of patient care—a measurement of change—the staging concept. Med Care 13, 467-473 (1975).

Hodgkin, K.: Towards earlier diagnosis. London: Churchill Livingstone (1973).

Hulka, B. S., Kupper, L. L., Cassell, J. C., et al.: A method for measuring physician's awareness of patient concerns. H.S.M.H.A. Health Project 86 (1971).

Hulka, B. S., Kupper, L. L., Cassell, J. C.: Practice characteristics and the quality of primary medical care: the doctor/patient relationship. Med Care 13, 808-820 (1975).

Hull, F. M.: Diagnostic pathways in rural general practice. J R Coll Gen Pract 22, 241-258 (1972).

King, L. S.: What is a diagnosis?. JAMA 202, 714-717 (1967).

Kleinmuntz, B.: The processing of clinical information by man and machine. New York: Wiley (1968).

Korsch, B. M., Guzzi, E. K., Francis, V.: Gaps in doctor/patient communication: I. Doctor/patient interaction and patient satisfaction. Pediatrics 42, 855 (1968).

Lamont, C. T., Hennen, B. K.: The use of simulated patients in a certifying examination in family medicine. J Med Educ 47, 789-794 (1972).

Leaper, D. J., et al.: Computer assisted diagnosis of abdominal pain using estimates provided by clinicians. Br Med J 2, 350-254 (1972).

Lipworth, L., Lee, J. A. H., Morris, J. N.: Case fatality in teaching and non-teaching hospitals. Med Care 1, 71-76 (1963).

Lloyd, J. S.: Definitions of competence in specialties of medicine. Chicago: American Board of Medical Specialties (1979).

Marsland, D. W., Woodward, M., Mayo, F.: A data bank for patient care curriculum and research in family practice. J Fam Pract 3, 25-48 (1976).

McDermott, J. F., McGuire, C. H., Berner, E. S.: A study of board certification in child psychiatry as a valid indicator of clinical competence. J Am Acad Child Psychol 16, 517-525 (1977).

McFarlane, A. H., Norman, G. R., Spitzer, W. O.: Family medicine—the dilemma of defining the discipline. Can Med Assoc J 105, 397-401 (1971).

McFarlane, A. H., O'Connell, B. P., Hay, J.: Demand for care model: its use in programme planning for primary physician education. J Med Educ 46, 436-442 (1971).

McNeil, B.: Primer on certain elements of medical decision-making. N Engl J Med 298, 211-215 (1975).

McWhinney, I. R.: Problem-solving and decision making in primary medical practise. Can Fam Physician 18, 109-114 (1972).

Miller, G. E.: The orthopedic training study. JAMA 206, 601-606 (1968).

Morrell, D. C.: Symptom interpretation in general practice. J R Coll Gen Pract 22, 297-309 (1972).

Moses, L. E., Mosteller, F.: Institutional differences in postoperative death rates. JAMA 203, 491-494 (1968).

National Center for Health Statistics: The national ambulatory medical care survey—1976. Washington, D.C.: U.S. Department of Health, Education and Welfare (1978).

Neufeld, V. R., et al.: Clinical reasoning of medical students: A cross-sectional and longitudinal analysis. Med Educ 15, 315-322 (1981).

Peterson, O. L. et al.: An analytic study of North Carolina general practice. J Med Educ 31, 1-165 (1956).

Price, P. B., et al.: Measurement and predictors of physician performance. Salt Lake City, Utah: LLR Press (1971).

Sackett, D. L.: Clinical diagnosis and the clinical laboratory. Clin Invest Med 1, 37-43 (1978).

Sanazaro, P. J., Williamson, J. W.: End result of patient care: A provisional classification based on reports by internists. Med Care 8, 299 (1970).

Scherger, J. E., et al.: Comparison of diagnostic methods of family practice and internal medicine residents. J Fam Pract 10, 95-101 (1980).

Senior, J. R.: Toward the measurement of competence in medicine. Philadelphia: National Board of Medical Examiners (1976).

Tumulty, P. A.: The effective clinician. Philadelphia: W. B. Saunders (1973).

Tyrer, J. H., Eadie, M. J.: The astute physician. Amsterdam: Elsevier (1976).

White, K. L.: The ecology of medical care. N Engl J Med 265, 885-889 (1961).

Williamson, J. W.: Validation by performance measures. In American Board of Specialties Conference on extending the validity of certification. Chicago: American Board of Medical Specialties (1976).

PART **II**

Methods

The first chapter in this section identifies and describes criteria to be applied to any method which purports to measure clinical competence. Each chapter following then focuses on one instrument (or class of instrument). Included is a synthesis of the strengths and weaknesses of the tool under discussion and suggestions for further research.

CHAPTER 3

An Introduction to Measurement Properties

VICTOR R. NEUFELD

Chapter 1 of this book explored the various reasons why clinical competence is worth studying. Chapter 2 reviewed the many attempts to define clinical competence, and the research approaches used in each case. Part II will focus on the methods used to assess clinical competence. In this section the word *method* will be used interchangeably with the nouns *tool, instrument, test, measure, observation, technique, examination, data source*, and so on, to refer to the means by which information about the competence of a physician is obtained. This section will review the more common methods used to assess clinical competence.

To begin this section on methods, we offer some introductory pages which will serve to clarify the major terms and concepts used and to list and define the properties that any evaluation instrument measuring competence would be expected to have.

The Terms *Measurement* and *Performance*

When "clinical competence" is referred to in this book, it is limited to those attributes displayed by a health professional in an encounter with an individual patient. We have arbitrarily excluded considerations of the physician in his responsibility to himself (for example, as a continuing learner), or the physician as a member of a group of some kind, such as a practice group, an interprofessional health care team, or even a committee member. Nor have we included the physician's interaction with social groups, such as families, schools, and community gatherings.

Chapter 2 has made it clear that clinical competence is a multidimensional, not a unidimensional, set of attributes. It follows that no one tool will adequately tap the range of competencies involved. The challenge then is to find the most appropriate tool for a specific purpose and the best set of tools for the spectrum of components of interest.

Measurement Properties of a Test

We come now to a brief review of what we have chosen to call measurement properties. These are sometimes called "criteria," implying that certain test standards have to be met before the instrument is ready to be used. We prefer the use of "measurement properties," because the term "criteria" is used in other contexts of measurement as well (for example, criterion-referenced scoring).

Contributors to this section were asked to review a given assessment method to determine whether it appears to measure what it claims to measure (credibility); whether it touches on important components of competence (comprehensiveness); whether it measures performance consistently (precision); whether it truly measures what it claims to measure (validity); whether it can be used in the real world (feasibility); and whether it is appropriate for use in an educational setting. This checklist may be useful in a general way to clinician-educators who read this book, particularly those who are the consumers (users) of the research on clinical competence. The aim of any clinical competence assessment is to obtain a true measure of an attribute. The use of this checklist of measurement properties may help sort out what sources of variation (other than the "true" score) contribute to the scores. These sources of variation include: the assessment situation (e.g., the physical setting, the time of day, the presence of fatigue or anxiety), the nature of the clinical problem (or perhaps several distinct problems considered in a given physician-patient interaction), the observer(s), and the method of assessment.

Similar checklists appear quite regularly in textbooks of educational, psychological, and biological measurement. An example is the well-known "Standards for Educational and Psychological Tests" published in 1974 by the American Psychological Association. Properties of good measurement instruments have also been described in connection with the interpretation and use of diagnostic tests (Sackett, 1978), as well as for process measures of the quality of care (Tugwell, 1979).

For clinicians who are concerned with the assessment of clinical competence, several problems arise when reading these publications. First, while the ideas may be similar in these various domains, the terms used may be quite different. For example, the evaluation of a test by common sense as being appropriate to assess a given attribute may be called "credibility" in the health care field, and "face validity" in educational research. Further, although an instrument may meet conventional standards of reliability and validity, the issue of feasibility is frequently not considered. Finally, there are several considerations that apply specifically to the use of these methods in an educational setting.

Our checklist is summarized in Table 3.1. Each property or attribute is defined briefly and synonyms are listed opposite. We have carefully selected words that will be understood by both those who read the health care research field and those more familiar with educational research. Thus, we are attempting to throw grappling hooks between ships that often pass in the night. These measurement characteristics are described in more detail, with some examples included, in the following section.

Credibility

This property simply requires the application of reflective common sense: "Does this instrument seem to test what I'm interested in measuring?" We have put this characteristic at the top of our list, because unless an instrument appears to be credible, it is unlikely to be used or considered. The synonym from the educational literature is face validity; that is, "On the face of it, does this instrument seem to be a valid measure for what I want to test?"

As an example, many licensing boards use performance on written multiple-choice examinations as a general reflection of clinical competence. But most clinicians suspect that, although knowledge of facts is one component of competence, there is an enormous difference between performance on multiple-choice questions and the competent care of patients (Eichna, 1980), and to some extent the research literature confirms this (Wingard and Williamson, 1973).

TABLE 3.1
Measurement Properties of Tests of Clinical Competence

Properties	*Synonym(s)*
1. Credibility	
A nonnumerical judgment of the degree to which a test appears to measure the attribute of interest.	Common sense Clinical credibility Face validity
2. Comprehensiveness	
The extent to which an instrument "covers" or samples all aspects of the attribute of interest (e.g., an educational objective).	Content validity
3. Precision	
A quantitiative expression of the reproducibility with which the instrument measures the same event on different occasions, with different observers, etc.	Reliability Repeatability Consistency Agreement Objectivity
4. Validity (Quantitative)	
Quantitative expressions to indicate the degree to which an instrument "truly" measures what is intended.	
(a) Concurrent Validity Statistical association with the "best" external measure available.	Criterion-related validity Concurrent criterion validity Accuracy
(b) Predictive Validity Association with some relevant outcome measure obtained some time in the future.	Predictive criterion validity Prognostic accuracy
(c) Construct Validity The demonstration of expected (hypothetical, theoretical) differences, using the test in question.	Substitution (direct measurement of attribute not available; a hypothetical approximation is used instead)

TABLE 3.1 (cont.)

Properties	Synonym(s)
5. Feasibility	
This includes consideration of costs, scheduling, and logistics.	Applicability Acceptability
6. Educational Considerations	

(a) Appropriateness
Does the test selected match with its intended educational purpose?
Such as: student learning
    certification
    decision making
    program modifications
	Test mismatch

(b) Use Are the users of the information provided by the test aware of its strengths and limitations?	
(c) Side Effects Are there ways in which the test does more harm than good?	Test anxiety

Comprehensiveness

Comprehensiveness describes the extent to which a test samples or "covers" the area of competence under consideration. It answers the question: "Have most of the important things been considered?" Most typically, it is used in reference to a body of knowledge which is sampled in an examination and is sometimes expressed in quantitative terms. The synonym from the educational literature is "content validity."

As an example, the Medical Council of Canada recently explored the comprehensiveness of its Part A multiple-choice examination by asking the 16 Canadian medical schools to rate each item on two dimensions: the degree of importance, and whether the topic was taught in the curriculum. The survey revealed that overall, 90 percent of items were seen as essential or important; in addition, 82 percent of items were considered to be taught somewhere in the curriculum (Park et al., 1981).

Another situation might be recalled where comprehensiveness is short-circuited. An oral examiner in a fellowship exam is famous for certain favorite questions, which he asks with predictable regularity. If a candidate, primed by this grapevine advance information, is lucky, he will be asked one of these predicted questions. The "content validity" of this situation, considering the overall range of areas of competence, is obviously low.

Precision

There are many synonyms for "precision," the most frequently used being "reliability." It is a quantitative expression of the extent to which an instrument measures the same component under different test situations, such as different occasions or with different observers.

There are many ways to check the precision or reliability of an instrument, dependent on the nature of the test and the way it will be employed. For example, to test whether a multiple-choice test is "balanced," it is common practice to compare performance on half the items on a test with performance on the other half. This is called "split-half reliability" or "internal consistency."

Another type of precision is illustrated in an example where two patient management problems (PMPs) are given to a class of final-year students. These are given to the same class a few days later, and the results are compared to see whether the performance is equivalent. This is a form of "test-retest reliability."

A third type of reliability is seen in the following situation: The oral examinations of three medical residents are videotaped. The three tapes are then viewed and rated by five other examiners. The correlations on the ratings provide an indication of interrater reliability. If the videotapes are seen again, and rerated by the original examiners one week later, the correlations provide an index of intrarater agreement or reliability.

The term *objectivity*, which implies freedom from bias, is commonly used in referring to the precision of a measuring instrument. The more objective a test, the better it is; the more subjective, the "softer" it is (Wilson, 1975). From a measurement point of view, the term *objective* is not particularly helpful, in that it does not add anything to our understanding of precision or bias.

To those unfamiliar with measurement terms, "objective" has a hallowed sound to it, often equated with quantification or instrumentation. A common example is the computer-marked multiple-choice examination, which is held up as the epitome of objectivity, yet it too is a victim of subjectivity. Human judgment (and therefore bias) is involved in the selection of the test-setter, in the selection of content areas, in the design and wording of the items and the multiple options, and in the designation of the most correct response. We suggest dropping the terms *subjective* and *objective* from the measurement glossary. Let us recognize that there always will be bias. The challenge is to recognize bias and to minimize it, and in particular to ensure that no one individual is unfairly affected by it. To quote a colleague, the late Dr. Gilles Cormier, "the task is to spread the bias around."

Validity

This is perhaps the most frequently used expression in the measurement vocabulary. It is the degree to which a test "truly" measures what it is intended to measure. Not only is this term the most common, it is also the most confusing. Dozens of adjectives have become affixed to the term, each purporting to contribute some shade of meaning to the concept. We have already disposed of two types of validity (face validity, content validity) by selecting other words (credibility, comprehensiveness).

There remain several expressions of validity which usually are quantitative. There are two basic types—those that involve comparison with some criterion or "gold standard," and those where no direct measures of the attribute are available (that is, there is no gold standard or criterion), so that a hypothetical construct must be substituted. The criterion-related validity determination can be made either at the same time as the new measure is applied (concurrent), or at some future time (predictive).

Let us look at these three forms of validity; two involve comparison with a criterion measure, and one does not.

Concurrent Validity. In this form of validity, performance on the measure of interest is compared with performance on the best existing external measure available. The performance on both measures should be obtained concurrently. Synonyms for this form of validity are "criterion-related validity" or "accuracy." As an example, Goran and colleagues compared the performance of physicians on patient management problems (PMPs) with their performance on actual patients in an outpatient clinic who had the same condition, urinary tract infection (1973). The latter measure (performance on actual patients) was the criterion or "gold standard." The researchers found considerable differences between performance in the two measures and concluded that the concurrent criterion validity of PMPs was questionable.

Predictive Validity. This is another form of criterion-related validity, but the criterion measure is applied at some point in the future. The question is, "To what extent does the new test predict performance on this attribute in the future?" Because prediction is the key idea here, the best term in our view is "predictive validity." Synonyms are "predictive criterion validity" or "prognostic accuracy" (a term borrowed from the clinical measurement literature). Predictive validity was being measured in the following example: A test of clinical reasoning ability in a card deck format was given to medical school applicants before entry into a medical school program (Tamblyn, 1981). The performance on this test was compared (for accepted applicants) with tutor ratings of problem-solving ability in the clerkship period two years later. A second criterion measure used was performance on the workup of standardized simulated patients, obtained during the clerkship.

As a second hypothetical example, the director of a medical residency program introduced a "structured oral" examination procedure, used mainly to provide feedback to residents. He wondered, however, whether it predicted performance on the national certification examination (which includes an oral examination). Perhaps residents who received an "unsatisfactory" rating in the structured oral should not be allowed to take the national examination. When the director looked at the performance of each of 22 residents on two structured oral examinations in the previous year, he found that 10 had one (and in some cases two) "unsatisfactories." He used this designation in his analysis. Of these 10, 7 passed the certification exam and 3 failed. Of the 12 with no unsatisfactory orals, all but one passed the national examination. Given these results, the director decided that the structured oral was useful in predicting who would pass but not who would fail.

This example illustrates a strategy of analysis which is similar to that used in the assessment of a new diagnostic test in clinical medicine (see Chapter 14 by Brian Haynes, David Sackett, and Peter Tugwell) which is appropriate when the criterion measure can be expressed in binary categories such as yes/no or pass/fail. The same measurement principles would apply in each case.

Construct Validity. This form of validity is used when there is no "gold standard" instrument with which a new test can be compared. A hypothetical construct is substituted. The construct validity exercise attempts to demonstrate *expected* differences in performance between individuals or groups differing on some other dimension which is hypothesized to be related to the competence being assessed.

Construct validity is demonstrated in an example in which a paper-and-pencil test of clinical problem-solving ability is given to three groups: second-year medical students, clinical clerks (fourth-year students), and second-year residents. It is expected that aggregate performance should improve with increased training and experience. If a difference is found, the test is validated. If no difference is found, the test may be inadequate or the hypothetical construct may be incorrect.

In a second example, the medical educator George Miller (Annual Report, 1963) tells the story of an anatomy professor who claimed that his examination was relevant for clinical practice. This examination was taken by first-year medical students, clinical clerks, residents, and practicing physicians. Aggregate performance *decreased* with more seniority, while the professor had expected increases. This test did not have construct validity.

Construct validity is often used to demonstrate validity, but it is a relatively weak approach, one fraught with dangers. A common problem is the ignoring of concomitant variables which also influence performance and attributing performance solely to the construct being tested.

Feasibility

An important nonnumerical consideration is feasibility. "Is this test affordable? Can it be administered in a way that is feasible, in terms of scheduling and other logistics? Are the arrangements for updating the test and maintaining its quality relatively simple?" An example in which feasibility was a problem involved the Royal College of Physicians and Surgeons of Canada, who introduced a set of computer-based patient-management problems into the certification examination for certain specialties. Although the candidates were rather intrigued with this test, it was difficult to arrange. The computer in the originating center was not compatible with the computer in one of the test site cities. Candidates took an unexpectedly long time to familiarize themselves with the mechanics of using the computer. The PMPs took a long time to develop, and this was very costly. Eventually it was decided to drop the test.

Educational Considerations

The last set of considerations are included because most tests of clinical competence are applied in an educational setting or have educational implications. For example, one of the main purposes of medical audit exercises in hospitals is the continuing education of the staff physicians in that hospital. Yet educational aspects are usually ignored when a new test instrument is introduced. We have selected three considerations: appropriateness, use, and educational side effects.

Appropriateness. There are several reasons why a given test may be used in an educational setting. The main purpose may be feedback to learners or the certification that a student has achieved the objectives of a given curricular unit or program; or an instructor or program director may wish to make changes in his program, and the test is applied to obtain an indication of aggregate student performance. It is important to specify the reason for using a given instrument and the manner in which the performance information will be used.

An example will illustrate some of the difficulties in designing an appropriate instrument in an educational setting. A department chief in an academic teaching hospital introduced the idea of a chart audit. Medical audit was a requirement for hospital accreditation, but he was also curious to see whether the attending physicians were using up-to-date concepts in diagnosis and management. He proposed using the results of the chart audit to select topics for future grand rounds, focusing on any deficiencies that might become apparent during the audit procedure. Many physicians in the department raised objections to this plan. Some said that the results would indicate the competence of the house staff, but not the attending staff. Others objected to the method of providing feedback. They would learn much more, they said, if they could receive specific and personal feedback on individual records. Still others said they did not see enough patients with any of the conditions proposed for the audit and so the sample size would be too small to give an indication of the competence of individual physicians. And so the chairman went "back to the drawing board," realizing that he could not meet all of the objectives with one procedure.

Use. The question needs to be asked whether the users are aware of the strengths and shortcomings of a given test. The booklet "Standards for Educational and Psychological Tests" (David, 1974), has an entire section on standards for the *use* of tests. These include the qualifications and concerns of users, the choice or development of a test or method (see section on "Appropriateness" above), the administration and scoring of a test, and the interpretation of scores. All of these features can usefully be applied to tests of clinical competence.

Side Effects. In clinical medicine, there has been growing awareness of the side effects of a drug or some other therapeutic procedure. Clinicians are now more often asking the question: "Are we possibly doing more harm than good?" The question can also be used in the assessment of a diagnostic test. "If I use this test, what will I do with the resultant information? Will it change what I do with this patient? Does the benefit clearly outweigh the risks to the patient in terms of discomfort and possibly morbidity? Is the cost worth it?"

An example where the application of an assessment measure may have done more harm than good was the case of Bob, a second-year medical student. He was certainly intelligent, but not particularly organized. He scraped through his first year of studies, but the second year almost did him in. The problem was the exams. He had some kind of written examination every three weeks or so. Typically, he would skip lectures and labs for a day or two before an exam, cram for it, and usually pass it. He then would borrow the lecture notes he had missed. At just about the time he caught up in his work, it was time to get ready for the next examination. And so this roller coaster pattern continued. Eventually Bob decided medicine might not be for him; the hassle of going through the training program did not seem to be worth it, and so he told his student advisor that he was dropping out.

Most clinicians have on their shelves a compendium of current pharmaceuticals. Each drug is described in detail: the chemical structure, the indications for its use, the dosage and route of administration, and the adverse effects. Perhaps all reports which introduce new tests of clinical competence should include a listing of the possible educational side effects.

Other Comments on Following Chapters

Each of the following chapters includes a synthesis of the strengths and weaknesses of the measure in question. Contributors have been asked to state their own view of how the measure can most appropriately be used, given the current state of development and experience with it. Finally, each contributor has been asked to list some relevant and practical questions which could be addressed in further research. We hope that this listing will serve at least two purposes: to prompt communication about studies which already address a given question, but were not cited, and to serve as a stimulus for future research.

References

American Psychological Association: Standards for educational and psychological tests (1974).

Annual Report, Center for Educational Development, University of Illinois, 1963.

David, F. B. (Chairman): Standards for educational and psychological tests. Washington, D.C.: American Psychological Association, (1974).

Eichna, L. W.: Medical-school education, 1975-1979: a student's perspective. N Engl J Med 303, 727-734 (1980).

Goran, M. J., Williamson, J., Gonnella, J.: The validity of patient management problems. J Med Educ 48, 171-172 (1973).

Park, C., Skakun, E. N., Kling, S.: A study of the relevance of the multiple choice section of the qualifying examination of the Medical Council of Canada. ACMC Forum 14, 16-18 (1981).

Sackett, D. L.: Clinical diagnosis and the clinical laboratory. Clin Invest Med 1, 37-43 (1978).

Tamblyn, R.: Evaluation of an aptitude test for medical problem-solving. Unpublished M.Sc. thesis, McMaster University, Hamilton, Ontario (1981).

Tugwell, P., A methodologic perspective on process measures of the quality of medical care. Clin Invest Med 2, 113-121 (1979).

Wilson, D. R.: Assessment of clinical skills: from the subjective to the objective. Ann R Coll Phys Surg Can 8, 109-118 (1975).

Wingard, J. R., Williamson, J. W.: Grades as predictors of physician's career performance: an evaluative literature review. J Med Educ 48, 311-322 (1973).

CHAPTER 4

Direct Observation

JACQUELINE WAKEFIELD

Introduction

Historical Perspectives

From writings of Hippocrates and Aristotle, there are suggestions that actual observations of student physicians working with patients have been part of the medical education process for millennia. In many respects, this is not surprising since this approach has certain theoretical attractions—especially in the development of basic clinical skills by learners.

It is also not surprising that this method would be used at some times for evaluation purposes. For decades, information obtained by watching student and resident physicians at work with patients has constituted a portion of the "raw material" synthesized by some supervising teachers of physicians into summary reports and ratings. Many medical schools have incorporated this method into their systems for evaluation of the clinical skills of their students, and various professional certifying organizations throughout the world have used some type of direct observation of candidates "working up" patients as part of their examination procedures. Also, in studies of general practice conducted in the 1950s and 1960s, observations of practicing physicians caring for patients in their offices were reported to provide the most important information about the nature and quality of the practitioner's work (Clute, 1963; Jungfer and Last, 1964; Peterson et al., 1956; Taylor, 1954).

Thus, in current times as well as in ancient times, direct observation of actual performance with patients has been used as a method for the teaching *and* the evaluation of physician performance at different levels of training and practice.

Description. The term *direct observation* is widely used (Barro, 1973). Fortunately, it usually is used to mean exactly what it says, a technique for gathering information about physician performance by directly observing the physician during a visit or consultation with a patient.

There are some variations on this theme, however, which relate to the location of the observer and the nature of the observation. The use of one-way mirrors and the taping (audio or video) of interviews are the more common variants. They have been introduced in efforts (1) to make the observations more valid by attempting to minimize "audience effect" on the actual behavior of the person being observed or (2) to make the observation more effective by having several observers and/or more controlled observational situations.

More details about these different approaches will be given below in the section about the precision of direct observation. For the purposes of this review, however, these will all be considered as types of direct observation.

Uses and Rationale

The strongest advocates for the use of direct observation in the health professions have been clinician educators, who have cited the importance of actually seeing the data-acquisition process used by medical students (Engel, 1976; Feinstein, 1967; Maguire and Rutter, 1976; Platt and McMath, 1979; Seegal and Wertheim, 1962; Weiner and Nathanson, 1976). Their studies have identified that medical students, interns and residents, and practicing physicians may often be deficient in their techniques of interviewing and examination. Many types of defects have been noted in both interview and physical examination. More details about frequent errors in examination are provided in the study by Weiner and Nathanson (1976).

At times, critics have claimed that too much attention is paid to these process variables and that the assessment of clinical competence should focus on health care outcomes. In his review of quality-of-care assessments, however, Donabedian (1968) advocated the promotion of quality of care through the evaluation of the process of care. This stance does not detract in any fashion from necessary and critical outcome studies of quality of care. On the other hand, information from outcome studies can lack the details necessary to explain why a particular outcome did, or did not, occur. For example, some of the deficiencies identified in direct observation studies cited earlier could be detected using other strategies. Case discussion and record review might identify the omission of important data. If an accurate data base was available from another source, errors in detection and interpretation might be identified. Problems in interpersonal skills might be detected in indirect ways, like the unsolicited complaint of an offended or frustrated patient. Unfortunately, the details of what actually occurred or why it occurred is frequently too unclear under these circumstances to be of assistance in helping the student or doctor make appropriate changes. When this is the case, corrective action cannot occur. In addition, outcome measures of quality of care often require numerous patient cases to detect meaningful differences; this requirement seriously limits its applicability in undergraduate and graduate education. Also, since outcomes are linked to identified morbidity or mortality, outcome information is *post facto*. For many medical educators and providers, this type of monitoring of quality of care is not the most desirable for their situations. Here the monitoring must be focused on the process of care for the benefit of the patient and the provider. Under these circumstances, direct observation is one method to gather such process data.

Measurement Properties

Credibility

Even the harshest critics of direct observation as an evaluation method have not challenged its face validity. When the target of the assessment is interviewing or history taking or physical examination, direct observation has acceptability and credibility as a method for obtaining information for such an assessment. With this method the observer actually witnesses the process of data acquisition. Other methods (record reviews, oral examinations based on patient cases, patient management problems) are indirect; they are either a step removed from the actual process or they are based on simulated situations.

Kent and Foster (1977) likened data obtained from direct observation procedures to pictures of a scene captured by photographs. In many ways they both mirror the original setting. However, just as the type of photographic equipment and the way it is used can significantly influence the final photograph, it has been recognized that different types of observational strategies and the way in which they are applied will affect the nature and accuracy of the information captured.

Comprehensiveness

Realism. Given that direct observation is a credible method for the assessment of process aspects of clinical competence, what can it sample or test? From the literature it appears that direct observation has been used to assess interviewing, history taking, physical examination, and interpersonal-relationship skills.

At times direct observation has also been used to assess problem-solving and management skills. It is an indirect measure of these latter skills, however, as the observer must *infer* certain thoughts or plans from what is said or done with the patient. Sometimes the student will explain his ideas clearly to the patient, and the observer can be fairly confident about some inferences. In most situations, however, these explanations to patients will encompass neither a full set of working hypotheses nor a list of specific investigations or prescriptions. Also, although students may collect important items on history or in examination, they may not recognize the significance of this information (Ekwo and Loening-Baucke, 1979; Wakefield and Norman, 1977).

To overcome these limitations, Ekwo and Loening-Baucke have used a technique combining direct observation and stimulated recall, based on the design described by Elstein et al. (1978). Using this format, medical students are videotaped while they conduct a visit with a simulated patient and are asked to think aloud during the problem-solving process with the patient, and then are asked to participate in a stimulated recall session after the interview, at which time the student watches the videotape of the visit and is encouraged to explore and explain the pathway of his clinical reasoning. Using this format, Elstein et al. were able to obtain interrater agreement for scores from two independent physician raters ranging from 86 to 95 percent for all the categories of data utilization and overall performance. This method certainly offers considerable promise over attempts to assess these dimensions of clinical performance via direct observation alone.

Information about management plans, both investigations and therapeutics, obtained from direct observation also needs supplementation—by either discussion or record review. Without this additional input, direct observation does *not* yield accurate or reliable assessments of these dimensions of performance (Finkel and Norman, 1973; Wakefield and Norman, 1977).

In summary, direct observation can tap the skills of history taking, physical examination, interviewing, and interpersonal relationships, but it alone cannot adequately sample the cognitive dimensions of clinical problem solving or the specific details of management plans.

Precision

Probably the major methodologic criticism of direct observation has arisen because of limitations in obtaining consistent, reliable quantitative expressions of the behaviors being measured. The potential sources of disagreement are many. Table 4.1 highlights some of these. As these are identified, often they can be eliminated, minimized, or taken into account in the measurement.

Expectation Bias. A number of studies in the psychological literature have reported that knowledge of predicted or expected outcomes can significantly influence the recordings of observers (Kent et al., 1975), especially those of overall or global ratings. However, the ratings of specific aspects of behavior, as applied in direct observation assessment, may or may not be substantially altered (Kent and Foster, 1977; Kent et al., 1975).

This expectation effect may come from a number of sources: (1) a knowledge of the outcome expected in a study or from a certain treatment, (2) the impact of repeated feedback about observations, or (3) a familiarity between observers and subjects. There may also be other factors operating in some situations and settings.

In educational settings, some of these sources of expectation effect may be essential to the learning experience. Feedback to a student or resident about his or her behavior in patient visits helps to identify problems and make appropriate changes. This process may also make him or her aware of the unique emphasis that various evaluating supervisors may apply to any observation. For example, at a Family Practice Unit at McMaster, residents on one clinical team clearly recognize the importance that their particular supervisor places on a focused closure to interviews—stating the assessments of the problem(s), explicitly checking these out with the patients, and specifically asking the patients if they have any

TABLE 4.1
Sources of Bias in Direct Observation Measurement

TASK	Nature of "Problem" Difficulty Complexity

OBSERVER	Expectation of Task
	  Outcome
	Expectation of observee
	  performance
	"Audience effect"

OBSERVEE	Expectation "Audience effect"
REACTIVITY OF OBSERVATION PROCESS	Nature of observation Nature of format/media Interaction between task and observer

questions. When this supervisor is observing residents with patients, the residents already are aware that this is one aspect of the patient visit that is likely to receive attention.

Similarly, a degree of comfort and familiarity often develops between teachers and learners that can contribute to an effective learning environment. This may involve the development of a relationship that includes other shared experiences—observations, discussions, joint consultations. Obviously, this type of familiarity may influence observational recordings or ratings done on a day-to-day basis because of an expectation of a certain type or level of performance. However, for reasons discussed later in the section on the influence of reactivity of the observation procedure, there still may be definite advantages in having personnel who are already present in a specific setting collect data as participant observers.

As any or all of these sources of expectation bias are likely to exist in many clinical settings where direct observations are done, they must be considered carefully in the design of a study or an evaluation system that involves the assessment of physician performance.

Audience Effect. Studies have also been done to determine whether the presence of an observer has a significant influence on the performance of individuals being observed. Several of these studies have cited a definite "audience effect" in various situations (Cohen and Davis, 1973; Cottrell, 1968; Webb et al., 1966). On the other hand, in their study of staff on a research ward of a mental hospital, Hagan, Craighead, and Paul (1975) found that neither the appropriateness nor the frequency of certain staff activities was significantly altered by the presence of an observer. Others (Mercatoris and Craighead, 1974; Roberts and Renzaglia, 1965) have reported changes in the frequencies of certain behaviors but not in the types of behaviors observed.

This "audience effect" has also been cited in studies done of observers (Reid, 1970; Romanczyk et al., 1973; Taplin and Reid, 1973). When observers are aware that *they* are being observed and evaluated, it affects their behavior as raters. Or perhaps stated more accurately, assessments by observers done on a day-to-day basis become much less reliable compared with those of another observer when no system of repeated cross-checking or validation is in effect. The introduction of a periodic overt assessment of one observer's rating performance by another observer can raise the interrater reliabilities for those sessions, but this will likely not persist in the sessions that are not evaluated. If the observers are involved in a system where they know that they may be assessed at any time in a random and covert fashion, however, the "audience effect" appears to prevail in all observation sessions and a consistently high level of agreement with another observer's ratings can be maintained (Taplin and Reid, 1973).

It is often stated that the result of this audience effect on performance is to alter the behavior in the person being observed such that the measurement is of the "capacity to perform rather than of the usual levels of performance" (Donabedian, 1975). This implies that the measurement will be artificially high if the "observee" is aware that the observation is taking place. While this was the case in the studies of observers cited above, Kent and Foster (1977), based on their extensive review of observational studies, indicate that this is not necessarily so.

Given the conflicting evidence about the impact of audience effect, what conclusions can be drawn? Clearly audience effect is another of the factors that must be considered in observational studies. As Kent and Foster (1977) caution, however, "The number of factors determining the magnitude and direction of behavior change may be so great that manifest reactivity is scattered and almost completely unpredictable." However, it should be recognized that this is a source of potential bias which is difficult to control and therefore should be minimized as much as possible.

Reactivity of Observation Process. Nature of the process of observation. Acknowledging that the presence of an observer may influence the behavior being studied, a number of investigators have highlighted approaches to make the process of observation as unobtrusive as possible. These procedures have included (a) arranging a period of habituation to the presence of an observer before observational data is collected; (b) minimizing distractions introduced by the observers through careful planning and with training of the observers; (c) utilizing observation mirrors or audio- or videotape or closed-circuit television when an observer will likely be distracting.

It had been postulated that performance would be more "natural" if observers were "hidden" or unseen while the observations are in progress, and this idea probably contributed to the introduction of one-way mirrors and videotape/television monitors in many settings. Studies have indicated, however, that in certain situations the influence of an observer is not changed appreciably simply by the introduction of such special audiovisual equipment (Corley and Mason, 1976; Kent et al., 1975; Wagner and Alper, 1952). In fact, some of these studies suggest that the noting of certain vocal behaviors may be lessened with the use of either mirror or television, due to inability to clearly discriminate speech with those methods. A similar possibility with certain types of nonverbal interactions (particularly facial expressions) has been suggested by Eisler, Hersen, and Agras (1973). It certainly seems that the greatest influence on performance is the knowledge that one is actually being observed—regardless of whether the observer is visible or hidden.

Thus, the effective sampling of "typical" clinical performance obviously requires more than just alterations in the media used in the observational process. There are other aspects to be considered. Although the studies indicate that special audiovisual equipment may not be a necessary prerequisite for the use of the observational method in some situations, the *degree* of "visibility" of the observer may be quite important in others. For instance, it is important for an observer not to interact with the person(s) being observed, because this will alter the event. In clinical situations when the observer may actually be the patient's regular doctor, it is often difficult not to distort the situation by simply being present. Also, it is important for an observer to be "unobtrusive," but this is very difficult when several observers are required. In both of these situations, it is best if the observers actually can be hidden from view.

Despite these specific indications, for many situations (especially those in which the observer can spend a period of time becoming "incorporated into the background" as habituation to being observed occurs) direct observation with the observer physically present in the same room or area may be quite acceptable. Indeed, there may be situations, such as an examination process, where the observations must take place without complication or delay. At these times observers *in vivo* are usually the least inclined to unexpected mechanical failure and thus are the preferred approach.

As outlined above, there are various factors that contribute to making one type of observation format more appropriate for certain situations than for others, and the selection of the most appropriate format can often reduce the most deleterious influences on the results obtained from the observations. Regardless of the particular strategy selected, both a period of habituation to the process of observation *and* a procedure to avoid advance announcement of the actual observation are important if the major goal is to sample typical performance.

Interaction between observational task and observer. In addition to factors related to the nature of the observation process, there appear to be factors related to the guidelines and formats used in documenting the observation that affect what is observed. Among these are the complexity of the rating code and the complexity of the problem or situation.

In work related to child development and behavior, Reid (1970), studied the influence of the complexity of the rating code on reliability. His work suggests that both more exhaustive or complex rating codes and more difficult or complex situations result in less reliable data.

In the health disciplines, similar problems have been encountered in the rating of performance observed in clinical encounters. For example, in the assessment of physical examination skills, extensive checklists developed for specific organs or systems have produced high levels of agreement among raters, with interrater reliabilities ranging from 0.82 to 0.94 (Andrew, 1977). This certainly is important in examination situations and fortunately is feasible when the patient encounter can be structured in advance.

The development of unambiguous checklists is often arduous, however, and in many clinical settings the observations cannot be controlled to the extent that they are in examinations. Under these circumstances, appropriate and concise checklists or codes are not available and the complexity of detailed checklists (especially those that do not match the clinical problems) can result in poor interrater reliabilities. Here, more general forms (using rating scales for various categories of performance rather than specific checklists) can be used. Interrater reliabilities (Norman et al., 1973) are then less impressive than those cited by Andrew (1977), and range from 0.66 to 0.84. To some degree, this may be the result of complexity *within* the categories used on such forms, as one category often encompasses a considerable number of specific behaviors.

Other studies support the conclusion that more difficult or complex *situations* lessen reliability. Several studies at McMaster have demonstrated considerable variation in interrater reliability from one patient problem to another. When standard rating forms have been used with perplexing cases, a degree of reliability that existed with more straightforward cases was lost. One of these studies (Wakefield and Norman, 1977) used the assessments of performance of a group of residents with predetermined evaluators, who remained constant from case to case. Despite this condition of "fixed" evaluators, considerable interrater variability in ratings of the same skill or dimension was evident for particular cases. If the results of these observations from the same evaluator are used as the basis for calculations of test-retest reliability, it can be seen in Table 4.2 that these estimates of reliability are lower than those for interrater reliability using the same case with different evaluators. Similar findings were reported by Corley (1975) with the performance of candidates in the Certification Examination of the College of Family Physicians of Canada.

It has been suggested that the nature of the task in any one patient encounter may be sufficiently different from that of other encounters as to result in different ratings; however, the sources of this variation are unclear. Is it due to true differences in the level of performance displayed, depending on the content of the problem? Is it due to a greater difficulty in accurately evaluating the performance with certain problems? Or is it due to other variables that we have not yet clearly identified? The answers to these questions remain a challenge for future research.

Traits/training of observers. Traits of the raters can also

TABLE 4.2
Direct Observation Evaluations

Category	Interrater Reliability	Inter-encounter Reliability
Interview Skills	.62	.34
History	.58	.41
Physical Exam	.75	.53
Problem Formulation	.55	.43
Management	.54	.41
Doctor-Patient Interaction	.72	.55

Using one-tailed test, all of the above are significant at $p < 0.005$ level.

influence the reliability of observational data. Raters are subject to a number of scoring errors—halo effect, specific rating tendencies (lenient, stringent, central), unique interpretations of the categories or the standards, and so on. To overcome some of these, observer training sessions have been advocated. However, data to support these ventures are limited.

The information from several studies with faculty in the Department of Family Medicine at McMaster University has suggested that there is some benefit in improved interrater reliability from sessions that orient faculty to the direct observation mode of evaluation and allow some practice (coupled with feedback) by these faculty raters. Studies done with examiners of the College of Family Physicians of Canada and by Wildman et al. (1975) reflect the same trend—that brief practice sessions, linked with feedback and discussions about ratings on direct observations, does improve interrater reliability.

These demonstrated benefits are unfortunately associated with significant limitations and potential problems with such training sessions. In a study of evaluators for a clinical skills program in medical school, Newble and co-workers (1980) found that extensive training of evaluators had no demonstrable benefit in improving subsequent interrater reliability. Mash and Makohoniuk (1975) reported a situation in which observer performance actually worsened with training. Thus, in their review, Kent and Foster (1977) stress the importance of carefully planned and coordinated training sessions.

In order to achieve the desired results, training sessions need certain essential ingredients: (1) There should be some standard with which observers can compare their ratings and (2) the training content needs to provide a variety of situations that are similar to those that will subsequently be rated. Without this, inter-rater reliability may be lessened and the pattern of subsequent ratings distorted by the training sessions.

In summary, it appears that brief tailored sessions for observers do have some merit and should be included systematically at the beginning of any observational work, although extensive training is unlikely to provide significantly greater benefit. In addition, the training sessions should be carefully planned, and short retraining sessions interspersed throughout a study may enhance the uniform application of a rating standard.

Validity

Probably in part because of the lack of adequate criterion measures and perhaps also because of the high degree of credibility of direct observation, few attempts to address questions of concurrent or predictive validity have been made.

In Canada, where direct observation is a method used in many Family Medicine residency programs, studies have been done using the Certification Examination of the College of Family Physicians of Canada as the criterion measure. The use of this examination as a criterion may be questioned, although it has been cited as a "state of the art" examination of clinical competence in family medicine (Corley, 1975) and it uses various different measures to collect test data.

Some studies conducted at McMaster (Wakefield and Norman, 1977) assessed predictive validity by determining whether performance in the Family Medicine residency program, based on approximately 20 direct observations per resident, accurately predicted performance on the College certification examination. Composite scores from the certification exams for "cognitive skills" and for "affective skills" did yield correlation coefficients of 0.65 to 0.73 for pooled scores for similar categories from in-training assessments (supervisor summary ratings and direct observation ratings). On the other hand, the direct observation ratings did *not* accurately predict certification performance on any of the individual, specific tests, although there were low but consistent correlations of about 0.3 for doctor-patient relationships and interviewing skills. The results were obviously poor. On the other hand, if each of the certification orals is considered as a separate item or "problem" (and this is consistent with their design around a specific patient case), then these findings are not particularly surprising. They reinforce the results of many studies that indicate that performance on one single case is *not* a good predictor of performance with a single different case. When the performance on a number of cases during residency training were pooled, and these pooled performance ratings were compared with the pooled scores from the certification exams, the correlation coefficients climbed to greater than 0.60, with those for affective or interpersonal skills being nearly 0.75.

Tests of concurrent validity have been done with medical records (Wakefield et al., 1978; Zuckerman et al., 1975) and with PMPs (Norman and Feightner, 1981). The comparisons with medical record audits suggest that direct observation is more accurate for identifying data elicited from and information given to the patient, while records are better for documenting diagnostic labels and details of management plans. Comparisons with performance on PMPs indicate that more data are elicited on history, in examination, and with investigations on written PMPs than in the clinical encounter with a patient. Although differences obtained with these three measures have been documented, the significance of these differences is unclear.

Tests of construct validity have rested on the theory that "with time and experience in a program, students/residents should become more competent and therefore perform better on any valid measures of clinical competence." This test of construct validity has been met for the direct observation assessments in the McMaster studies (Wakefield and Norman, 1977), since the performance of more than 60 percent of the residents showed significant improvement over the two to three years in the residency program for all categories except physical examination. Similar results have been obtained in the Family Medicine Residency Program at the University of Western Ontario, where improvements were noted in all dimensions, with the most striking change occurring in the categories of management (Molineux et al., 1976).

In summary, studies of the validity of direct observation have been limited in number and the results tentative. This is definitely another area where future research is needed.

Feasibility

Although direct observation offers the potential for obtaining valuable and at least moderately reliable information about a range of clinical competencies, issues of feasibility and cost have been major constraints in certain settings.

There is little doubt that direct observation is a time-intensive method, although the time actually required may encompass a considerable spectrum. At one end of this time spectrum is the type of assessment described by Ekwo and Loening-Baucke (1979). A similar technique, combining direct observation with stimulated recall, has been used for various purposes at McMaster University and it does require considerable time. Despite this, it has definite attractions and advantages, as it allows one to collect information about a greater range of clinical problem-solving strategies, including those cognitive processes in the clinical method that direct observation alone cannot tap.

Near this same end of the spectrum is the observation of a "complete workup" of a patient. In various clinical specialties this is often the initial assessment of a new patient. In addition to being perceived as very time consuming (one observation may require from 30 to 60 minutes), it is also often tedious work for busy clinician-teachers. When additional time for discussion and feedback is required, as it would be for educational settings, this type of direct observation becomes too impractical and too costly to be done very frequently. Here again, though, the information so obtained in certain situations may be worth much more than the costs.

In other situations and in some disciplines, less time is involved. For example, in family practice, patient visits tend to be relatively brief, as the patient is usually already known to the physician and the focus is on one or two specific problems. Under these conditions, periodic observation of an entire patient visit is more feasible. Indeed, direct observation is more commonly done in these settings.

Farther along the spectrum comes a "sampling" approach. This is commonly used in the teaching or evaluation of some particular technique in physical examination or of a specific investigational or therapeutic procedure (for example, joint aspiration or suturing). Harden et al. (1975) describe this approach in their structured clinical examination. A "selective sampling approach" need not be limited to just these types of observations.

In the 1960s, G. L. Engel (1971) developed an approach to clinical teaching which he advocated as one way to overcome deficiencies in the case presentation method. This approach, which involved having a small group observe the first 15 to 20 minutes of a patient consultation, was a type of sampling that focused on interviewing and enquiry strategies. It also facilitated subsequent discussion about the interpretation of data and the generation/ testing of clinical hypotheses. From studies of clinical reasoning (Barrows et al., 1978; Elstein et al., 1978), there is theoretical support for such an approach—since clinical hypotheses do develop early in an interview, with learners as well as with practitioners. In fact, observing the first five to ten minutes of a patient visit and then briefly discussing the ideas that have arisen can yield information about both interview skills and early clinical reasoning. In similar fashion, the selective observation of the termination of patient visits can provide information about some management plans and about other interviewing skills (explanations to the patient, attention to patient's concerns, and so on). This type of approach is used by some clinical teachers at McMaster and appears to have merit.

From this review of the various formats for direct observation, it can be seen that there are ways to adjust some of the time factors involved in direct observation. If these adjustment are to be effective, it is important (1) that the specific aspects of clinical performance to be evaluated are identified in advance and (2) that any "sampling" is guided by a knowledge of the process of clinical reasoning. Otherwise, the sample may not contain the behavior that the observer wishes to capture.

Even when the time can be appropriately adjusted, other obstacles to the use of direct observation may exist. These are often related to those aspects of the *process* of observation described earlier—particularly the nature of the observational format.

As outlined above, many of the problems inherent in observational methods can be minimized. For example, if observers are to be physically present, they will be less obtrusive if they receive some guidelines and training about how not to intrude. If it is difficult to arrange to have observers in place at the correct times for interviews (especially if a sampling approach is used), capturing the interviews via audiotape or videotape may circumvent this problem. In fact, for most of the problems in this area, there fortunately are some potential solutions.

Educational Effect

Student Learning. As noted earlier, direct observation is a method that is particularly suited to the teaching and the evaluation of various clinical skills—the process variables of patient care. It is for these purposes that its educational use has been advocated.

Seegal and Wertheim (1962) and Weiner and Nathanson (1976) have stressed the importance of direct observation in physical examination. Engel (1971), Maguire and Rutter (1976), and Platt and McMath (1979) have discussed it in relation to history-taking skills. It has also been recommended for developing general communication skills (Sanson-Fisher and Maguire, 1980). Indeed, a national survey in the United States (Kahn et al., 1979) revealed that most medical schools there have programs for the teaching of interpersonal skills and that direct observation (live or via tape) with feedback was the predominant teaching method for "skill practice."

Although direct observation with feedback has been widely advocated, too few studies have been done assessing its effectiveness as an educational strategy. One of the pioneering studies in this area (Hing, 1966), in addition to investigating the dimensions of the assessment of clinical performance of students with direct observation, did attempt to address the question of educational impact. Unfortunately, unavoidable limitations in the study obviated conclusions about this aspect. Work by Maguire and colleagues (Maguire et al., 1977; Maguire and Rutter, 1976) has indicated that feedback to students based on observations of interviews with patients (live or audiotape or videotape) can improve the clinical performance of these students.

Thus, while this use of direct observation has a sound rationale (Sanson-Fisher and Maguire, 1980), some cautions are warranted. First, the process of direct observation does not, alone, ensure educational effectiveness. The process of *feedback* is also involved. Since this feedback is based on an assessment made via direct observation, efforts to improve the accuracy and reliability of that prerequisite assessment are vital. The nature of the feedback (as well as its substance), however, may have a significant impact on subsequent learning and efforts to study and improve that step are important, too.

Second, it is necessary to avoid unjustified extensions into areas beyond those shown to be reliably assessed by direct observation. Ekwo and Loening-Baucke (1979) have cautioned against using direct observation alone for the assessment of dimensions such as hypothesis generation and interpretation of clinical data. Work at McMaster (Wakefield and Norman, 1977) supports this and also indicates that similar cautions apply to the assessment of various aspects of patient management.

Decision Making. Direct observation is one of the preferred methods used in the evaluation of clinical skills, including interpersonal skills. Thus, it is not infrequently used to evaluate performance in introductory clinical medicine courses and in clinical clerkship and residency training programs. When used for such purposes, it is important that the measurement properties of direct observation in these situations be recognized. For example, given the variation in observed performance from encounter to encounter, little confidence should be placed on an evaluation based on a single observation.

The need for multiple observations represents a major obstacle to general acceptability. Despite this, direct observation is used in many programs and by some certifying bodies because of the invaluable information that is provided about aspects of clinical performance for which other valid and more reliable measures do not exist. Thus, if assessments of the *processes* of clinical performance (interviewing, history taking, physical examination, etc.) are desired, some type of direct observation will likely be needed.

Conclusion

In summary, there are definite constraints in the use of a direct observation method. If the usefulness of direct observation in a program is clear, however, many of these obstacles can be overcome through careful planning and judicious implementation.

References

Andrew, B. J.: The use of behavioral checklists to assess physical examination skills. J Med Educ 52, 589-591 (1977).

Barro, A. R.: Survey and evaluation of approaches to physician performance measurement. J Med Educ 48, 1051-1093 (1973).

Barrows, H. S., Feightner, J. W., Neufeld, V. R., Norman, G. R.: Analysis of the clinical methods of medical students and physicians. Report to Ontario Department of Health and PSI Foundation, (1978).

Clute, K. F.: The general practitioner. Toronto: University of Toronto Press, (1963).

Cohen, J. L., Davis, J. H.: Effects of audience status evaluation and time of action on performance with hidden-word problems. J Pers Soc Psychol 27, 74-85 (1973).

Corley, J. B.: The college certification examinations: A preliminary study. Can Fam Physician 21 118-124 (1975).

Corley, J. B., Mason, R. L.: A study on the effectiveness of one-way mirrors. J Med Educ 51, 62-63 (1976).

Cottrell, N. B.: Performance in the presence of other human beings. Social facilitation and imitative behavior. Boston: Allyn & Bacon (1968).

Donabedian, A.: Promoting quality through evaluating the process of patient care. Med Care 6, 181-202 (1968).

Donabedian, A.: Medical care appraisal, Part III: Issues of method and technique. A guide to medical care administration. Volume II. American Public Health Association (1975).

Eisler, R. M., Hersen, M., Agras, W. S.: Videotapes: A method for controlled observation of non-verbal interpersonal behavior. Behav Ther 4, 420-425 (1973).

Ekwo, E. E., Loening-Baucke, V.: Clinical problem solving and clinical knowledge. Med Educ 13, 251-256 (1979).

Elstein, A. S., Shulman, L. S., Sprafka, S. A.: Medical problem solving: An analysis of clinical reasoning. Cambridge Mass.: Harvard University Press (1978).

Engel, G. L.: The deficiencies of the case presentation as a method of clinical teaching—another approach. N Engl J Med 284, 20-24 (1971).

Engel, G. L.: Are medical schools neglecting clinical skills? JAMA 236, 861-864 (1976).

Feinstein, A. R.: Clinical judgment. Baltimore: Williams & Wilkins (1967).

Finkel, A., Norman, G. R.: The validity of direct observation. Proceedings 12th Annual Conference on Research in Medical Education. Washington, D.C. Association of American Medical Colleges (1973).

Hagen, R. L., Craighead, W. E., Paul, G. L.: Staff reactivity to evaluative behavioral observations. Behav Ther 6, 201-205 (1975).

Harden, R. M., Stevenson, M., Downie, W., Wilson, G. M.: Assessment of clinical competence using objective structured examination. Br Med J 911, 447-451 (1975).

Hing, C. G.: Direct observation as a means of teaching and evaluating clinical skills. J Med Educ 41, 150-161 (1966).

Jones, R. R., Reid, J. B., Patterson, G. R.: Naturalistic observation in clinical assessment. Advances in psychological assessment. San Francisco: Jossey-Bass (1974).

Jungfer, C. C., Last, J. M.: Clinical performance in Australian general practice. Med Care 2, 72-83 (1964).

Kahn, G. S., Cohen, B., Jason, H.: The teaching of interpersonal skills in U.S. medical schools. J Med Educ 54, 29-35 (1979).

Kent, R. N., Dietz, A., Diament, C., O'Leary, K. D.: A comparison of observational recordings in vivo, via mirror, and via television. Child Dev 76, (1975).

Kent, R. N., Foster, S. L.: Direct observational procedures: Methodological issues in naturalistic settings. Handbook of Behavior Assessment, New York: Wiley (1977).

Maguire, G. P., Rutter, D. R.: History-taking for medical students: I. Deficiencies in performance. Lancet 2, 556-560 (1976).

Maguire, G. P., et al.: An experimental comparison of three courses in history taking. Med Educ 11, 175-182 (1977).

Mash, E. J., Makohoniuk, G.: The effect of prior information and behavioral predictability on observer accuracy. Child Dev 46, 513-519 (1975).

Mash, E. J., McElwee, J. D.: Situational effects on observer accuracy: Behavior prediction, prior experience, and complexity of coding categories. Child Dev 45, 367-377 (1974).

Mercatoris, M., Craighead, W. E.: The effects of non-participant observation on teacher and pupil classroom behavior. J Educ Psychol 66, 512-519 (1974).

Molineux, J., Hennen, B. K., McWhinney, I. R.: In training performance assessment in family practice. J Fam Pract 3, 405-408 (1976).

Newble, D. I., Hoare, S., Sheldrake, P. F.: The selection and training of examiners for clinical examinations. Med Educ 14, 345-349 (1980).

Norman, G. R., Feightner, J. W.: A comparison of behavior on simulated patients and patient management problems. Med Educ 15, 26-32 (1981).

Norman, G. R., Wakefield, J. G., Pineo, G.: Experience with a single encounter assessment of clinical skills. Abstract, Royal College of Physicians and Surgeons Canada Meeting, Edmonton (1973).

Peterson, O. L., Andrews, L. P., Spain, R. S., Greenberg, B. G.: An analytical study of North Carolina general practice. J Med Educ 31, 1-64 (1956).

Platt, F. W., McMath, J. C.: Clinical hypocompetence: The interview. Ann Intern Med 91, 898-902 (1979).

Reid, J. B.: Reliability assessment of observation data: A possible methodological problem. Child Dev 41, 1143-1150 (1970).

Roberts, R. R., Renzaglia, G. A.: The influence of tape recording on counselling. J Counselling Psychol 12, 10-16 (1965).

Romanczyk, R. G., Kent, R. N., Diament, C., O'Leary, K. D.: Measuring the reliability of observational data: A reactive process. J Appl Behav Anal 6, 175-184 (1973).

Sanson-Fisher, R., Maguire, P.: Should skills in communicating with patients be taught in medical schools? Lancet 2, 523-526 (1980).

Seegal, D., Wertheim, A. R.: On the failure to supervise students' performance of complete physical examinations. JAMA 180, 476-477 (1962).

Taplin, P. S., Reid, J. B.: Effects of instructional set and experimenter influence on observer reliability. Child Dev 44, 547-554 (1973).

Taylor, S.: Good general practice. London: Oxford University Press (1954).

Wagner, S., Alper, T. G.: The effect of an audience on behavior in a choice situation. J Abnormal Soc Psychol 74, 222-229 (1952).

Wakefield, J. G., Norman, G. R., Barnes, R., Reynolds, J. L.: The validity of the medical record: A comparison of elicited and recorded clinical data.

Proceedings of the 17th Annual Conference on Research in Medical Education, New Orleans, La. (1978).

Wakefield, J. G., Norman, G. R.: The relationship between in-training assessment and certification performance. Report to the College of Family Physicians of Canada October (1977).

Webb, E. J., Campbell, D. T., Schwartz, R. D., Sechrest, L.: Unobtrusive measures: Non-reactive research in the social sciences. Chicago: Rand McNally (1966).

Weiner, S., Nathanson, M.: Physical examination—frequently observed errors. JAMA 236, 852-855 (1976).

Wildman, B. G., Erickson, M. T., Kent, R. N.: The effects of two training procedures on observer agreement and variability of behavior ratings. Child Dev 46, 520-524 (1975).

Zuckerman, A. E., Starfield, B., Hochreiter, C., Kovasznay, B.: Validating the content of pediatric outpatient medical records by means of tape-recording doctor-patient encounters. Pediatrics 56, 407-411 (1975).

CHAPTER 5

Oral Examinations

LINDA J. MUZZIN
LAWRENCE HART

Current and Historical Importance

The oral examination survives as an ultimate "rite of passage" to a postgraduate degree in the academic disciplines or to a specialization in medicine. There is also still an oral component in the M.B. examination administered by London medical schools (Buckley-Sharp and Harris, 1972) and in other schools following the British model. In the United States, however, the National Board of Medical Examiners discontinued the use of the oral in 1963 based on the results of a study undertaken by them in 1960 (Hubbard et al., 1963). Satisfied with the reliability of its objective tests (Parts I and II), the Board had turned its attention to the Part III "clinical." When three years of data and 10,000 examinations yielded a correlation of only 0.25 for independent evaluations of a single candidate by two examiners, the Board decided to discontinue the oral.

Prior to the study done by the National Board, very little had been published regarding the reliability and validity of oral examinations. In the United States there had been two simple demonstrations of the wide variations that can occur among raters in grading an oral examination in a general academic setting (Barnes and Pressey, 1929; Trimble, 1934) and a study undertaken in a medical setting that reported high variability in grading of oral exams (Goldstein, 1958). In Britain, Hartog and Rhodes

(1935) had also reported low intercorrelations between grades assigned by oral examiners for the same candidate. A study by Bull (1959) of medical orals and clinicals was the only paper at that time that reported reasonably high correlations between the grades assigned by pairs of examiners. Appearing when it did, the Hubbard study marked a significant point in the evaluation of the oral examination. The National Board replaced its Part III oral with a patient management problem (PMP) exercise and some of the specialty boards in the United States and Canada began to re-design their orals in an attempt to make them more reliable. In 1970, the American Board of Internal Medicine dropped its oral examination in favor of a written examination (Petersdorf and Beck, 1972). By 1975, the year in which the American specialty boards held a major conference on oral examinations (ABMS, 1975), two more of the 22 American Boards had joined the National Board in abandoning the oral. This was not only due to concern over unreliability, but also due to the increasing adminis-tration costs of final orals. Futcher et al. (1977), in discussing the experience of Internal Medicine, reported that the number of candidates for certification by that Board had risen from 1,429 in 1967 to 4,455 in 1975; the cost of a technique with dubious reliability for this number of candidates could not be justified.

A number of those speciality and subspecialty boards that have opted to retain the oral have undertaken studies of the re-liability and validity of their methods, and, in some cases, have developed new standardized forms of their examinations (Carter, 1962; Foster, 1969, 1975; Kelley et al., 1971; Kittle, 1975; Maatsch, 1980; Meskauskas, 1975). Perhaps the most ambitious of these projects has been undertaken in Illinois by the Center for the Study of Medical Education and the University of Illinois College of Medicine, in cooperation with the American Board of Orthopedic Surgery (Levine and McGuire, 1970a, 1970b). These efforts by the American specialty boards, together with those of a number of medical schools, provide much of what is known about the oral examination; altogether there have been about 20 different attempts to explore the measurement properties of the oral examination.

The results of these research efforts will be described and summarized in this chapter. Unfortunately, the studies, although many were rigorously done, differ enough in significant procedural detail and analysis to make comparison difficult. They suggest that longevity of the oral examination in medical evaluation cannot entirely be attributed to the stubborn and illogical persistence of a culturally established tradition; despite its shortcomings, the oral may be as good (or bad) a method as any other to assess clinical competence.

Measurement Properties of Oral Examinations

Credibility

Faith in the power of the oral examination as a measure of clinical competence is related to its face validity as a measurement technique. The "clinical," in particular, has been singled out as the best method for observing the candidate in the physican role, aside from direct observation itself (Abrahamson, 1975; Kittle, 1975; Levine and McGuire, 1970a; Van Wart, 1974). It has been claimed that the technique measures three areas of competence: a candidate's fund of knowledge, capacities for solving problems, and personal characteristics (Colton and Peterson, 1967; Levine and McGuire, 1970a; Rosinski, 1975).

In the cognitive domain, Lipscomb has suggested that orals can measure better than written examinations "breadth as well as depth," "to some degree cognitive aspects of technical capability," and "whether the candidate has maintained his information over a period of time" (1975, p. 42). The second domain thought to be measured by oral exams has been variously termed "problem-solving ability," "clinical judgment," "ability of the candidate to think on his feet," and the "ability to respond to a change in situation" (Abrahamson, 1975; Bonfiglio, 1975; Cox, 1978; Levine and McGuire, 1970a; Waugh and Moyse, 1969). The third area that advocates of oral examinations feel the technique measures might be summarized under Abrahamson's general term, "interpersonal skills." Under this rubric it has been claimed that orals could measure: "the candidate's ability to communicate verbally," his or her "interviewing technique," and "disabilities or incompetencies that are related to stressful or emergency situations" (Lipscomb, 1975, p. 42); "traits that could not be tested in writtens, such as personality, alertness, stress tolerance, etc. . . ." (Doyle, 1980, p. 1); and "the student's appearance, manner, personality, alertness, confidence, honesty, self-awareness and other aspects of values and attitudes" (Cox, 1978, p. 476).

The oral has both strong advocates and those who argue that it is merely a ritual, involving a judgment as to whether the student "is or is not fit to become a member of the club." On the other hand, it has been pointed out that even a ritual (Abrahamson, 1975) is not unimportant, in that it is associated with achieving another level of competence and admission to a professional group.

Precision

Barnes and Pressey, in 1929, were the first to draw attention to the unreliability of oral exams. Using graduate students in Psychology, they found that the average range of variation among judges rating the same candidate was 9 points on a 17-point scale and that even after committee discussion, the correlation between committee ratings of the same candidate was only 0.30. In 1932, Pressey, Pressey, and Barnes followed this up with a demonstration in which a candidate for a master's degree in Psychology underwent four oral examinations. The ratings of the judges ranged from 40 to 88 on a scale of 100; two committees failed the candidate and two passed her.

In the 50 years since the Barnes and Pressey demonstrations, many sources of variability in grades assigned in medical oral examinations have been identified: those due (1) to the examiner; (2) to the type of oral, the material it attempts to cover, and the situation or context in which it is administered; and (3) to the candidate's personality and reaction to the exam, as well as his or her ability or competence. Each source of error is reviewed in this section.

Variation due to Examiners. A few researchers claim that grades assigned by oral examiners are so inconsistent that they show no patterns whatsoever (e.g., Marshall and Ludbrook, 1972). Other investigators, on the contrary, claim that oral examiners are unreliable, but that their biases follow a pattern. Two specific types of examiner bias across candidates that have been identified include the tendency for one examiner to "spread" his marks more widely than another examiner—for example, grading within a range between 35 and 75 percent as compared to a range of 45 to 65 percent. Another source of bias may be the tendency for one examiner to be more lenient than another—the "dove/hawk" dimension (Foster et al., 1969). These two sources of bias were identified by an early researcher (Bull, 1959), who dismissed them because they could be eliminated by converting examiner grades to standard grades.

Another source of examiner bias that may occur between candidates is the so-called halo effect, or the tendency to rate a candidate high (or low) in all areas being evaluated in a session if he scores high (or low) in one area. On this question it should be noted that if the skills being evaluated reflect a unitary trait or ability, as Maatsch (1980) has suggested, then there should be high correlations between subscores or internal consistency in an oral evaluation. Thus a demonstration of "halo effect" may mean that there is an examiner bias; alternatively, it may reflect the true ability of the candidate. We need to know more about the nature of the skills being evaluated.

In spite of these various charges made against oral examiners, the evidence shows that studies using *pairs* of examiners in the same examination tend to report positive correlations between the grades assigned by each member of the pair, even when these grades are independently assigned. In an early study of this type by Carter (1962), 250 candidates who had passed the written examinations for certification by the American Board of Anesthesiology underwent oral examinations by three pairs of examiners in different rooms. Examiner pairs independently assigned grades on a five-point scale. Results showed correlations between 0.25 and 0.45 between individual raters, but the agreement between pairs who saw the same performance was better, with correlations ranging from 0.55 to 0.67. This corresponded to a reliability coefficient of 0.89 for the total oral examination, using all six examiners, which led Carter to conclude that ". . . these oral examinations are very much more reliable than one would expect oral examinations to be" (p. 150). Carter speculated that this was because his examiners were briefed and questions were similar, although not standardized, from candidate to candidate. Hubbard (1971), however, questioned these high correlations because the pairs of examiners were in the same room and unlikely to be independent. The National Board study that he had reported on had found a correlation of 0.25 between totally independent ratings of a candidate, which is at the lower end of the spectrum of correlations found by Carter between individual raters.

The finding that the scores of raters agree more closely on candidates when the raters examine in pairs is a common thread that runs through the studies on the reliability of the oral back as far as Bull (1956, 1959), who found that the correlations between marks assigned by pairs of examiners (who were asked to try not to influence each other's marks) were 0.69 and 0.51 on the "major

case"; 0.82 and 0.89 on the "minor case"; and on the "oral,"[1]
0.83 and 0.74. Wilson et al. (1969) found, in a similar study, correlations between examiners of a pair of 0.78 for the "long case"
and 0.835 for the "short case." Evans et al. (1966) found that
reliability within three pairs of raters in the same setting, grading
independently, was 0.772, 0.852, and 0.824, respectively. Holloway et al. (1967), who also recorded grades assigned by pairs of
examiners grading independently, found a between-examiner correlation of 0.67. And O'Donohue and Wergin (1978), who had
examiner pairs grade independently and then assign a joint grade,
found a correlation of 0.754 between the independent ratings.

Even Ludbrook and Marshall, who were unable to find significant overall correlations between grades assigned by individuals
to candidates on "short cases," found positive correlations between the grades of examiners working in pairs. In an initial study
(1971), they chose 16 faculty members from the University of
Adelaide staff and "trained" half of them for oral grading by using
videotape review and group discussion. Two pairs of examiners
then saw each candidate (final-year medical students), half of the
candidates being seen by "trained" pairs and half by "untrained"
pairs. The correlations between grades assigned by co-examiners
were 0.55 for trained and 0.49 for untrained pairs. However, comparing the mean grades assigned by the first pair of examiners with
those for the second pair yielded correlations of only 0.10 and
0.14, respectively, for trained and untrained examiners. In a second study (1972), when Marshall and Ludbrook used eight examiners to score each candidate *individually*, correlations between scores assigned by the two individuals for each candidate
ranged between -0.04 and 0.46. Overall correlations were not significant.

By contrast, studies that have not used examiners working
in pairs—but instead have used individual raters or teams of three
or more raters—have tended to report problems with rater reliability. Meskauskas (1975), for example, found an average reliability coefficient obtained between individual examiners of 0.39

---

[1] The conventional clinical usually consists of a "long case" and a number of
"short cases." In the long case, the candidate has an hour to take a history
and carry out a physical examination on a selected patient before being
questioned by a pair of examiners for 15 minutes on diagnosis and plans
for treatment. In the short cases, the student has only to demonstrate his
ability to elicit and elucidate physical signs or to recognize various clinical
conditions (Wilson et al., 1969).

(ranging from 0.29 for "history taking" to 0.44 for "evaluation of skill in synthesis") for independent ratings of candidates for certification in Cardiology. Goldstein (1958), who studied the evaluation of students in pharmacology at Harvard (1952-1955) and Stanford (1955-1957) by teams of oral raters, found a level of reliability which was "so imprecise as to be meaningless." Colton and Peterson (1967), who had teams of three medical faculty members at Harvard Medical School rate medical students, found an average intrateam reliability of 0.56. Reliability by team varied considerably, however, from a low of 0.20 for one team to a high of 0.95 for another. In the case of the low-reliability team, analysis showed one member to be "nonconformist" in his ratings. A third American study using teams of raters was done by Pokorny and Frazier (1966). In their study, psychiatric residents were subjected to oral exams by four teams, two giving "clinicals" and two "oral interviews." When the coefficient of concordance was calculated (to determine agreement among the teams on the rankings of the residents by the teams), it was found to be only 0.303, which was not significant.

McGuire (1966) has argued that consultation or some type of "subtle communication" underlies the high interrater reliability of pairs of raters. But if this is the crucial factor, why do the three studies that used teams of raters find low rater reliability within and between the teams in some cases? Does examiner rapport break down when the number of examiners exceeds two? One confounding factor between the studies using individual raters and those using pairs is that the individual raters are seeing different performances, while the pairs are seeing the same performance. In cases where examiners grade different performances independently, it is clearly difficult to identify inconsistencies as due to the examiners or to variations in what is observed (e.g., Ludbrook and Marshall, 1971).

Variation due to Candidates. Any demonstration that the oral exam measures something other than "knowledge," "clinical judgment," and "interpersonal skills" is a demonstration of error. For example, variation due to candidate anxiety might be considered a deviation from valid measurement. Cox (1978) claims that "oral examinations can be more highly threatening to some students than to others, with a consequent poorer performance by the threatened students" (p. 477). Pokorny and Frazier (1966) found evidence for this pattern among psychiatric residents who underwent an oral examination. The average examination grade ranged from 80.8 for those who said they had "minimal anxiety" to 74.9 for those who reported "severe anxiety." The average grades of the sessions rated by the residents as "friendly" or "hostile" were 79.0 and 67.4, respectively. The importance of a sympathetic examiner to help set the candidate at ease has been identified by Waugh and Moyse (1969) in a study in which videotapes of oral sessions were reviewed by examiners and examinees.

Another study that found some evidence for an inverse relationship between anxiety and performance in the oral examination was done by Holloway et al. (1967). They concluded that this was a reasonable finding in that "candidates who are less anxious (whether they show it or not) should perform better in the rather frightening situation of confronting their examiner face-to-face . . ." (p. 231). In a second study (Holloway et al., 1968), they found some suggestion that the anxious candidates did better in an MCQ test and were more coherent with their essay answers in an essay test. It has also been found that introverts perform better in examinations than extroverts (Bligh et al., 1975). However, it might be expected that the extrovert would convey a greater sense of confidence in the interview situation and thus perform better.

Small differences in grades due to candidate anxiety or slight introversion can be tolerated. But how should the finding that a student's oral grade is correlated .668 with the percentage of words he contributes to an oral (Evans et al., 1966) be interpreted? Evans and his colleagues interpreted this finding as meaning that "many students with higher grades were able to organize their thoughts while speaking fluently and so used more words"— in other words, a true reflection of ability. But perhaps the ability to speak fluently should not influence scores on a medical oral to this degree. Doyle (1980), for example, expresses concern that one candidate "who considers orals as life-threatening may become speechless, while the bewitching, well articulated, sophisticated test taker may lead the questioning and get his certificate" (p. 6). Pokorny and Frazier (1966), in this vein, identify verbal fluency in oral examinations as a form of "testmanship" on the part of the candidate. While they relate fluency to general intelligence and sensitivity, they note, contrary to the observations of Evans et al., that "verbal fluency appeared to be a two-edged sword. Certain examiners seemed to correct, even overcorrect, for this, so that they were overly critical of such 'glib' residents" (p. 33). This two-edged sword is illustrated in a study of candidate behavior during orals by Green, Evans, and Ingersoll (1967).

They observed that in response to a difficult question, since a prolonged silence tended to irritate the examiner, it was better for the candidate to give a vague answer rather than a categorical one, which would have to be defended. Further, they observed that some students engaged in aggressive speaking, even "filibustering" their examiners. Others would attempt to speak more by broadening the issue or deviating into esoterics. Still others showed guilt, incoherence, and even anger.

There is very little evidence that the sex of a candidate, appearance, or various personality characteristics affect oral grades (but see Easton, 1968; Holloway et al., 1968). The best evidence that oral examiners are influenced by the personal characteristics of students in grading clinicals appears in a tightly designed demonstration by Wigton (1980). He coached five medical students to present each of five prepared case summaries which varied significantly in content and organization, and then had 15 experienced faculty view and evaluate the presentations by ranking. Cases were presented in a sequence that allowed comparisons of grades given to the same case by different students, although no examiner saw the same student or case twice. Results clearly showed that the ranking given each case was affected by which student presented it. Interestingly enough, the ranking at graduation in clinical courses for the five students was the same as the ranking they received in the experiment. Wigton commented that "it was not apparent . . . what these personal factors [that influenced grading] were: the students all were groomed and could express themselves well" (p. 457). Participating faculty later suggested that it might be the "degree of self-assurance of the presenters," but they were unsure about this.

A demonstration by Holloway et al. (1967) deepens the mystery about what the personal characteristics measured in oral examinations might be. Holloway had 17 final-year medical students interviewed by a psychologist with special experience in the field of personality assessment. The psychologist attempted, without success, to predict who would do well on an oral by assessing their verbal fluency and social ease. Neither were assessments of the students' "overall professional qualities" made by their school tutor correlated with the *viva* scores.

These findings raise questions about the extent to which true ability is measured in oral examinations and how such measurement is contaminated by unsystematic judgments about other characteristics of students. Resolution of these issues must await further research.

Variation due to Oral Type and Content. The oral examiner has often been faulted for inconsistencies in his questioning from candidate to candidate and for his lack of agreement with other examiners on what is to be tested (McGuire, 1966; Pressey et al., 1932). Without guidelines, however, the oral examiner might be expected to have some difficulty living up to expectations, first, that he maintain consistency in the quantity, quality, and difficulty of his questions from candidate to candidate; and second, that he ensure that he accurately samples the candidate's clinical competence (Evans et al., 1966).

To reduce inconsistency of the first type—that due to variation in questions asked or cases presented from candidate to candidate—one approach has been to develop checklists of questions that the examiner must cover for each candidate. A number of such checklists and rating forms for guidance of the examiner in the "clinical" now exist (e.g., Harden and Gleeson, 1979; Littlefield et al., 1977; Maatsch, 1980; Newble et al., 1980; Petersdorf & Beck, 1972). Reliability appears to be improved using these lists: for example, Littlefield et al. reported generalizability coefficients from 0.79 to 0.92; and Maatsch has reported interrater reliability ranging from 0.61 to 0.85 on his "simulated patient encounters" and from 0.79 to 0.89 on his "simulated situation encounters" (p. 75). The more rigid the structure of the oral, it seems, the higher the reliability.

On the other hand, even with structured orals using rating lists, McGuire and others, in perhaps the most exhaustive work on this problem, have had some difficulty in achieving high reliability. Their "problem-solving" or "cognitive" oral requires teams of examiners to rate each candidate on four dimensions (recall of factual information, analysis and interpretation of data, problem-solving ability, and attitude) in three half-hour sessions. The instrument yields a combined sampling and rater reliability that the authors estimate to be about 0.50, and reliability is not significantly increased by a three-fold increase in the length of the test (Levine and McGuire, 1970a). Another type of oral developed by these researchers, called the "role-playing oral," consists of three or four standardized oral simulations over a half-hour period, administered by two trained examiners who alternate in taking the role of specified patient, colleague, or allied health professional. The reliability values for this instrument are somewhat higher: The reported correlation between raters observing the same examination has been 0.73 and the reported overall reliability using the Spearman-Brown formula has been 0.84 (Levine and McGuire, 1970b).

Why are such relatively high reliability figures obtained for McGuire's role-playing orals as compared to the cognitive orals, which are three times longer? Levine and McGuire suggest that this occurs because the role-playing orals "presuppose much less specific content than do the tests of cognitive skills . . . " (1970b, p. 702). This is an important point. There is some supporting evidence for it in the data presented by other researchers but this has not been commented on or analyzed by them. Bull (1956), for example, found lower correlations between grades assigned by raters in the "major case" of a clinical oral (0.69 and 0.51) than on "minor cases" and traditional orals (0.82 to 0.89). Also in the "clinical," Wilson et al. (1969) found lower correlations between grades assigned by examiners on the "long case" than on the "short case" (0.78 and 0.835, respectively). Trimble (1934) found the reliability of "composite" ratings among three examiners in a 12-minute oral to be quite high (0.821, using the Spearman-Brown formula). If all of these findings reflect the same underlying process, it seems that the more behavior the examiner has to score, the lower the reliability. As O'Donohue and Wergin (1978) demonstrated, in their study of the orals of 175 medical students, reasonably reliability (0.754) can be obtained based on one sample of behavior. They feel, however, that this "may represent a very biased sample of the student's overall clinical competence" (p. 58). In a longer oral or a longer sequence of oral evaluations, a more valid measure might be obtained.

There has been some suggestion in the literature that a less serious problem, variation in grading by time of day, may also occur in oral examinations (Colton and Peterson, 1967; Marshall and Ludbrook, 1972; Platt, 1961). The trends are small and inconsistent, however, and have not been found in at least one study (Pokorny and Frazier, 1966).

Validity

Oral Examinations and Other Measures of Clinical Competence. The MCQ is widely acknowledged as the best measure of factual knowledge as well as the most reliable for the assessment of clinical competence (see Chapter 6). The extent to which the results of oral and MCQ assessments in medicine correlate, then, might be taken as an indication of the extent to which orals measure cognitive skills or knowledge. Although it is not legitimate to compare the correlations between written and oral grades reported in the literature, since the types of orals and the scores being correlated were derived differently, Table 5.1 gives some indication of the range of correlations that have been reported.

If scores on MCQ exams and orals were highly correlated, it might be assumed that both measured factual recall or "knowledge." Only two of the studies listed in Table 5.1 have come to this conclusion. One was a study of the final MB examination at London University in which correlations among the scores obtained by candidates on an MCQ, essay exam, oral, and "clinical" were calculated (Tomlinson et al., 1973). Correlations between the MCQ and oral grades were 0.47 and 0.53 and between MCQ and clinical grades were 0.17 and 0.39, leading the researchers to conclude that "the oral is primarily assessing recall of knowledge" (p. 9), while the clinical is not. The second study was reported by Maatsch (1980), who found an overall correlation of 0.77 between scores obtained by candidates on a Part I MCQ exam and scores obtained on a Part II structured "oral." He argued that Part I measures "clinically relevant knowledge," Part II measures "clinical performance," and the two overlap across the broad range of clinical competence. He estimates, in fact, that "the true relationship approaches 0.92, a virtual identity . . ." (p. 17). As can be seen from Table 5.1, three other investigators have obtained reasonably high correlations between written and oral scores (Anderson, 1979; Pokorny & Frazier, 1966; Young and Gillespie, 1972). However, these investigators made no claims about what was being measured.

All other investigators have found small positive or insignificant correlations between the results of MCQ and oral examinations, but not all have interpreted these findings in the same way. The most common interpretation is that orals and writtens measure different aspects of clinical competence (Carter, 1962; Holloway et al., 1968; Littlefield et al., 1977; McGuire and Levine, 1970b; O'Donohue and Wergin, 1978; Taylor et al., 1976) although a few researchers have suggested that low intercorrelations might also be obtained because of low reliability (Levine and McGuire, 1970a; Marshall and Ludbrook, 1972; Meskauskas, 1975). Thus there is disagreement about whether orals and writtens measure different aspects of competence or whether the orals measure the same dimension as writtens, but unreliably. A third possibility, little discussed, is that orals and writtens measure different aspects of clinical competence but that "case specificity"

TABLE 5.1
Reported Correlations Between Written and
Oral Examinations Scores*

Study	Reported Correlation
Barnes & Pressey (1929)	.47
Trimble (1934)	.49
Bull (1956)	.123 to .358
Carter (1962)	.45
Evans et al. (1966)	.314
Pokorny & Frazier (1966)	.736 (oral)
	.070 (clinical)
Colton & Peterson (1967)	.29
Holloway et al. (1967, 1968)	not significant, values not reported
Levine & McGuire (1970b)	.19 (role-playing orals)
	.23 to .35 (cognitive orals)
Ludbrook & Marshall (1971)	.23 to .35
Marshall & Ludbrook (1972)	.28 and .34
Young & Gillespie (1972)	.71 and .54
Tomlinson et al. (1973)	.17 and .39 (clinical)
	.47 and .53 (oral)
Meskauskas (1975)	.32
Taylor et al. (1976)	.31
Littlefield et al. (1977)	.27
O'Donohue & Wergin (1978)	.19
Anderson (1979)	.58 (clinical)
Maatsch (1980)	.77

*The "oral" here is defined as an interview-type situation in which the candidate is quizzed on general topics, while the "clinical" involves questioning regarding diagnosis and treatment plans for a particular patient. McGuire's "cognitive" orals involve problem-solving around specific cases, while "role-playing" orals involve students in assuming various "roles" with the examiner.

affects the aspect measured by orals, making them appear unreliable.[2]

While it is impossible to choose among the three interpretations discussed above, it is possible to detect some patterns in the data. Orals of the brief "interview" type, for example, appear to

---

[2] One difficulty in interpreting many studies of correlations between oral exams and other measures is the possibility of contamination. For example, the practice of having a candidate's written grades in front of the oral examiner is probably widespread, but its effects remain to be determined (e.g., Bull, 1956).

correlate more highly with MCQ grades than orals of the "clinical" type. Referring to Table 5.1, it can be seen that three early studies, using the "interview" format, all found intermediate correlations between written and oral grades (Barnes and Pressey, 1929; Carter, 1962; Trimble, 1934). The Bull study (1959) assigned grades in both clinicals and orals but, unfortunately, correlated a composite of these with MCQ results, thus perhaps canceling out any effect. The Evans study (1966) also used an unstandardized interview format and achieved intermediate correlations. Pokorny and Frazier (1966) were the first to compare grades on a clinical and an interview type oral with written grades. They found a correlation of 0.736 between the averaged grade of two oral interview exams and a written examination, but a correlation of only 0.070 between the averaged grade on two clinicals and the written grade. This was related to the fact that the scores on the two clinicals were only intercorrelated -0.160, while the two interview scores were correlated 0.573. Pokorny and Frazier argued from these data that the clinical "did not seem to be an effective evaluative tool" unless it could be suitably standardized.

Pokorny and Frazier were also the first to report correlations between interview oral scores and clinical scores and another measure of clinical competence, the supervisor's ratings on various dimensions. They found no significant correlations between subscores on the clinical orals and the ratings. The average score of the interview orals, however, did approach a significant correlation with the supervisor's rating of the candidate's "knowledge of theory" (.486), which is comparable to the correlations of a similar order found with the early interview-type orals and written exams. Colton and Peterson (1967) also attempted to show the intercorrelations among various measures of academic performance and an "oral consensus grade" assigned by interviewing teams. They found that the "oral consensus grade" correlated about the same level with the three other measures—a preclinical index, assigned before the student entered his Principal Clinical Year (PCY); a PCY index, based on his work in that year; and his scores on the National Boards. The correlations were 0.39, 0.34, and 0.29, respectively. As might be expected, the highest intercorrelation was between the preclinical index and the National Board scores (0.61). However, the correlation between the oral score and the PCY index was higher than that between the PCY index and the National Board scores (which was only 0.22).

At about this time, Levine and McGuire (1970a) and Miller (1968) reported that, in contrast to the traditional orals which emphasize recall, their "cognitive" orals put the emphasis on problem solving. Perhaps this is why they have found correlations of only 0.23 to 0.35 between these orals and multiple-choice scores, which reflect recall of factual information. These orals, in fact, seem to be closer to clinicals or oral PMPs than interview orals and appear to have all of the problems that these measures have with reliability. The other type of oral developed by McGuire and Levine—the "role-playing oral"— shows an even lower correlation with MCQ scores (0.19). Levine and McGuire (1970b) say that this is to be expected, since this type of oral is designed to measure something different than recall and since it depends to a lesser extent on specific content than do the other orals.

Two other sets of studies that appeared at about this time reported difficulty establishing correlations between scores given in orals and MCQ scores (Holloway et al., 1967, 1968; Ludbrook and Marshall, 1971; Marshall and Ludbrook, 1972). Holloway and colleagues were unable to find correlations between oral scores and any other measures in their studies, except with the neuroticism scale of the Eysenck Personality Inventory and with a visual impression score assigned by one examiner; these results led him to conclude that not only did the *viva* fail to measure recall of factual information, but that what it did measure was questionable. Ludbrook and Marshall expressed the same type of frustration. The correlation that they observed between clinical grades and written grades was lower with "trained" than "untrained" examiners (0.23 and 0.35, respectively). Interestingly enough, they note that the "trained" group had "agreed to avoid introducing questions about theoretical knowledge into the clinical examination" (1971, p. 154). Perhaps this is the reason that they then observed lower correlations with the MCQ—a measure of theoretical knowledge.

Two recent studies (Maatsch, 1980; Taylor et al., 1976) have added another dimension to what has been observed so far (that the interview-type oral is correlated with MCQ scores to the extent that it measures factual recall, while the clinical shows lower correlations with MCQ scores). The Taylor study, in which four CPMPs (computerized patient management problems) were administered along with the traditional orals and MCQs to candidates for certification in pediatrics, showed a higher correlation between the orals and the MCQ results (0.31) than between the CPMP results and the MCQ results (0.24). A similar pattern is reported by Maatsch, who found higher correlations between his "orals" (that appear more "cognitive" than most orals) and this MCQ results (0.43) than between PMP and MCQ results (0.30). (The PMP and "oral" results were intercorrelated 0.16). The authors warn that these results should be interpreted with caution, but one cannot help but speculate that CPMPs, PMPs, McGuire's "oral PMPs," and traditional clinicals may have something in common. Further research may show that, unlike the traditional interview-type oral, they do not measure factual recall, but instead some other aspect of clinical competence that is prone to unreliability due to "case specificity."

Another recent study by Skakun et al. (1976) raises new questions concerning the correlation between in-training evaluation reports (ITERs) and scores achieved on orals. In their study of candidates for certification in various specialties, 152 candidates who had achieved good or excellent ITERs failed the orals (while only 32 of 657 who passed the orals had poor or marginal ITERs).

The results of other studies listed in Table 5.1 also tend to show low correlations between orals and clinical ratings. O'Donohue and Wergin (1978) obtained reasonable reliability with the oral they had administered, but have expressed skepticism, given its tight structure and standardization, about whether it measures the broad spectrum of clinical competence. They note only a small positive correlation between written examination scores and oral examination results (0.19) as well as small positive correlations between oral and written scores and a clinical rating given by preceptors (0.254 and 0.208, respectively). They comment that the clinical ratings are very unreliable, being the summary of ratings given in very different situations by different raters. These findings are similar to those of DeNio et al. (1975), who found correlations of only 0.17 and 0.12 between oral and written scores, respectively, and global ratings. Only the Littlefield et al. (1977) study has found an intermediate correlation between composite oral exam scores and composite ward ratings, that being 0.39.

The key to determining what is going on in the oral exam will probably lie in resolving the nature of what we have been calling "case specificity." What is "case specificity"? Is it unreliability in measurement? Is it a reflection of clinical competence which is composed of a number of skills or traits? Or does it mean that some "cases" are more difficult than others, and that some cases measure skills that are more clinically relevant than others? This issue will be discussed further in Chapter 17.

Performance on Orals and Level of Medical Training. Although Levine and Noak (1968) report statistically significant differences in the expected direction between levels of medical training and performance on an oral exam, a paper by Miller (1968) showed that differences in performance within levels of training were greater than differences between those levels. The mean scores achieved in orals for candidates in this study were lowest for those in the first year of residency and highest for those in the fourth year. The range of scores within each year, however, were such that "some residents in the middle of the first year of training have acquired more than others in the middle of the fourth year." Even more variation was found with PMP scores, which led Miller to suggest that this might be because "the elements of problem solving tested by this procedure are neither a central element of residency training, nor uniformly improved by the residency experience" (p. 605).

The only other report on performance on orals by groups with different training is from Maatsch (1980). His analysis of the scores of "practice-eligible" and "residency-eligible" candidates on Part II of his exam shows a great deal of overlap, although he states that there are differences between the groups.

Feasibility

Valberg and Firstbrook (1977) list a number of serious problems in using a final oral evaluation system. First, it is usually impossible to examine all candidates at the same hospital, on the same patients, and by the same examiners, even though this type of standardization has been demonstrated to be crucial for establishing the reliability of the technique. Second, the oral testing period is short and stressful, thus not entirely mirroring real life. Third, it is difficult to marshal, or even find, sufficient numbers of patients in the large specialties for clinical orals. And, finally, the actual cost of the system is considerable. There are several cost factors, not the least of which is that of "volunteer examiners who travel great distances and spend several days of very valuable time doing the examinations" (Abrahamson, 1975, p. 27). In 1976, Taylor et al. calculated the cost of an oral as $250 per candidate compared to a cost of $280 per candidate for a CPMP and a $62 per candidate for an MCQ.

Educational Considerations

Abrahamson has suggested that the oral might be "a great teaching device" even if "it is not a very sound measurement device" (1975, p. 25). Similarly, Halio (1963) has speculated that, under the correct circumstances, the oral could be "a teaching situation, a true dialogue of learning through which the student discovers what he does know and begins to augment his knowledge, even the knowledge of his examiners" (p. 152). In the same vein, Colton and Peterson (1967) have called orals a potentially "useful feedback mechanism" on the strengths and weaknesses of a curriculum (p. 1013).

Rosinski (1975) points out the similarity between orals and teacher-student dialogue at the bedside (for example, during "rounds") and during conferences. It is difficult to estimate to what extent the oral technique is used in teaching situations, although Littlefield et al. (1977) suggest that it is a widely used method for evaluating the performance of students in clinical clerkships. At McMaster, an oral called a "triple jump exercise" (Painvin et al., 1979) has been developed for evaluation of student learning progress. The student performs an initial analysis of a problem in the presence of an assessor and then proceeds with an independent search for additional information for a limited period such as two hours. He then describes his search and problem analysis to the assessor. Acceptable interobserver reliability and positive acceptance of the technique by students and tutors have been demonstrated, and further investigation of the approach is going on (Powles et al., 1981).

A recent report has appeared on the orals being used as evaluation instruments as part of the clinical clerkship program at the Southern Illinois University School of Medicine (Vu et al., 1981). There have been some difficulties scheduling these oral sessions and students have complained about the time involved in the evaluations and differences in evaluator's styles. On the other hand, the advantages most commonly cited by the students were "the learning-teaching experiences which occurred during the oral evaluations, the immediate feedback provided by the faculty, a better understanding and fairer evaluation of students' data base, an opportunity for discussions and explanations of data misinterpretations and the motivation for students to keep up their study" (p. 666).

Summary

Summing up a 1971 conference at the University of Alberta, John Ellis, then editor of the *British Journal of Medical Education* and Secretary to the Association for the Study of Medical Education, lamented that the oral examiner, "along with respect for husbands and fathers and cucumber sandwiches on the lawn at tea time" would play "a less dominant role" in medical education (1971, p. 418). He compared traditional methods to "making doctors by hand," which is not appropriate in our need to "mass-produce" doctors. Dr. Ellis' judgment, in retrospect, appears to have been too hasty. Oral examining techniques have not only survived the last decade, they are appearing in new forms and are being researched rigorously.

Oral examinations are appealing because of their high face validity, their flexibility, and the possibility that they measure aspects of clinical competence that are perhaps not tapped in written examinations. The reliability of the technique may be affected by various factors, such as the anxiety of the candidate, inconsistency of the rater, and various situational factors. However, reasonable reliability has been demonstrated with structured, standardized orals using hand-picked examiners. The range of competency assessed by the technique and its validity are highly dependent upon the type of oral. The evidence suggests that general interview-type orals may measure, to a large extent, factual recall. "Clinical" type orals may measure something else, such as "problem-solving ability" or "interpersonal skills" but there is, as yet, no hard evidence that this is so (nor is there for any other technique). On the negative side, orals are costly and logistically difficult to administer. More research is needed on what is being measured in order to justify using the technique for large numbers of candidates.

Research on the reliability and validity of oral techniques has raised some interesting questions that should be pursued over the next decade. The effects of examiner training may be one promising area of research. Why does training appear to reduce rater reliability in some cases? Further, why do some raters appear to be consistent and others nonconformist, even without training? A second area for research might focus on what personality variables affect oral examination scores. There has been much talk but little evidence on this point. A third area needing attention is the issue of whether performance on orals improves with the level of medical training. But the research question of most importance has to do with the nature of "case specificity." This mysterious variable may be the source of most of the unreliability in orals which is usually attributed to examiner error. Can it be demonstrated that "case specificity" appears more regularly with some types of orals than with others? Is it due to the nature of clinical competence or to some artifact of test construction? The answer to this question is probably the key to understanding the basic nature of clinical competence.

References

Abrahamson, Stephen: The oral examination: the case for and the case against. In: The American Board of Medical Specialties. Proceedings: Conference on the oral examination. pp. 25-27. Des Plaines, Ill. (1975).

American Board of Medical Specialties. Proceedings: Conference on the oral examination. Des Plaines, Ill. (1975).

Anderson, J.: Controversy: For multiple choice questions. Med Teacher 1, 37-42 (1979).

Barnes, E. J., Pressey, S. L.: The reliability and validity of oral examinations. School and Society 30, 719-722 (1929).

Bligh, D., Ebrahim, G. J., Jaques, D., Piper, D. W.: Teaching students. Exeter University Teaching Services, Devon, England (1975).

Bonfiglio, M.: American Board of Orthopedic Surgery. In: The American Board of Medical Specialties. Proceedings: Conference on the oral examination, pp. 31-33. Des Plaines, Ill. Summary of Proceedings (1975).

Buckley-Sharp, M. D., Harris, F. T. C.: An assessment of a final qualifying examination. Brit J Med Educ 6, 201-211 (1972).

Bull, G. M.: An examination of the final examination in medicine. Lancet August, 368-372 (1956).

Bull, G. M.: Examinations. J Med Educ 34, 1154-1158 (1959).

Carter, H. D.: How reliable are good oral examinations? California J Educ Res 13, 147-153 (1962).

Colton, T., Peterson, O. L.: An assay of medical students' abilities by oral examination. J Med Educ 42, 1005-1014 (1967).

Cox, K.: How to improve oral examinations. Med J Aust 2, 476-477 (1978).

DeNio, J. N., Holmes, F. F., Pierleoni, R. G., Greenberger, N. J.: Evaluation of internal medicine clerkship students. Proceedings, 14th Annual Conference on Research in Medical Education, Washington, D.C. (1975).

Doyle, M.: Oral examinations—the current state of the art: where do we go from here? Unpublished paper submitted to the R. S. McLaughlin Examination and Research Center (1980).

Easton, R.: Differences between oral examination grades given by doctor-nurse pairs. Brit J Med Educ 2, 301-302 (1968).

Ellis, J.: Proceedings of an international conference on oral examinations. Edmonton, Alberta (1971).

Evans, L., Ingersoll, R. W., Smith, E. J.: The reliability, validity and taxonomic structure of the oral examination. J Med Educ 41, 651 (1966).

Foster, J. T., Abrahamson, S., Lass, S., Girard, R., and Garris, R. Analysis of an oral examination used in specialty board certification. J Med Educ 44, 951-954 (1969).

Foster, J. T.: The examination in pediatric cardiology. In: The American Board of Medical Specialties. Proceedings: Conference on the oral examination, pp. 17-18. Des Plaines, Ill. (1975).

Futcher, P. H., Sanderson, E. V., Pusler, P. A.: Evaluation of clinical skills for a specialty board during resident training. J Med Educ 52, 567-577 (1977).

Goldstein, A.: An inquiry into the value of rank grades in the medical course. J Med Educ 33, 193-199 (1958).

Green, E., Evans, L. R., Ingersoll, R. W.: The reactions of students in the oral examination. J Med Educ 42, 345-349 (1967).

Halio, J. L.: Ph.D.'s and the oral examination. J Higher Educ 34, 148-152 (1963).

Harden, R. M., Gleeson, F. A.: Assessment of clinical competence using an objective structured clinical examination (O.S.C.E.). Med Educ 13, 41-50 (1979).

Hartog, P., Rhodes, E. C.: An examination of examinations. London, England (1935).

Holloway, P. J., Hardwick, J. L., Morris, J., Start, K. B.: The validity of essays and viva voca examining techniques. Brit Dental J 123, 227-232 (1967).

Holloway, P. J., Collins, C. K., Start, K. B.: Reliability of viva voce examinations. Brit Dental J 125(5), 211-214 (1968).

Hubbard, J. P., Levitt, E. J., Schumacher, C. F., Schnabel, T. G.: An objective evaluation of clinical competence. N Engl J Med 272, 1321-1328 (1963).

Hubbard, J. P.: The oral examination. Measuring medical education. Chapter 11, pp. 93-99. Philadelphia: Lea and Febiger (1971).

Kelley, P. R., Matthews, J. H., Schumacher, C. F.: Analysis of oral examination of the American Board of Anesthesiology. J Med Educ 46, 982-988 (1971).

Kittle, C.: American Board of Thoracic Surgery. In: The American Board of Medical Specialties. Proceedings: Conference on the oral examination, pp. 35-36. Des Plaines, Ill. (1975).

Levine, H. G., McGuire, C. H.: The validity and reliability of oral examinations in assessing cognitive skills in medicine. J Educ Measurement 7(2), 63-73 (1970a).

Levine, H. G., McGuire, C. H.: The use of role-playing to evaluate affective skills in medicine. J Med Educ 45, 700-705 (1970b).

Levine, H. G., Noak, J.: The evaluation of complex educational outcomes. Office of the Superintendent of Public Instruction, State of Illinois (1968).

Lipscomb, P. R.: Summary: Conference on oral examinations. American Board of Medical Specialties (1975).

Littlefield, J. H., Harrington, J. T., Garman, R. E.: Use of an oral examination in an internal medicine clerkship. Proceedings, 16th Annual Conference on Research in Medical Education, Washington, D.C. (1977).

Ludbrook, J. H., Marshall, V. R.: Examiner training for clinical examinations. Brit J Med Educ 5, 152-155 (1971).

Maatsch, Jack L., Model for a criterion-referenced medical specialty test. Office of Medical Education Research and Development, Michigan State University in collaboration with the American Board of Emergency Medicine, December (1980).

Marshall, V. R., Ludbrook, J.: The relative importance of patient and examiner variability in a test of clinical skills. Brit J Med Educ 6, 212-217 (1972).

McGuire, C. H.: The oral examination as a measure of professional competence. J Med Educ 41, 267-274 (1966).

Meskauskas, M. S.: A study of the oral examinations of the Subspecialty Board of Cardiovascular Disease of the American Board of Internal Medicine. In: The American Board of Medical Specialties. Proceedings: Conference on oral examination, pp. 19-23. Des Plaines, Ill. (1975).

Miller, George: The orthopedic training study. JAMA 206, 601-606 (1968).

Newble, D. I., Hoare, J., Sheldrake, P. F.: The selection and training of examiners for clinical examinations. J Med Educ 14, 345-349 (1980).

Nunnally, J. C.: Introduction to psychological measurement. New York: McGraw-Hill (1970).

O'Donohue, W. J., Wergin, J. F.: Evaluation of medical students during a clinical clerkship in internal medicine. J Med Educ 53, 55-58 (1978).

Painvin, C., Neufeld, V. R., Norman, G. R., Walker, I., Whelan, G.: The "triple jump" exercise—a structured measure of problem-solving and self-directed learning. Proceedings, 18th Conference on Research in Medical Education, Washington, D.C. (1979).

Petersdorf, R. G., Beck, J. C.: The new procedure for evaluating the clinical competence of candidates to be certified by the American Board of Internal Medicine. Ann Intern Med 76, 491-496 (1972).

Platt, J. R.: On maximizing the information obtained from science examinations, written and oral. Am J Physics 29, 111-122 (1961).

Pokorny, A. D., Frazier, S. H.: An evaluation of oral examinations. J Med Educ 41, 28-40 (1966).

Powles, A. C. P., Wintrip, N., Neufeld, V. R., Wakefield, J. G., Coates, G., Burrows, J.: The "triple-jump exercise—further studes on an evaluative technique. Proceedings, 20th Conference on Research in Medical Education, Washington, D. C. (1981).

Pressey, S. L., Pressey, L. C., Barnes, E. J.: The final ordeal. J Higher Educ 3(5), 261-264 (1932).

Price, P. B., Taylor, C. W., Richards, J. M., Jacobsen, T. L. Measurement of physician performance. J Med Educ 39, 203-211 (1964).

Rosinski, E. F.: The oral examination as an educational assessment procedure. In: The American Board of Medical Specialties. Proceedings: Conference on the oral examination, pp. 7-9. Des Plaines, Ill. (1975).

Skakun, E., Wilson, D. R., Taylor, W. C.: A comparison of performance on multiple choice tests, oral examinations and in-training evaluation reports. Ann R Coll Phys Surg (Canada) (1976).

Taylor, W. C., Grace, M., Taylor, T. R., Fincham, S. M., Skakun, E. N.: The use of computerized patient management problems in a certifying examination. J Med Educ 10, 179-182 (1976).

Tomlinson, R. W., Pettingale, K. W., McKerron, C. G., Anderson, J.: A report of the final MB examination of London University. Brit J Med Educ 7, 7-9 (1973).

Trimble, O. C.: The oral examination: its validity and reliability. School and Society 39, 550-552 (1934).

Valberg, L., Firstbrook, J.: A project to improve the measurement of professional competence for specialty certification in Internal Medicine. Ann R Coll Phys Surg (Canada) 10, 278-282 (1977).

Van Wart, A. D.: A problem-solving oral examination for Family Medicine. J Med Educ 49, 673-679 (1974).

Vu, Nu V., Johnson, R., Merta, S. A.: Oral examination: A model for its use within a clinical clerkship. J Med Educ 56, 665-667 (1981).

Waugh, D., Moyse, C. A.: Medical education II: Oral examinations: a video study of the reproducibility of grades in pathology. Can Med Assoc J 100, 635-640 (1969).

Wigton, R. C.: The effects of student personal characteristics on the evaluation of clinical performance. J Med Educ 55, 423-427 (1980).

Wilson, G. M., Harden, R. McG., Lever, R., Robertson, J. I. S., MacRitchie, J.: Examination of clinical examiners. Lancet Jan 4, 37-40 (1969).

Young, S., Gillespie, G.: Experience with the multiple choice paper in the primary fellowship examination in Glasgow. Brit J Med Educ 6, 44-52 (1972).

CHAPTER 6

Written Examinations

VICTOR R. NEUFELD

This chapter will address the role of paper-and-pencil tests in the assessment of clinical competence. The discussion will focus predominantly on multiple-choice questions (MCQ), but will begin with a brief scrutiny of essay examinations and conclude with a consideration of the modified essay question (MEQ) approach and its variants, a sequence which reflects the historical appearance of these three forms of written examinations. Testing items of the true-false (TF) variety will be included in the discussion of multiple-choice questions. Paper simulations of clinical problems (i.e., patients) are considered in Chapter 9 and will not be considered here.

It is important to understand what this chapter is not. It is not a comprehensive review of paper-and-pencil testing in medical education. Documents of this nature are available elsewhere (Hubbard, 1978). Nor is it a "how to do it" manual; again, there are useful works for both test makers and test takers (Pappworth, 1975). This chapter will not deal in any depth with issues of scoring and standard setting. Admittedly, these are important topics and much of the discussion of these topics is based on experience with paper-and-pencil tests, but these issues are addressed in textbooks of educational evaluation.

Essay Examinations

The earliest record of essay examinations can be found in China more than 4,000 years ago (Coffman, 1971; Wilson, 1975). Until well into the twentieth century, they were the only form of written examination used in medicine. However, in the middle of this century questions began to be raised about their credibility, reliability, and validity in the assessment of clinical competence (Bull, 1956; Lipton and Huxham, 1970), and today they have been largely superseded by other testing methods. Let us take a brief look at the essay examination as it has been used to assess clinical competence.

Credibility

On the face of it, writing an essay question bears little resemblance to what a clinician does in his work with patients. Proponents of essay examinations may argue, however, that physicians are professionals and, as such, should demonstrate that they can display their analysis of a problem in clear, logical, and accurate prose. It is further argued that a good performance on an essay question demands the capacity to integrate information, to synthesize, to weigh arguments and justify choices, and perhaps even to be creative and original. While all these claims have some appeal, the evidence suggests that most of them have not been substantiated.

There are occasional intriguing descriptions of adaptations of the essay format for testing clinical problem solving. An example is an integrated examination used in Tromso, Norway (Naeraa and Lundgren, 1980). For several reasons—the perceived importance of written communications skills, student resistance to "MCQ-like" tests, and the low number of students—Naeraa and Lundgren selected the essay format. A typical examination consists of several clinical cases; specific questions are asked and criteria are specified. (On average, 150 questions are covered in a three-day examination which might involve 10 cases, some short and some long.) For second-year students, morphologic case-problems based on pathoanatomic specimens are used; this exercise includes pathologic-clinical correlation questions. Another form of these examinations has been adapted for physiology (Naeraa and Huxham, 1980). On closer inspection, these examinations resemble the "modified essay question" (MEQ), which is considered later.

Comprehensiveness

The nature of essay questions suggests that their comprehensiveness is limited. Only a small number of topics can be discussed in a single examination, due to limitation of time and "writer's cramp." While there are some scattered descriptions in earlier literature about attempts to systematically select topics for essay questions from a specified set of objectives, this approach has been rare. In general, it can be concluded that essay questions fare poorly on the criterion of comprehensiveness (content validity).

Precision

Precision is a major stumbling block in the use of essay questions. Wilson (1975) describes the interjudge reliability of markers of essay examinations in various specialties of the Royal College of Physicians and Surgeons of Canada over a period of four years. Using a correlation coefficient of 0.7 as a minimum level of acceptable agreement, the proportion of pairs of examiners who reached this level in any specialty group ranged from 50 percent down to 10 percent. From the general education literature, Ebel (1979) cites several studies that show wide variations in grades assigned to essays. There is some evidence that when written instructions are specified in detail, when scoring criteria are made more explicit, or when the assessors are carefully trained and monitored, precision can be improved (Naeraa and Lundgren, 1980), and occasionally an article will appear in the medical literature with suggestions along these lines (Bandaranayake, 1978).

Validity

What is the evidence that performance on essay questions truly measures clinical competence? The evidence is weak, primarily because the criterion measures against which essay examinations have been compared have themselves been suspect as "gold standards" (for example, multiple-choice questions, or oral examinations). Most of the studies on essay examinations, as used in medical education or quality assurance, were conducted more than a decade ago, before the emergence of more sophisticated (and hopefully valid) indicators of competence were available. One exception was Clute's classic study (1963) of Canadian practitioners, which showed no correlation between his measures of performance in practice and grades in medical school—the latter based mostly on essay examinations.

Several studies have compared performance on essay and multiple-choice questions (Cowles and Hubbard, 1952; Lipton and Huxham, 1970). In general, substantial differences in scores have been found for these two methods. Huxham, Lipton, and Hamilton have gone on to explore why these differences might be present in second-year medical studies (1975). Using a battery of psychometric tests, they found that introverted students scored higher on multiple-choice tests and students with "high scores in a factor associated with emotional maturity and illegible writing" performed higher on essay examinations (p. 271).

Feasibility

Essay examinations are easy to prepare and relatively easy to mark, particularly if there is a specified scoring key. It is quite inexpensive to mail examinations to examiners, but as every schoolteacher knows, marking dozens of essay examinations can be a tedious task.

Educational Considerations. Although there is little written about the educational aspects of the use of essay questions, there are general statements to the effect that essay examinations can be used for testing organizing and integrating ability. No studies are available about essay examinations used specifically for purposes of feedback to the learner. Other than minor consequences of marker boredom and writer's cramp, the educational side effects are probably minimal.

In general, it can be concluded that typical essay examinations have little place in the assessment of clinical competence. They fall short on most criteria: credibility, comprehensiveness, precision, and validity. Modifications of classical essay examinations, however, may be promising, as will be seen later.

Multiple-Choice Questions (MCQ)

Although it had been used earlier, the MCQ examination came to the attention of the medical community in the early 1950s. Two publications are frequently cited as pivotal contributions to the sweeping trend that became established. In Britain, Professor Bull (1956) threw great doubt on the reliability of the essay question while, at the same time, introducing the MCQ idea. A few years earlier, the work of Cowles and Hubbard (1952) had a similar impact in the United States. In fact, MCQ examinations were frequently equated with the term *objective*, because of the demonstrated increase in reliability obtained in scoring (Illingworth, 1963). This was possible, of course, because examinees simply marked a box indicating their best answer and examiners simply compared these check marks against predetermined correct answers. The scoring was no longer "subjective"; the bias and variability of the individual assessor was removed from the scoring procedure. This move to objectivity was extended to the use of computer-marked systems.

The numerous publications on MCQ examinations in the last two decades attest to the popularity of this format. MCQs are the main component in many certification procedures, intended to provide evidence that an adequate level of clinical competence has been achieved. A number of item types have been devised, sometimes referred to by letter (A-type, K-type, and so on) and sometimes by description, for example the "simple association" item or B-type. These types were described two decades ago (Hubbard and Clemans, 1961) and have themselves been the focus of various analyses (Skakun et al., 1979). Other streams in the MCQ literature have been concerned with test construction, the use of confidence weighting, item analysis techniques, and approaches to standard setting. This literature will be referred to selectively as we begin our analysis of the question: "Do MCQ examinations measure clinical competence?"

Credibility

On the criterion of credibility, the MCQ format has been the target of erudite and persistent criticism. Sir George Pickering (1978) listed a number of disadvantages of this format in his personal survey of medical education in Great Britain. More recently, Ludwig Eichna, a professor of medicine who on his retirement went back as a student through four years of medical school, had this to say about MCQ examinations: "They glorify facts, many of which are detailed, and some not necessary for a medical student but only for an expert in the field. Only minimal thinking is needed. Problem solving is virtually absent" (p. 732, 1980). In contrast, Robert Ebel, a doyen of educational measurement in the United States, stated: "They [multiple choice items] are adaptable to the measurement of most important educational outcomes: of knowledge, understanding and judgment; of ability to solve problems, to recommend appropriate action, to make predictions," (p. 149, 1979).

There are several specific features of MCQ testing that limit its credibility. Since these represent general criticisms of the use of MCQs, and are not special to considerations of clinical competence, they will be mentioned only briefly. First, persons taking an MCQ test either receive full credit or no credit in a given item; there is no opportunity to display partial knowledge. Strategies such as the use of confidence scales for each item have been proposed to offset this problem. This has been an area of extensive study but, although the evidence is somewhat conflicting, it appears generally that confidence testing and other strategies do not substantially improve test reliability or validity (Hakshan and Kansup, 1975).

Second, the MCQ format "cues" the test taker, thereby introducing a source of error. A recent study by Newble (1979) demonstrated a systematic difference in performance on multiple-choice and "free-response" items, with the students scoring significantly lower on the free-reponse items; it was concluded that the differences were produced by the cueing effect of MCQ items, thereby overestimating the students' abilities. There are also "style" features of MCQ tests, unrelated to the content of the items, that can be learned; the mastery of these features may contribute to a falsely elevated score. In fact, a considerable literature on "test wiseness" exists. It has been demonstrated that interventions designed to enhance test wiseness can result in improved scores on MCQ examinations (Wile, 1978). Various forms of test wiseness have been used for decades for all kinds of testing formats; any physician who has been a candidate in a classic oral examination will recall special advice he received about length of his haircut and the modesty of his suit for the occasion!

While the role of the MCQ examination continues to be a matter of debate (Anderson, 1979; Pickering, 1978), some general statements can be made about its credibility as a tool for assessing clinical competence:

1. It has low "face validity." There is little resemblance between the writing of MCQ examinations and the work of a clinician.
2. Most critics would agree that its role in medical education is limited to testing factual knowledge.
3. The main criticism of this tool concerns its dominance in current assessment procedures of clinical competence; in many situations, it is the major and sometimes the only instrument that is used.

The issue of the relationship between demonstrated factual knowledge and actual clinical performance will be addressed in a later section.

Comprehensiveness

How extensively do MCQ examinations assess clinical competence? This is a question relating to comprehensiveness or content validity. It can be answered only if there is a clear statement about assumptions underlying the examination or assessment system under scrutiny. Three examples will be offered to illustrate the importance of stating the assumption before analyzing the "content validity" or comprehensiveness of the MCQ instrument.

In the mid-1950s, Benjamin Bloom and colleagues published their classic "taxonomy" document (1956), which clustered cognitive or "knowledge-related" educational objectives into various categories and subcategories and soon became influential in medical education. This influence affected both the style of writing educational objectives and the construction and analysis of examinations. In a landmark study, McGuire (1963) analyzed the 1961 certifying examination of the National Board of Medical Examiners. The assumption was that this MCQ exam tested the full range of "cognitive skills" in medicine, including clinical problem solving, critical thinking, and the understanding of concepts and principles. He used a "process approach," a system of examination analysis that was popularized in general education in the United States. Twelve subject-matter experts (three in each of four disciplines) categorized each MCQ item using the eight-level classification of intellectual activity of Bloom, which ranges from isolated recall (level 1) to synthesis (level 8). With an adequate degree of interrater agreement, the results clearly demonstrated that 78 percent of items measured isolated recall and fewer than 8 percent required data interpretation or application of principles. None required overall synthesis.

In summary, given the assumption that a comprehensive certifying examination should test a full range of intellectual activities, this study, done 20 years ago, showed that this clearly was not the case. Observations such as these stimulated the development of other measures of competence, such as the patient management problem.

A second example of a content validity study began with a somewhat different assumption. Kling and his collegues at the R. S. McLaughlin Examination and Research Centre recently conducted a nationwide survey of the Medical Council of Canada MCQ examination (1980). Successful performance on this examination is required by every province in Canada for a license to practice medicine. In 1979, Part A of this examination, which constitutes about three-fourths of the total examination, contained 516 MCQ items in six specialties. Each of the 16 Canadian medical schools were asked to designate specialty committees to rate each item as "essential," "important," or "unimportant." Standard definitions were offered. The assumption was that the content of the examination was consistent with the content of curricula in Canadian medical schools.

The results indicated that half (50.6 percent) of the items were "essential," another 40 percent were important, and less than 10 percent were unimportant. Just over 82 percent of all items were taught; interestingly, 250 item ratings (with a limit of one rating per item per school) were unimportant items that were taught. Similarly, there were 206 ratings of essential items that were not taught. However, the study did not ask faculty members to indicate whether there were important areas of knowledge *not* included in the examination. (As an example of a missing content area thought to be important, see Chapter 14, "The Assessment of the Use of Diagnostic Tests.") This study demonstrated a reasonably high level of agreement among Canadian medical educators on the relative importance of the content of MCQ items on a national licensing examination. Similar studies have been done on an institutional basis (Garrard, McCollister, and Harris, 1978; Wile, 1978).

A third example illustrates the importance of understanding the underlying assumptions in a content validity study. The directors of a medical residency program were concerned about the degree to which various examination techniques corresponded to the range of competencies that medical residents in training were expected to demonstrate. These competencies were listed on a global rating scale called the "in-training evaluation" (ITE) report. Tugwell (1978) surveyed all the faculty members of the Department of Medicine at McMaster University. Each respondent was asked to match an evaluation instrument with a stated competency. The assumption here was that an examination technique should correspond to a stated objective. The results indicated, as might be expected, that MCQ tests were matched with an objective that included the application of medical knowledge to clinical problems. MCQ tests were not matched with the majority of competencies listed on the evaluation form, including history taking, physical examination skills, management of emergencies, and several others.

To return to our original question on how extensively MCQ examinations assess clinical competence, the answer depends upon the assumptions behind the question. A large MCQ examination can sample a broad spectrum of knowledge. And appropriate sampling methods can ensure that it is representative of a designated "universe" of knowledge—for example, the curricula of Canadian medical schools. In this sense, MCQ examinations have considerable content validity. It appears, however, that they are not usually representative of the full range of intellectual activities which it is assumed medical students and physicians should demonstrate. Similarly, when looking at any list of the components of clinical competence, it is soon acknowledged that MCQ tests can be used with confidence for only knowledge-related components.

Precision

Several forms of reliability (repeatability) have been devised to analyze multiple-choice item examinations. Given the nature of multiple-choice items, in particular the characteristic that the test setters agree in advance about the "correct answer" option of a question, it is no great surprise that the MCQ format is reasonably precise. The reliability formulas that are most commonly in use were devised by Kuder and Richardson more than 40 years ago (1937).

Reliability is expressed as a correlation coefficient where two sets of performance scores of the same examinees are compared. These may be the scores on two equivalent tests, on the same test taken on two different occasions, or most commonly by splitting an examination into two halves and determining the correlation coefficient of the scores on the halves. It is not surprising that most multiple-choice tests consisting of upwards of 50 or 100 items demonstrate a high degree of internal consistency or "split-halves" reliability. It should be noted, however, that there have been no quantitative studies on the degree of agreement or disagreement that may exist at other stages of MCQ test development. These stages include:

1. The selection of the disciplines or topics within disciplines to be included.
2. The selection of particular items to represent these topics.
3. The designation of the correct option.

A systematic look at those issues would be of considerable interest, particularly since MCQ examinations are used so extensively to assess clinical competence.

Validity

To what extent to MCQ tests truly measure clinical competence? It is this question of validity ("truth") that gives rise to the most serious reservations about the use of MCQ items (Levine, McGuire, and Nattress, 1970). To explore this issue, we will look at examples of three kinds of validity studies: those on concurrent validity, on predictive validity, and on construct validity. The first two categories of studies require a criterion test of performance against which MCQ performance can be compared. A range of criterion measures have been used, including global rating scales (for example, during internship or residency training), clinical oral examinations, direct observation of physician-patient encounters, and medical record reviews (the results of a medical audit). Unfortunately, there is a considerable range of opinion as to which of these measures is the best "gold standard" or which is the best indicator of the competent physician. This question will be addressed in some detail elsewhere (see Chapter 15). Here, we will simply describe some relevant studies and state a conclusion on the specific question of validity of MCQ tests.

Concurrent Validity. Studies of the concurrent validity of MCQs have been described at various points along the "continuum of medical education"—undergraduate training, certification at the end of postgraduate training, and continuing medical education.

Typical studies from the undergraduate area compare the MCQ results of classes of students with performance on other measures. In England, Anderson (1979) correlated the results of various components of the 1977 Newcastle-Upon-Tyne final MB BS examination. These components included a clinical exam (oral examination) and an in-course (global rating) assessment, in addition to MCQ examinations. Anderson found statistically significant correlations between MCQ scores and all other components: the total exam score (+0.698), the clinical exam score (+0.582), and the in-course score (+0.611).

A Canadian study of an examination in a second-year pathology course at Toronto (Rothman and Kerenyi, 1980) included correlations between MCQ and two other components. The correlation with performance on short essay questions was 0.51, and with a practical examination was 0.46. Both studies concluded that the MCQ format was a legitimate and valid component of a multiple-component assessment procedure.

A number of studies have analyzed performance on multiple-component certification procedures, where MCQ examinations are included. In an analysis of the performance of 1,304 candidates on the certifying examinations of the Royal College of Physicians and Surgeons of Canada, Skakun and colleagues (1978) found low correlations between MCQ performance and global ratings on an In-Training Evaluation Report (ITER). It was found that of 130 candidates who had poor or marginal global ratings, 77 had passed the certifying MCQ examination and 53 failed. Of 1,174 candidates who had good or excellent global ratings, 950 passed the MCQ examination, but 224 failed. Using a Kappa correlation statistic, the relation between the two data sets was poor (K = +0.05); however, this may be a reflection of the inadequacy of global rating scales (see Chapter 7).

More recently, Maatsch at Michigan State University has reported a series of studies performed in connection with devising a new multiple format certification examination for the American Board of Emergency Medicine (1980). This two-part examination includes MCQ items, pictorial MCQ items, and patient managment problems (PMPs) in Part I and simulated clinical encounters (SCE) in Part II. The SCE is a patient-based structured oral examination in which the candidate asks for clinical information from the examiner. The examination was first administered in a field test and then in a first administration for certification purposes. The correlation between MCQ and SCE performances in the field test was +0.83, and in the first administration was +0.43. Maatsch also found that PMPs did not appear to assess any unique aspect of competence vis-à-vis traditional MCQs. The report concludes that the cognitive aspects of clinical competence can be understood to have two main components, a knowledge factor and a performance factor, and that these two factors are quite highly correlated. The authors recommend that the measurement of both factors is preferable for specialty certification. They also state that MCQ tests based on clinical-relevant medical content serve as an adequate method to test the knowledge factor (and that other paper-and-pencil tests such as PMPs are not necessary).

From the area of continuing education, a recent study reported by Sibley and colleagues (1982) provides some relevant insights. In this educational trial, family physicians in Ontario were randomly allocated to experimental and control groups.

Experimental physicians received individualized educational packages consisting of patient management problems, selected readings, and self-administered MCQ tests; each package focused on a common clinical condition. The packages were further categorized into high and low preference designations, depending on the physician's choice from a list of available packages. Before the packages were distributed, and again 18 months later, an intensive medical record audit (using an "indicator condition" approach) was conducted in the practices of both groups. The main results of the study showed significant increases in quality of care (the "indicator condition" scores) in the experimental physician group for low preference packages only. Of particular interest, for the purposes of this chapter, was the fact that there was no significant correlation between MCQ-based pre- and post-test scores and the quality-of-care scores. This was despite the demonstration that, on the whole, experimental physicians gained in their knowledge and achieved mastery of the concepts in the packages.

The findings from these various examples of concurrent validity studies of MCQ tests therefore seem to be mixed. This may be, in part, a reflection of the various criterion measures that were used.

Predictive Validity. How well do the results of MCQ tests predict future performance? Again the choice of an appropriate criterion measure is a fundamental question in any predictive-validity study. A landmark report which raised this issue of predictive validity was the review by Wingard and Williamson (1973) on the degree to which grades in undergraduate medical education were predictors of physician performance. Of the 27 studies cited, six were studies of medical practitioners. Although not specified, it can be assumed that some of the data reflected in undergraduate grades came from MCQ examination scores. The six studies showed low or no correlations between grades and a variety of performance measures, including direct observation in a practice situation, board certification, and global ratings of internship performance.

There have been no recent studies to shed more light on this difficult question.

Construct Validity. As defined in the introductory chapter to this section, a construct is hypothesis or assumption that can be stated with reference to a test or examination. Where MCQ tests have been used to assess clinical competence, the two most commonly analyzed constructs are the following:

MCQ exam performance will be higher with an increasing level of training.

MCQ examinations can test all cognitive levels, including problem solving.

Let us look at some examples of studies which explore these assumptions.

In the studies by Maatsch (1980) tests of clinically relevant knowledge of emergency medicine were administered to subjects at various levels of training. It was shown that MCQ tests in particular (and to some extent other tests also) discriminated between final-year medical students, emergency medicine residents, and eligible candidates for the certification examination; the latter group included those eligible by practice experience and those eligible by virtue of having successfully completed an approved residency program in emergency medicine. It was observed that the "residency-eligible" group scored somewhat higher than the "practice eligible" group.

In contrast, McLeskey and Ward (1978) analyzed the results of the American College of Anesthesiologists' Annual Certification Written Examination. Using percentile ranks against a standard score, they displayed the aggregate results of three groups of candidates: those with less than two years of residency, those with two years of residency or more, and those who had completed a residency program. They found, to their surprise, that those with more training performed less well on this MCQ examination. The authors concluded that "the degredation in test results among individuals with more training and experience reflects the decrease in knowledge of specific facts that may occur during the time medical judgment is developing."

These two studies exemplify other similar studies, where it would seem that MCQ tests which measure medical knowledge yield the highest scores in the early postgraduate period. They can, in general, discriminate between undergraduate and postgraduate groups. However, performance on medical knowledge tests (typically MCQ examinations) progressively deteriorates with the increasing time interval from medical school graduation (Burg, 1979).

Do MCQ tests measure all the cognitive levels of clinical

competence? We have already referred to the analysis by McGuire (1963) of a comprehensive examination at the undergraduate level. The analysis revealed that a large majority of the items were at the "factual recall" cognitive level. A similar finding was reported in a factor analysis study of a physiology examination, where the majority of MCQ items were at the "look up" (factual recall) level (Huxham and Naeraa, 1980).

A similar study, but with interesting additional features, was described by Cox (1978). The MCQ examination under review was a 150-item surgical examination for final-year medical students. A three-level cognitive taxonomy (Knowledge Recall; Comprehension; and Problem Solving) was used. It was hypothesized that the three levels were in a hierarchy and represented stages of increasing difficulty. Hence, the "highest" taxonomy items should be more difficult and the percentage correct should decrease. This did not occur; each of the three levels had similar aggregate scores. Of additional interest was an analysis of the degree of agreement in allocations of items to taxonomic levels. Three experienced surgical teachers agreed on only 44 percent of the items; barely more than random. Percentage agreement among six senior students was even lower, with students tending to allocate more items to higher taxonomic levels. The authors concluded that it is generally unproductive to "fuss about a classification," and that clinical problem-solving skills should be assessed using the tool of confrontation with a patient.

What can be concluded about the validity of MCQ tests as measures of clinical competence? The following conclusions are warranted:

1. The evidence from various studies is far from uniform; considerable disagreement exists in the available literature.
2. At best, MCQ examinations test the "clinically relevant knowledge" component of clinical competence.
3. There is some evidence that performance on clinically relevant MCQ examinations is moderately (and positively) related to well-constructed simulated clinical encounters; clearly, however, they are not sufficient in themselves to assess all the cognitive components of clinical competence.
4. There are no convincing studies that demonstrate the predictive validity of MCQ examinations.

Feasibility

In general, it is relatively easy to prepare, administer, and score MCQ tests. Their preparation requires a degree of expertise, but various books, instructional manuals, and workshops are available for this purpose. A typical item might require 15 to 30 minutes to prepare. Most institutions who use MCQ tests use a staged sequence of MCQ preparation including "double-check" and "second opinion" procedures. All of this requires a considerable amount of faculty time and, therefore, is costly. Other costs have to do with test administration, test marking and scoring, and item analysis, including the time of technical and administrative staff, as well as direct computer costs. Item storage and "security" (particularly for items used in certification procedures) are further considerations. When all the required resources are added up, the costs to an institution are considerable; however, it is apparent that the cost and effort is usually considered to be justified.

Educational Considerations

Like any examination, MCQ tests have been used for various purposes. Most commonly, of course, they are used in connection with student learning—for example, to grade students in a course or to certify competence using comprehensive examinations at various points along the medical education continuum. Less has been written about their direct use for feedback to students than about their use for grading and certification. This may be because MCQ items take time to prepare; they can be "banked" and reused by an institution. If extensive feedback is provided to students, the answers will become generally known; the items are, therefore, not longer reusable for testing purposes. (Of course, the students are more likely to learn the content represented in these items!)

Three areas of experience with MCQs are worth noting. First, the MCQ format has been used increasingly in physician self-assessment programs. Examples are the Medical Knowledge Self-Assessment Program (MKSAP) of the American College of Physicians (Burg, 1979) and the National Self-evaluation Program of the College of Family Physicians of Canada (Rosser, 1975). Similar programs are available for other specialties in North America, Britain, and Australia. Some of these are quite elaborate; for example, MKSAP VI (the sixth trienniel program of the American College of Physicians), in addition to MCQ items in nine medical subspecialties, also has a manual of correct answers with annotations and references, as well as written synthesis of recent advances in each specialty. Rub-out patient management problems are included. More than 30,000 physicians have participated in MKSAP IV.

A second educational use of MCQs involves having students construct MCQ items themselves and then administer them to their peers (Hoffman et al., 1975). By preparing these MCQs, it is claimed that students gain a sound understanding of the topic in the question. Third, there have been a few reports of MCQ examinations completed in a "permissive" setting, typically with textbooks available (Mankun et al., 1973). A specific example is the report by Schumacher and his colleagues (1978), who assessed the effect of "open versus closed book" testing conditions, with volunteer groups of practicing pediatricians and medical students. It was found that while "open book" conditions significantly raised mean student scores, the mean score for the practitioners did not change appreciably.

MCQ tests have been used for purposes other than student learning. An obvious example is the use of scores to analyze the "performance" of the examination itself, or of individual items—the difficulty and discrimination indices. MCQ examination scores have been used to provide feedback to teachers (Cox, 1978) and to assess the impact of curricular change (Shapiro, 1974).

Reports are available describing MCQ item banks organized for multiple purposes: feedback to students; feedback to teachers in relation to specific topics which were taught; and feedback to a department or institution—for example, comparing aggregate student performance in a given discipline from one year to the next (Masden et al., 1977). A variety of research studies using MCQ tests have been reported. For example, the performances of final-year medical students from three British medical schools were compared, using a common item pool in general medicine and therapeutics (Ricketts et al., 1974); this report displays the mean or scores for three consecutive years in 11 specialties.

Summary

The MCQ format is probably the most widely used method for assessing clinical competence at the present time. The following conclusions can be made in response to the initial question, "Do MCQs measure clinical competence?" using our six measurement criteria:

Criterion	Comment
Credibility	Low; little apparent resemblance between clinical performance and test-taking performance.
Comprehensiveness	Depends on the underlying assumption; MCQ tests are particularly useful for efficiently testing knowledge from a broad range of topics.
Precision	Once the "correct" answers have been agreed upon, MCQ test scoring is highly reliable.
Validity	Available evidence inconclusive; MCQ test validity for clinical competence likely limited to the "clinically relevant knowledge" component
Feasibility	In general, the processes of MCQ test preparation, administration, scoring, and storing are all feasible.
Educational Considerations	Given the limitations of credibility and validity (as above), MCQ tests can be efficiently used for many purposes: grading, direct feedback to students, feedback to teachers, and educational research.

Modified Essay Questions

Having reviewed traditional essays and multiple-choice questions as formats for measuring clinical competence, we come now to the modified essay question (MEQ). Our basic query is unchanged: "Does this format measure clinical competence?"

Most of the experience with the MEQ is British and Australian. It was originally used in the fellowship examinations of the Royal College of General Practitioners (Board of Censors of the Royal College of General Practitioners, 1971) and later described by Hodgkin and Knox as a device for stimulating problem-based learning in undergraduate education (1975). The MEQ has become the main assessment device in the problem-based curriculum of the

University of Newcastle, New South Wales, Australia (Feletti and Engel, 1980).

What is the MEQ? Knox describes it as "an account of a series of events in the evolution of a case study, narrated as they occur" (p. 20, 1980). At frequent junctures, specific questions are asked which require a short written (essay) answer. The MEQ is based on an actual patient. It was originally introduced in order to assess components of competence "appropriate to the personal doctor providing primary and continuing medical care" (Board of Censors of the Royal College of General Practitioners, 1971). Dissatisfaction with available methods (which tended to test factual recall) had also been expressed; the traditional essay was considered to be unreliable and the multiple-choice format invalid.

It is interesting that a similar approach, but using a different name, was developed by Barrows and Mitchell (1975) at McMaster University. They described a learning package called a "problem box," which was used in a problem-based undergraduate neuroscience course. The primary purpose was the encouragement of problem-based learning, but the format was also used for assessment purposes. Barrows developed the problem box specifically as a result of insights obtained through research into the nature of clinical reasoning (Barrows and Bennett, 1972). The problem box consists of a case protocol based on an actual patient, with descriptions of events arranged serially as they occur in real life. Also in the box are items of information derived from the original case (for example, photographs of a skin rash, a short film of a gait disorder, a slide of a blood smear, an electrocardiogram, a miniature X-ray)—all available to help students think through the problems of the patient. Since it was not used for formal assessment purposes, the problem box was not extensively developed in terms of its potential use as measure of clinical competence.

There are similarities between the MEQ and other short-answer testing formats including short essay questions (Wakeford and Roberts, 1979), free-response tests (Newble et al., 1979), and other "open-ended" formats (Langdon, 1978). There are also similarities to standard patient-management problems, in that a case is presented and the examinee proceeds through the case in a sequential manner. In this discussion only the original concept of an MEQ will be considered. The key features of the MEQ are that it is based on an actual case and laid out in sequential fashion, and that it requires short written responses to "open-ended" questions.

Measurement Properties of the MEQ

Because the technique is relatively new, and because relatively little systematic psychometric development has been done, the review of the MEQ as a measure of clinical competence will be limited. On first pass, the MEQ is a credible approach. Actual cases are used, the protocol is arranged in sequential fashion to reflect real life, and the examples displayed in the literature contain questions that are wide-ranging and practical. No systematic reports of "face validity" are available, however.

It is claimed that the MEQ can sample from a much wider range of knowledge than essay questions; this is logical, since short answers are required. It is also stated the MEQ can measure abilities, such as attitudes, not assessible by other methods. In his recent description, Knox (1980) lists objectives of a behavioral science course and provides an example of an MEQ that tests abilities at various (cognitive) levels: factual recall, application, and synthesis. The "content" includes patient-doctor communication, antenatal care, and patient management, including the involvement of a health visitor. Again, no systematic reports of content validity or comprehensiveness are available.

With respect to precision, the original reports on the MEQ described procedures wherein acceptable performance of an examiner on a given case was agreed upon by experienced practitioners. In his report of the psychometric properties of the MEQ at Newcastle, Feletti (1980) showed that the estimated reliability or internal consistency lies between 0.57 and 0.91, using Cronbach's alpha coefficient. No interexaminer agreement correlations are provided in this report, although it is implied that the degree of agreement is satisfactory, once the "model answers" have been worked out. In their report on short essay questions, Wakeford and Roberts (1979) report interexaminer agreement (between two examiners, working independently without model answers) at 0.54. This increased to 0.83 when one of six short essays, which was obviously aberrant, was excluded.

Few MEQ validity studies are available. Feletti (1980) reports on two forms of construct validity, both based on models of problem solving. The models were a variant of Bloom's taxonomy and the clinical reasoning process described by Barrows and Bennett (1972) and Elstein et al. (1978). The results of these analyses are difficult to interpret. In general, the taxonomy-level model is of questionable value for MEQ; the clinical reasoning model is perhaps more useful (particularly for remediation purposes), but more work is required. On the hypothesis that

MEQ performance should improve with experience and training, several British reports are available. Freeman and Byrne (1973) provide some evidence that high MEQ scores are correlated with experience in practice, unlike the MCQ. Murray and his colleagues from Glasgow (1978) report that significantly higher MEQ scores were obtained by practitioners who had completed one year of a general practice residency than by those who had not.

We found no reports of predictive validity, although the original paper by the Board of Censors of the Royal College of General Practitioners (1971) included a simplified concurrent validity table. The examination included three written papers (MCQ, MEQ, and traditional essay) and two oral exam sessions. MEQ scores were more highly correlated with a candidate's overall examination score than were traditional essay examination scores.

From the perspective of feasibility, the main drawback of MEQs is the requirement that they be hand marked; they cannot be computer scored. It would not appear that they are otherwise more time consuming to prepare than MCQ examinations. Since they are sequential in their structure, each succeeding page may provide further clinical data; examinees are, therefore, not allowed to go back (to the past) or look ahead (to the future). It may not be feasible to expect compliance with this rule. A "sequential management problem" approach has been described by Berner, Hamilton, and Best (1974) in which an examinee hands in a completed section to a proctor and picks up the next segment to complete.

General statements are made in several reports of the value of the MEQ as a learning tool in a small group tutorial or a plenary session or as a method of self-assessment.

To sum up, the MEQ appears to be a practical and credible paper-and-pencil format for assessing aspects of clinical competence, but much more work on its precision and accuracy is required.

Overall Conclusions

Written tests are the most common form of assessing clinical competence. In this chapter we have focused on three types: essays, multiple choice questions, and the modified essay question.

Table 6.1 displays a summary of these three formats on the criteria of interest. An informal and somewhat arbitrary comment rating is included, which summarizes this review.

TABLE 6.1
Summary of Measurement Properties of
Three Paper-and-pencil Formats

Measurement Attribute	*Format*		
	Essay	*MCQ*	*MEQ*
Credibility	Low	Low	Fairly high
Comprehensiveness	Low	Fairly high (knowledge)	Modest; not well studied
Precision	Low	High	Fairly high
Validity	Low	Mixed situation; may be relatively high on clinically relevant knowledge	Not well studied
Feasibility	Fair (additional problem of hand marking)	Fair	Fair (additional problem of hand marking)
Educational Considerations	Not particularly useful	Useful for self-assessment of knowledge if annotations provided; some considerable side effects on study habits	Potentially useful for teaching and learning; not widely explored

More research is required on issues such as:

1. The predictive validity of clinically relevant MCQs when compared with actual practice performance.
2. The reliability and validity (all types) of MEQs.

References

Anderson, J.: Controversy: For multiple choice questions. Med Teacher 1, 37-42 (1979).

Bandaranayake, R.: Can I really grade essays fairly? Med J Aust June, 595-596 (1978).

Barrows, H. S., Bennett, K.: Experimental studies on the diagnostic (problem-solving) skill of the neurologist, their implications for neurological training. Arch Neurol 26, 273-277 (1972).

Barrows, H. S., Mitchell, D. L. M.: An innovative course in undergraduate neuroscience: experiment in problem-based learning with "problem boxes." Brit J Med Educ 9, 223-230 (1975).

Berner, E. S., Hamilton, L. A., Best, W. R.: A new approach to evaluating problem-solving in medical students. J Med Educ 49, 666-672 (1974).

Bloom, B. S.: A taxonomy of educational objectives: Handbook I—The cognitive domain. New York: Longmans, Green (1956).

Board of Censors of the Royal College of General Practitioners: The modified essay question. Proc Roy Coll Gen Practit 21, 373 (1971).

Bull, G. M.: An examination of the final examination in medicine. Lancet ii, 368 (1956).

Burg, F. D.: A national self-assessment program in internal medicine. Ann Intern Med 90, 100-109 (1979).

Clute, K. F.: The general practitioner. Toronto, Ontario: University of Toronto Press (1963).

Coffman, W.: Essay examinations. In: R. L. Thorndike, (Ed.), Educational measurements. Washington, D.C.: American Council on Education (1971).

Cowles, T., Hubbard, J. P.: A comparative study of essay and objective examinations for medical students. J Med Educ 27, 14-17 (1952).

Cox, K.: How did you guess: What do MCQ's measure? Med J Aust 1, 884-886 (1978).

Ebel, R. L.: Essentials of educational measurement (3rd ed.). Englewood Cliffs, N. J.: Prentice-Hall (1979).

Eichna, L.: Medical school education, 1975-1979: a student's perspective. N Engl J Med 303, 727-734 (1980).

Elstein, A. S., et al.: Medical problem-solving: an analysis of clinical reasoning. Cambridge: Harvard University Press (1978).

Feletti, G. I., Engel, C. E.: The modified essay question for testing problem-solving skills. Med J Aust 1, 79-80 (1980).

Feletti, G. I.: Reliability and validity studies on modified essay questions. J Med Educ 55, 933-941 (1980).

Freeman, J., Byrne, P. S.: The assessment of postgraduate teaching in general practice. London: Society for Research into Higher Education (1973).

Garrard, J., McCollister, R. J., Harris, I.: Review by medical teachers of a certification examination: rationale, method and application. Med Educ 12, 421-426 (1978).

Hakshan, A. R., Kansup, W.: A comparison of several methods of assessing partial knowledge in multiple choice tests: II. Testing Procedures, J Educ Measurement 12, 231-239 (1975).

Hodgkin, K., Knox, J. D. E.: Problem-centered learning. London: Churchill Livingstone (1975).

Hoffman, K. I., Solina, J., Marshall, J. G.: Student-constructed examination items. Proceedings, 14th Annual Conference on Research in Medical Education, Washington, D.C. (1975).

Hubbard, J. P., Clemans, W. V.: Multiple choice examinations: A guide for examiner and examinee. Philadelphia: Lea & Febiger (1961).

Hubbard, J. P.: Measuring medical education: The tests and experience of the National Board of Medical Examiners (2nd ed.). Philadelphia: Lea & Febiger (1978).

Huxham, G. J., Lipton, A., Hamilton, D.: Reasons for difference in performance in multiple choice and essay tests. Brit J Med Educ 9, 264-272 (1975).

Huxham, G. J., Naeraa, N.: Is Bloom's taxonomy reflected in the response pattern to MCQ items? Med Educ 14, 23-26 (1980).

Illingworth, C.: The "multiple choice" or objective examination: A controlled trial. Lancet ii, 1268-1271 (1963).

Kling, S., Skakun, E., Park, C.: A study of the content validity of the Medical Council of Canada multiple choice examinations. Unpublished document (1980).

Knox, J. D. E.: How to use modified essay questions. Med Teacher 2, 20-24 (1980).

Kuder, G. F., Richardson, M. W.: The theory of the estimation of test reliability. Psychometrika 2, 151-160 (1937).

Langdon, L.: An open-ended examination format to assess interpretive skills. In: A.B.M.S. Conference on Research in Evaluation Procedures, Chicago, Ill. (1978).

Levine, H. G., McGuire, C. H., Nattress, L. W.: The validity of multiple-choice achievement tests as measures of competence in medicine. Am Educ Res J 1, 69-82 (1970).

Lipton, A., Huxham, G. J.: Comparison of multiple-choice and essay testing in pre-clinical physiology. Brit J Med Educ 4, 228-238 (1970).

Lipton, A., Huxham, G. J.: Examination design and preparation. Med Educ 12, 159-167 (1978).

Maatsch, J. L.: Model for a criterion-referenced medical specialty test. Office of Medical Education Research and Development; and the American Board of Emergency Medicine, East Lansing, Mich. (1980).

Mankun, H., et al.: The effect of permissive environment on scoring of the orthopedic in-training examination. J Bone Joint Surg 55A, 1100-1111 (1973).

Masden, B. W., et al.: The development of a computer assisted instruction and assessment system in pharmacology. Med Educ 11, 13-20 (1977).

McGuire, C.: A process approach to the construction and analysis of medical examinations. J Med Educ 38, 556-563 (1963).

McLeskey, C. H., Ward, R. J.: Validity of written examinations. Anesthesiology 49, 224 (1978).

Murray, T. S., et al.: Evaluation of structured and unstructured training for general practice. J R Coll Gen Practit 28, 360-362 (1978).

Naeraa, N., Lundgren, T.: Essential features of a criterion-based, integrated examination at Tromso, Norway. Med Educ 14, 267-272 (1980).

Naeraa, N., Huxham, G.: Criterion-based open book examinations in physiology. Med Educ 14, 113-118 (1980).

Newble, D. I., Baxter, A., Elmslie, R. G.: A comparison of multiple-choice tests and free-response tests in examinations of clinical competence. Med Educ 13, 263-268 (1979).

Pappworth, M. H.: Passing medical examinations. London: Butterworth (1975).

Pickering, G.: Quest for excellence in medical education. London and Oxford: Oxford University Press for Nuffield Provincial Hospital (1978).

Pickering, G.: Controversy: against multiple choice questions. Med Teacher 1(2), 84-86 (1979).

Ricketts, B. S., Anderson, J., Richmond, J., Wood, W. A.: Multiple choice questions in medicine: comparison of performance of M.B. candidates from three universities. Brit J Med Educ 8, 209-217 (1974).

Rosser, W. W.: A national self-assessment program for Canadian family doctors. Can Med Assoc J 112, 982-985 (1975).

Rothman, A. I., Kerenyi, N.: The assessment of an examination in pathology consisting of multiple-choice, practical and short essay questions. Med Educ 14, 341-344 (1980).

Schumacher, C., et al.: The effect of open versus closed book testing conditions on MCQ performance. In: Conference on research in evaluation procedures. Philadelphia: American Board of Medical Specialties (1978).

Shapiro, A. P.: The impact of curricular change on performance on National Board Examinations. J Med Educ 49, 1113-1118 (1974).

Sibley, J. C., Sackett, D. L., Neufeld, V. R., Rudnick, K. V., Fraser, W., Gerrard, B.: A randomized trial of continuing medical education. N Engl J Med 306, 511-515 (1982).

Skakun, E. N., Wilson, D. R., Taylor, W. C.: A comparison of performance on multiple choice tests, oral examinations and in-training evaluation reports. Ann R Coll Phys Surg Can 11, 284-285 (1978).

Skakun, E. N., Nanson, E. M., Kling, S., Taylor, W. C.: A preliminary investigation of three types of multiple choice questions. Med Educ 13, 91-96 (1979).

Tugwell, P.: Evaluation methods for objectives in an internal medicine residency programme. Unpublished report, McMaster University, Hamilton, Ontario (1978).

Wakeford, R. E., Roberts, S.: A pilot experiment on the inter-examiner reliability of short essay questions. Med Educ 13, 342-344 (1979).

Wile, M. Z.: External examinations for internal evaluations: the National Board, Part I, as a case. J Med Educ 53, 92-97 (1978).

Wilson, D. R.: Assessment of clinical skills from the subjective to the objective. Ann R Coll Phys Surg Can 8, 109-118 (1975).

Wingard, J. R., Williamson, J. W.: Grades as predictors of physicians' career performance: An evaluative literature review. J Med Educ 48, 311-322 (1973).

CHAPTER 7

Global Rating Scales

DAVID L. STREINER

Introduction

The process of judging the competence of students in any educational program is based on evaluations by the teacher. Throughout a person's career in school, it is expected that he or she will receive a final grade at the completion of each course or area of study. While this may suffice to indicate how much knowledge has been acquired, it has long been recognized that there are other aspects of education which cannot be measured through written examinations. Even in grade school, the summary of academic performance is fleshed out on the report card by teacher comments in such areas as "Deportment" or "Works and plays well with others."

This need is acutely felt in medical education, where much of what makes a good physician is described in terms of "problem-solving ability," "judgment," or "rapport with patients." These qualities are not readily amenable to evaluation through written examinations, and other techniques have had to be devised to measure and quantify these attributes. Many medical schools have opted to use global rating scales to supplement, and in some cases even to replace, formal written examinations and course grades. These scales most often consist of a series of adjectives or descriptive terms, each of which can be graded along a continuum from very poor to superlative performance (see Figure 7.1 for an example of a global rating scale used by the Royal College of Physicians and Surgeons of Canada).

FIGURE 7.1

The Royal College of Physicians and Surgeons of Canada
Le Collège Royal des Médecins et Chirurgiens du Canada
74 Stanley, Ottawa, Canada K1M 1P4   Telephone (613) 746-8177

FINAL IN-TRAINING EVALUATION REPORT
(Please read the attached Explanatory Notes before completing this report).

NAME OF CANDIDATE: (Please print SURNAME first):

NAME OF SPECIALTY:

REPORT COVERS PERIOD FROM

UNIVERSITY: 19   TO   19
                          NAME OF PROGRAM DIRECTOR:
HOSPITAL(S):

CRITERIA*	UNSATISFACTORY	BORDERLINE	GOOD	VERY GOOD	OUTSTANDING	NOT APPLIC.
A. FUNDAMENTAL SKILLS						
1. DATA-GATHERING: e.g. HISTORY & EXAMINATION	☐	☐	☐	☐	☐	
2. CHOICE & USE OF ANCILLARY TESTS: e.g. LABORATORY TESTS	☐	☐	☐	☐	☐	
3. SOUNDNESS OF JUDGEMENT & DECISIONS	☐	☐	☐	☐	☐	
4. PERFORMANCE UNDER EMERGENCY CONDITIONS	☐	☐	☐	☐	☐	
5. RECORDS & REPORTS (INCLUDING ORAL REPORTS)	☐	☐	☐	☐	☐	
B. PROFESSIONAL ATTITUDES						
1. PHYSICIAN-PATIENT RELATIONSHIPS	☐	☐	☐	☐	☐	
2. TEAM RELATIONSHIPS	☐	☐	☐	☐	☐	
3. SENSE OF RESPONSIBILITY	☐	☐	☐	☐	☐	
4. ATTENTION TO PREVENTIVE MEASURES	☐	☐	☐	☐	☐	
5. SELF-ASSESSMENT ABILITY (INSIGHT)	☐	☐	☐	☐	☐	
C. TECHNICAL SKILLS						
1. TECHNICAL SKILLS RELATED TO SPECIALTY	☐	☐	☐	☐	☐	
2. USE AND CARE OF EQUIPMENT	☐	☐	☐	☐	☐	
D. KNOWLEDGE						
1. BASIC SCIENCE	☐	☐	☐	☐	☐	
2. CLINICAL	☐	☐	☐	☐	☐	
E. SPECIAL CRITERIA	☐	☐	☐	☐	☐	
	☐	☐	☐	☐	☐	
F. OVERALL COMPETENCE	☐	☐	☐	☐	☐	

Do you consider that this final-year candidate has demonstrated sufficient professional ability to practise
effectively and responsibly and act as a consultant in the stated specialty?

Do you consider this candidate's moral and ethical standing satisfactory?   yes* ☐   no* ☐

Was this evaluation done by: yes ☐   no ☐
      a committee ☐   one individual (please name) ☐

      other (please explain) ☐

*COMMENTS: (Please use other side of this page.) Your comments are very important. They should summarize the candidate's strengths and
weaknesses.

_____   _____   _____
      (date)   (title)   (signature)

The history of this rating method can be traced back to two sources—attempts by psychologists to measure attitudes and job performance, and efforts within the American Armed Forces to evaluate the performance of trainees in their various training programs. In 1922, Paterson developed a rating form which consisted of a solid line, with different adjectives below certain segments of it. The rater would put a mark on the line corresponding to his evaluation of the worker. The distance between the adjectives on the continuum was quite arbitrary, however. To get around some of the psychometric difficulties, Thurstone (1929, 1931) devised the technique of "equal appearing intervals," in which all points were more or less evenly spaced along a continuum. This had the decided advantage that the scale could be considered to have the properties of interval data, and more powerful statistical methods could be used. The procedure for deriving a Thurstone scale is quite laborious, however, involving a large number of statements to be rated and a recommended minimum of 100 judges. A simpler technique was developed by Likert (1932), whereby subjects respond to each item by stating whether they "strongly agree," "agree," are "undecided," "disagree," or "strongly disagree" with it. A numerical value can then be assigned to each category for scoring purposes. In one form or another, this method has since served as the mainstay of subsequent scales.

The second source was the "critical incident" technique developed by Diederich (cited in Dielman et al., 1980) to assess Air Force pilot trainees (see Chapter 2). This was modified by Cowles and Kubany (1959) for application to medical students. They interviewed 12 experienced faculty members to determine "the most important characteristics for a student to possess or acquire in preparing for general practice" (p. 140). These statements were reduced to eight categories: (1) knowledge of medical information; (2) the ability to gain and maintain the patients' confidence; (3) assumption of responsibility; (4) observing, recording, and reporting skills; (5) the ability to develop and verify hypotheses from clinical data; (6) stability in difficult situations; (7) integrity, honesty, and ethics; and (8) interest in the profession and in self-improvement. Students were rated on a three-point scale along these dimensions. Global rating scales used today in medical education frequently consist of some variation of Cowles and Kubany's eight characteristics, combined with the more sophisticated scaling techniques borrowed from attitude measurements.

The choice of descriptors, the number of points along the continuum, the frequency of the evaluations, or even the status of the evaluator (e.g., peer, supervisor, or patient) can be varied. Given this degree of flexibility, it is hardly surprising that global rating scales have achieved a high degree of acceptance. The question remains, however, whether the scales warrant this acceptance, or whether their advantages are outweighed by their shortcomings. The purpose of this chapter is fourfold: (1) to review the positive features of global rating scales; (2) to examine some of the measurement properties, such as precision and validity; (3) to discuss some of the factors which may affect these properties; and (4) to suggest ways in which they may be improved.

Advantages of Global Rating Scales

While all medical schools share the common goal of producing graduates who are knowledgeable in medicine and skilled in its practice, the philosophies advocating the best means to achieve this end differ widely. At the one extreme are schools that emphasize the retention of as many facts and techniques as can be taught during the student's tenure, reflecting the belief that medicine is a body of knowledge and skills which must be learned and mastered. On the other hand, there are schools that feel that the corpus of medical knowledge is simply too large to be learned in a reasonable length of time, and that, in addition, these "truths" have a very short life span. Consequently, the emphasis is more on teaching problem-solving and self-directed learning skills. Even within the same faculty, various departments stress different attributes, with "Rapport" being more valued in some clinical areas, and "Completeness of the Physical Examination" in others. This diversity presents two problems. First, it is unlikely that any examination developed in one setting will completely meet the needs of another school or department. Second, many of the end points, like "Empathy" or "Communication Skills" are "soft" and do not readily lend themselves to evaluation through traditional paper-and-pencil tests (cf. Goldberg, 1972).

Global rating scales are ideally suited to cope with these problems. It is possible to rate different attributes simply by choosing various defining adjectives or descriptive phrases. For example, technically oriented subjects could stress the acquisition of specific skills, such as history taking or thoroughness of the physical exam. Without changing the format of the scale, a different department could substitute its own end points, such as working appropriately with other professionals. At the same time, the scales could overlap in areas which are common to various subspecialties, such as ethical or professional conduct.

Attributes such as reliability or maturity are frequently deemed as important in a physician as knowing the cranial nerves or being able to detect a flow murmur. Although we may be hardpressed to define these explicitly, or even to provide exemplars of them, we all feel that we can tell whether they are possessed by a student. (Whether or not this confidence is warranted will be discussed later.) Written examinations or simulations require that specific examples be given and, in a formal testing situation, these can often appear contrived with self-evident answers. A rating scale, though, allows the preceptor to indicate the degree to which he or she feels a student demonstrates these traits.

A third benefit is the relative cost of completing a rating scale as compared with other forms of evaluation. Gallagher et al. (1977) estimated that evaluating 20 residents in their setting cost $10 using a rating scale, $15 if multiple-choice tests were used, $60 for patient management problems (PMPs), and $1,600 to videotape and score clinical interviews. While the first three techniques are relatively comparable in terms of financial cost, the advantage of rating scales is made more evident when the time needed to develop each is taken into account. They estimated 68 hours for the scales, 195 hours for the multiple choice tests, 400 hours for PMPs, and 1,200 hours for the videotaped interviews.

Moreover, rating scales can be far less intrusive than other grading techniques. The artificiality or contrivance of videotaping, having a rater present during an exam, or PMPs may bias the performance of the student. For example, Donnelly and Gallagher (1978) have shown that a laboratory test was ordered 85 percent of the time on a PMP, but in only 39 percent of actual clinical cases. Rating scales, on the other hand, can be completed based on the preceptor's knowledge of the student gained over time. Used in this way, the evaluation of the student does not produce a "Hawthorne effect," where the very process of measurement affects what is being measured.

The last advantage of the technique is that it can be used quite readily to provide feedback to the student. Because of its low development and administration costs, a global rating scale can be completed many times during a course or rotation, while these factors may limit the use of more objective examinations. Furthermore, the end result is, not simply a percentage of items answered correctly, but a profile showing the student's performance across a number of areas, written in terms easily understood by the student. This makes it easier for him or her to see exactly which areas need improvement and may facilitate discussion with the faculty about these deficiencies. Although this potential exists, there is unfortunately a dearth of research indicating whether feedback using global rating scales actually enhances learning or performance.

Thus, the major advantages of the global rating scale technique are (1) flexibility; (2) ability to tap "soft" areas; (3) cost; (4) unobtrusiveness; and (5) potential for feedback.

Measurement Properties

Before any test instrument is adopted for use, it must meet certain minimum criteria of precision (also called "reliability" in educational and psychological usage) and validity. In this section we will examine how well global rating scales do in achieving these criteria.

Precision

A test's precision is an index of how repeatable the results are. There are many different ways of measuring precision, each tapping a different aspect of the instrument's performance. Test-retest reliability reveals how closely the scores agree if the test is given to a person on two separate occasions. With alternate-form reliability, the test has two purportedly interchangeable forms; the index shows whether scores on one form are similar to scores on the parallel form. Objectivity is an index of the similarity in scores when two independent raters observe and rate the same events. Internal consistency, as measured by split-half reliability, the Kuder-Richardson 20 formula, or Cronbach's alpha, indicates whether all of the items on a test are measuring the same domain. It may be inappropriate to apply all of these tests of precision to a single questionnaire or scale; however, it should perform well on at least some of these tests, since precision imposes an upper limit on the validity of an instrument (Murstein, 1963).

There has been relatively little work done on assessing test-retest or alternate-form reliabilities of rating scales. Linn et al. (1975), having derived two summary scores from their 16 items through factor analysis, reported that the test-retest reliabilities of the factor scores over a one-week period ranged from 0.68 to 0.91. Erviti et al. (1979) randomly divided their pool of items into two forms. They mention in passing that these alternate forms differed in terms of their means and standard deviations, although they did not indicate by how much. It is regrettable that such an important index of the precision of a test has received so little attention by its users.

Considerably more work has been done looking at interrater agreement. However, the results are far from consistent. Some studies have reported quite high levels of agreement between observers. For example, Weissman et al. (1975) had untrained raters check off whether or not medical students elicited certain information or performed various tasks. They found 50 percent agreement between two raters in assessing the depth of the history taken, and 93 percent for the completeness of the physical examination, with an overall agreement rate of 83 percent. Brumback and Howell (1972) found a correlation of 0.86 between raters using a 20-point scale of clinical effectiveness, while Printen and Chappell (1973) reported an interrater correlation of 0.64 between two judges. Cowles (1965) said that agreement between raters was high on some items (how "high" was not stated), but fell precipitously when the items were ambiguous or "double barreled" (e.g., "Quick to seek advice but not unduly dependent").

On the other hand, there are as many studies reporting low levels of agreement. Although Hammond and Kern (1959) found interrater correlations as high as 0.85 on some items, the median was only 0.37, with some ratings dropping as low as -0.20. Negative reliability coefficients are almost unheard of and reflect very serious deficiencies in the instrument, implying that two raters, having observed the same event, reach opposite conclusions about it. Erviti et al. (1979) found that the mean Cohen's kappa between faculty and house staff rating the same student was 0.26, with some values as low as -0.01. Goldberg (1972) reported that, based on over 10,000 candidates sitting for board certification, the average agreement between independent examiners was 0.25.

Validity

One of the major ways of testing the validity of a new instrument is to correlate it with existing, accepted criteria, either measured at the same time (concurrent validity) or at a later date (predictive validity). However, the rating scale technique was developed primarily because there did not seem to be any other way to tap some important aspects of medical training. Consequently, in many cases, no other criterion exists against which the performance of global rating scales can be judged. Measures must therefore take the form of correlations with other performance indices which may be as subjective or are only tangentially related to the areas of interest. These measures have usually been standardized tests of "potential" or performance, such as the MCAT or the National Boards; premed or medical school grade point averages (GPAs); or other, nonstandardized evaluations of performance.

The correlations between faculty evaluations made during the last two years of medical school and preadmission criteria have been uniformly low. Gough and Hall (1964) reported correlations with the MCAT ranging from -0.18 to 0.01; and from -0.18 to 0.08 with premed GPA. Eleven years later, Kegel-Flom (1975) reached a similar conclusion that ratings of internship performance were not related to MCAT scores, premed GPA, or admission interview ratings. While these findings initially seem very disappointing, it would have been more surprising if the correlations were higher. As numerous authors have pointed out (e.g., Gough and Hall, 1975; Wingard and Williamson, 1973), there is a major shift in orientation between the first two and the last two years of medical school. The preclinical courses are primarily academic, while the final years emphasize clinical effectiveness and the utilization of knowledge. Thus, rating scales completed during the end of a student's career which focuses more on clinical performance need not necessarily bear any relationship to the more academic performance tapped by the MCAT and premed GPA.

Perhaps more disturbing are the low correlations between rating-scale evaluations and other concurrent indices of medical school performance. With few exceptions (e.g., Gough et al., 1964), the association between rating-scale scores and medical school GPA have been uniformly low (Gardner, 1972, 1973; Korman and Stubblefield, 1971; Linn et al., 1975). A similar picture emerges when we look at other examinations which the students take in medical school, often in the same year in which the rating scales are filled out. One study (De Nio et al., 1975) reported a moderate correlation of 0.50 between written exam scores and the average of various ratings completed during an internship experience on an inpatient ward. However, the same study yielded much lower correlations with oral exam scores

(0.33) or between the oral and written exams and performance when the clerks were rated in an outpatient clinic setting (0.17 and 0.12, respectively). These smaller correlations are more consistent with the results of the majority of other studies (e.g., Dowaliby and Andrews, 1976; Gardner, 1972, 1973; Nerenberg et al., 1978; O'Donohue and Wergin, 1978; Pierleoni et al., 1978; Skakun et al., 1976).

One of the most important hurdles a medical student must overcome in the United States is the National Board examination. Are rating scales able to determine who will do well on these? Again, the results are mixed, but not overly encouraging. De Nio et al. (1975) reported correlations in the low 0.40s with ratings done on a ward, but clinic performance correlated only 0.15 with scores on the Medicine subtest, and 0.06 with the Total Score. Similarly low correlations were found by Nerenberg et al. (1978). Alarmingly, Gardner (1972) indicated that evaluations by residents or interns working under them correlated -0.65 with the interns' later scores on the Boards!

It could be argued that the same objections that apply to premed GPA also apply here: medical school GPA, written or oral examinations, and the National Boards are all academically oriented, whereas the rating scales are designed to tap a different set of skills. The test, then, would be to see whether rating scales correlate well with other measures of performance. The two criteria most commonly studied are patient management problems and other indices of clinical performance. Both Dowaliby and Andrews (1976) and Pierleoni et al. (1978) have found only very modest correlations between PMPs and rating scales, never exceeding 0.29 in either study. Gardner (1972) found a correlation of 0.07 between a rating-scale score of interns' performances and an average of four case report grades, 0.30 with the residents' evaluations of the interns, and -0.09 with the attending physicians' ratings of them. Donnelly and Gallagher (1978) compared faculty ratings of residents with proficiency scores of their clinical workups. They sadly concluded that, "while the lack of correlation between rating scales and clinical performance is not too surprising, it is surprising to find such consistently negative correlations. . . . Ratings of clinical performance appear to be inversely related to measures of actual clinical performance" (p. 212).

In summary, it appears that global rating scales, with few exceptions, correlate quite poorly with measures of academic performance, either before or during medical school; other indices of clinical performance in school; or the National Boards. We will leave until a later section discussion on whether the few positive results are merely the results of poor research and statistical artifact, or whether they offer a ray of hope about the actual potential of this technique.

Sources of Imprecision

The generally low correlations between global rating scales and other indices of performance tend to cast doubt upon their ability to accurately measure differences among students or within the same student from one time to another. This forces us to take a closer look at the scales themselves and to examine their psychometric properties to determine whether they are able to do what we ask of them. The first place to look is their precision. There are generally considered to be three sources of imprecision (or unreliability) which affect scores on a test—imprecision within the test itself, variability among the people using the test (the raters), and properties inherent in what is being rated. (The term *test* is used here in a broad sense, covering not only paper-and-pencil questionnaires but any instrument used to estimate the value of an attribute of interest.)

All three sources of error are present every time we make an assessment, but the proportion of the imprecision attributable to each varies with the type of test, the raters, and what it is that we are measuring. In this section we will examine the potential error in the first two areas: the rating instruments and the raters.

The Items

To briefly recapitulate, a global rating scale consists of a list of attributes, each of which is evaluated by a rater along a continuum. We will first examine how each individual item is constructed and then turn to the scale as a collection of these items.

In constructing a questionnaire or a test of any type, one of the key steps is selecting the items. Not only must they tap the area of interest, they must also be understandable to the user, be unambiguous in what they are asking, and elicit a range of responses. A question of which everyone answers "True," or an attribute on which everyone is rated as "Satisfactory" does not help at all in differentiating among people. No useful information is gained over omitting the item entirely and simply assuming that all people agree with it or are performing at a satisfactory level on it. As Cowles (1965) found, ambiguity in the item results in lower reliability. Jackson (1970) has outlined an iterative procedure that should be followed to determine if an item contributes anything to a test, if it should be rewritten, or if it is unsalvageable and should be dropped completely. While few questionnaires have been devised in keeping with all of the steps Jackson has recommended, global rating scales used to assess clinical competence seem almost singularly notorious in their disregard of these steps.

With few exceptions, no rationale is usually given as to why a specific attribute was included on the scale. Turner et al. (1972) are almost unique in having preselected their items on the basis of high interrater agreement. More typical are the methods used by Geertsma and Chapman (1967), who chose items "on an intuitive and *a priori* basis" (p. 946); or of Erviti et al. (1979), who had an advisory committee decide which of 400 items "represented a major component of clinical competence and whether medical students might be expected to vary on the item" (pp. 185-186). These latter procedures help ensure that the scale appears credible (or has "face validity," in the psychological jargon). This is often a very desirable property, especially when the test is to be used by raters with little background in psychometric theory. By itself, however, it does not guarantee that the test is either precise (reliable) or valid.

Having decided which items to include, the next step is to determine how many points there should be on the continuum. This could range from just two or three (Satisfactory-Unsatisfactory; Below Average-Average-Above Average) to simply labeling the two extremes and placing 20 or 30 boxes between them. (One can simply draw a long line and allow the rater to put an "X" anywhere along it. This does not solve the problem, but merely postpones it, since the person scoring the results would now have to decide how finely the line should be divided for scoring purposes.) Among the various scales which have been reported, the preference seems to be to use four or five points (e.g., Dielman et al., 1979, 1980; Gough et al., 1964; Linn, 1979), although as few as three (Cowles and Kubany, 1959; Geertsma and Chapman, 1967) and as many as 20 (Brumback and Howell, 1972) have been employed.

Are four or five points sufficient to accurately differentiate among students? We can look to two sources of information for an answer: psychometric test theory and the actual performance of the scales.

For many years, test construction theorists have debated the optimal number of points for a scale. If there are too few divisions, then the test may not be fully utilizing the rater's ability to discriminate fine gradations in performance from one person to another. Too many points, though, may be beyond the rater's powers of discrimination. If the interval between the steps is very small, for example, three or four boxes may fall within the range which a rater wants to mark and the actual box chosen would be somewhat arbitrary. The next time the same rater observes the same behavior, he or she may indicate a different box within that range, thus introducing some degree of error variance into the final score.

In 1924, Symonds concluded that, on theoretical grounds, the optimal number of steps was seven. This number remained almost as a magic talisman, unquestioned but untested. Three decades later, Guilford (1954) stated, "The optimal number is a matter for empirical determination in any situation. . . . It can be said, however, that the number 7 . . . is usually lower than optimal and it may pay in some favorable situations to use up to 25 scale divisions" (p. 291). Nunnally (1967), also on theoretical grounds, stated that the reliability of a scale increased rapidly as the number of divisions increases to about seven, and then rises more slowly until there are 11 points. Beyond 11 steps, he contends, the increase in reliability becomes vanishingly small, although it never decreases. This, though, was disputed by Bendig (1953, 1954), who empirically found a drop in reliability when there were fewer than 4 or more than 10 categories. Thus, while the actual optimal number of steps is still a matter of some conjecture, it is probably between 7 and 11—more than the 4 or 5 divisions commonly used.

It may seem that arguing for at least seven points to be used rather than five is quibbling over a minor matter. It is commonly felt, however, that there is a "central tendency" bias, in that raters tend to avoid the extremes of a scale, thus reducing a five-point scale to effectively three points (cf. Guion, 1965). This problem becomes more acute when the ends of the continuum are defined with terms which are so extreme that the raters would seldom use them (Guilford, 1954). This was, in fact, found by Printen and Chappell (1973), who noted that "raters are reluctant to use the full breadth of the one to five rating scale" (p. 347).

Another consequence of this restriction in range is manifested in the "ceiling effect." Since applicants to medical school must pass a rigorous screening procedure before they are accepted, there will be relatively few poor or unsatisfactory students. This effectively eliminates the lower half of a scale, and if the upper end is not made high enough, most of the people will cluster near the top. For example, Erviti et al. (1979) found a mean score of 3.3 on a four-point scale; and Linn (1979), using a five-point scale, reported a mean of 4.11. He also stated that the scores ranged from 3.30 to 4.56—over 50 percent of the scale was never used.

Compounding this problem even further is the seeming reluctance of many raters to use the low end of the scale, even when it is appropriate to do so. Rather than using the traditional "Unsatisfactory-Satisfactory-Superior" three-point scale, Cowles and Kubany (1959) asked raters to assign students to the "Top one-fifth" of the class, the "Middle three-fifths," or the "Lowest one-fifth." With this scheme, students were not judged against some absolute criterion, but against others in their year, thus allowing the whole scale to be used. Although one would expect 20 percent to fall at each extreme, with 60 percent in the middle, they actually found that 31 percent were rated as being in the top one-fifth, and only 5 percent in the lowest one-fifth.

One of the advantages mentioned for this technique is that it allows for the evaluation of "soft" areas, those that are difficult to define, such as "responsibility" or "professional standards." The other side of the coin, however, is that this vagueness is a major source of poor reliability. Although most clinicians feel that they can detect the "Ability to gain the patient's confidence," there is no assurance at all that any two supervisors are necessarily responding to the same behavior in the student, or even assigning it a similar degree of import. Levine et al., (1975) comment that the reliabilities of ratings are low because "the raters observe different experiences, rate on different criteria and have difficulty in agreeing on the meaning of particular numerical scores" (p. 38).

This problem is especially acute when the rater is asked to evaluate a vague concept on a scale in which the four or five points are similarly undefined and open to interpretation, such as "Above Average" or "Usually Characteristic." "Above" what average—the "average" medical student in that class? As compared with previous classes (and all were better than the present one)? Or in relation to how the average medical student is *expected* to perform? In short, the severe penalty paid for ease in writing an item is the susceptibility of that item to varying interpretations.

Fortunately, there has been a trend in recent years to use "anchoring," whereby each point along the continuum is defined by a phrase which attempts to explain the intent of that particular value. An example of this is seen in Figure 7.1. This does not totally solve the problem, since the description itself may contain words that are open to interpretation. Dielman et al. (1980) define the low end of their Ward Responsibilities item as, "Needs repeated reminders of assignments; does less than prescribed work." How many reminders constitute "repeated"? One supervisor may feel that anything more than one is "repeated," while a more lenient colleague may allow five or six before his patience is exhausted. This is definitely a move in the right direction, however, as it allows these differences in opinion to be aired and potentially resolved with adequate training.

A more sophisticated procedure was introduced by Smith and Kendall (1963), in which the general descriptions are replaced by concrete examples of actual behavior. While these "behaviorally anchored rating scales" show increased reliability over other formats (Borman and Vallon, 1974; Burnaska and Hollmann, 1974; Campbell et al., 1973), they have not been widely adopted in the area of assessing clinical performance. In their review of these scales, Landy and Farr (1980) point out some of the difficulties with this technique, such as expense of preparation, limited generalizability across settings, and difficulties defining the center of the scale, which may account for its low utilization.

The Scale

With almost every scale used, the number of items on the scale is equal to the number of areas covered. That is, there is one item for "Ward Responsibility," one for "Judgment," one for "Problem-solving Ability," and so forth. Let us compare this with scales commonly used in psychology or education.

Many scales used in these fields are unidimensional: they are meant to measure only one attribute or characteristic, such as depression, creativity, or short-term memory. Yet the scale may consist of 20, 30, or even 60 items. The reason for this can be found in psychometric theory. As the number of items in a scale decreases, so does its reliability (Cronbach, 1970). For example, let us assume that a 20-item anxiety scale has a reliability coefficient of 0.80, which is quite good in this field (and higher than is found in most global rating scales). If we randomly delete half of the items, then its maximum reliability drops to 0.67; with only five items in the scale, the maximum is 0.50; and with only one item, the reliability can never exceed 0.17. Since the aim of most global rating scales is not to sum the various items into a total score, but to use each item separately to provide feedback (cf. Dielman et al., 1979), the results is that there are 10 to 20 separate scales, each with poor reliability.

The Raters

As was seen in the section on the measurement properties of rating scales, agreement between raters varies considerably from one study to another, reaching acceptable values in some (e.g., Weissman et al., 1975) and unacceptable levels in others (e.g., Hammond and Kern, 1959). Part of this difficulty obviously lies in the scales themselves. Let us now turn our attention to another potential source of variability, the raters using the scales. We will examine two factors: who does the evaluating and whether raters do what we ask of them.

Clinical training in medical school often takes the form of a pyramid: interns are supervised primarily by junior residents, the junior residents are supervised by more senior residents, and the senior residents by the faculty, with the faculty member, though, still having ultimate responsibility for those under him or her. Although most evaluations are done by the faculty, this hierarchical structure allows an intern, for example, to be evaluated by both peers and residents. Does this make any difference? The evidence is sparse but quite consistent in answering "yes." To begin with, peers and supervisors appear to be responding to different attributes. Kegel-Flom (1975) found that supervisor (as well as self) evaluations were most highly correlated with previous ratings by the faculty, while peer evaluations were associated more with personality characteristics of the intern. After reviewing a large number of articles in the industrial psychology area, Landy and Farr (1980) concluded that, "supervisory and peer ratings may represent two distinct views of a common individual's job performance and may be equally valid, even though they are not highly correlated" (p. 76). This appears to be the case in assessing clinical competence as well. Cynically (perhaps accurately), Gardner (1973) stated that the chief resident's evaluation "usually reflects the student's availability to the ward and his willingness to perform menial tasks ("scut work") necessary to the running of a surgical service" (p. 81). Moreover, house staff have more direct day-to-day contact with the intern than do faculty. This is reflected in the ratings in terms of higher levels of interrater agreement (Dielman et al., 1979, 1980) and fewer items answered "Don't

Know" (Erviti et al., 1979). In fact, Erviti and her colleagues found a high negative correlation (-0.52) between the amount of time spent with a student and the number of "Don't Know" responses.

Rating scales usually consist of between 10 and 20 items, but are the raters responding to this many discrete dimensions? Again, the evidence seems to point in one direction, that they cannot. For example, in 1964, Gough et al. asked raters to use a 10-item scale. Eleven years later, though, they (Gough and Hall, 1975) had lowered their expectations since, they said, "faculty raters could make only two basic distinctions: a factor of general medical competence and a factor of clinical effectiveness with patients" (p. 305). Dielman et al. (1980) similarly found that two factors—problem solving and interpersonal skills—accounted for between 59 and 71 percent of the variance of 12 initial items. Hammond and Kern (1959) were even more pessimistic, feeling that students were being evaluated "in terms of each staff member's single-dimensioned, unique concept of good performance" (p. 496).

Evidence exists from other sources as well. We would expect "good" students to be performing well across a number of areas. If each item on the scale is meant to tap a different aspect of performance, however, then there should be some degree of variability from item to item within a given student. Thus, we might expect moderate, but not overly high, correlations among the items. The pattern seems to be, though, that very high inter-item correlations are found (e.g., Gough et al., 1964; Kegel-Flom, 1975; Pierleoni et al., 1978). In fact, Brumback and Howell (1972) found that the internal consistency of their 37-item scale was 0.98, indicating that all of the items were measuring just one area. Results such as this have led researchers such as Levine et al. (1975) to despair that "it is not clear whether the ratings reflect genuine achievement on the part of the student in managing patient problems or global impressions of personality inferred from observations of the student's interactions with the rater" (p. 38).

That this should be true is not surprising; what is surprising is that it has been ignored for so long by designers of global rating scales and that it comes as a shock to them when it rears its head. It was first noted around the turn of the century (Wells, 1907), and more than 50 years ago, Rugg (1922) said that we "rate or judge our fellows in terms of a general mental attitude toward them" (p. 37). Thorndike (1920) referred to this phenomenon as the "halo effect." Its effects, and the circumstances under which it is most clearly evident, were best described by Allport (1937):

> The halo effect appears with monotonous uniformity in nearly all studies of ratings, and its magnitude is often surprisingly great. The judge seems intent on reporting his final opinion of the strength, weakness, merit, or demerit of the personality as a whole, rather than on giving as discriminating a rating as possible for each separate characteristic. Whenever the variables have moral connotation the halo effect is larger, for it is a striking fact that a general attitude of approval or disapproval toward the subject colors every single judgment concerning his vices and virtues. The halo effect is also large when any single variable is not easily observed in action or when it is ill-defined: in such cases the judge substitutes his general impression for the variable that he cannot rate directly [p. 447].

Thus it seems unlikely that raters can accurately assess more than one or two dimensions of performance. Rather, they seem to reach an overall impression of the student, which then influences each item on the scale.

Recommendations

Global rating scales have a number of distinct advantages over other evaluation techniques: flexibility, cost, unobtrusiveness, potential for feedback, and the ability to tap soft areas. Counterbalancing this, however, is the technique's poor track record with respect to precision and validity. Should we abandon the technique entirely and rely on other methods, or are there ways to improve the instrument?

It is our feeling that the full potential of the technique has not been realized and that there are changes which can be implemented that would result in improvement. In this section, which relies heavily on an excellent chapter by Holt (1965), we will list some recommendations which we believe will increase the reliability and validity of global rating scales.

Recognize Its Limitations

Perhaps the major problem underlying global rating scales is that they held out the promise of being able to do more than was actually possible. They seemed to offer an inexpensive method of evaluating students along a number of separate and distinct dimensions. As we saw in the section on the "halo effect," though, raters are probably not able to make a large number of independent ratings. The overall impression that the student makes on the rater influences most of the evaluations on the form, resulting in high correlations among the individual items. Thus, the scale may be quite useful for conveying the supervisor's global impression of the student, but not for providing valid feedback in specific areas.

Anchoring

To the extent that it is feasible, the area that is being evaluated should be defined concretely and explicitly. Further, each point on the continuum should be described in concrete terms. If it is possible, examples of performance that do and do not meet the criteria should also be given. It may be necessary to provide this on a separate sheet, if they cannot be placed under each point. If behavioral anchors cannot be defined, it is still preferable to use adjectives rather than simply numbers. The end cues, either behavioral or adjectival, should not be so extreme that they will never be applied. To do so effectively reduces the scale by two points.

Use of Checklists

When the behavior being rated is observable, as in performing an examination, checklists are preferable to global rating scales. These are usually more difficult to construct, as the scale designer must include everything the student must do, as well as procedures he or she may do unnecessarily. However, the interrater reliability of checklists is usually significantly higher than for global scales. Both Turner et al. (1972) and Weissman et al. (1975) used versions of checklists completed while the raters observed the student. These two studies report among the highest interrater correlations, ranging from 0.45 to 0.75 with two observers and as high as 0.92 when four raters were used. Thus, the use of global rating scales should be restricted to those areas where checklists are not feasible.

Number of Points

Rating scales appear to suffer from two deficiencies in terms of the number of points used for each item: the number often seems to be chosen arbitrarily, and there are usually too few of them. While it is often convenient or esthetic to have the same number of points for each item, it is better to choose the fineness of the scale on the basis of the raters' ability to discriminate among levels of performance in different areas. This may result in some items having only 5 divisions, while others may have 11, but this seems preferable to either losing precision from too coarse a scale or adding error variance from too many points. The tendency in the literature, though, seems to have been to err in the former direction. It would appear that raters may be able to draw finer distinctions than the existing scales allow. A good criterion to use was proposed by Tukey (1950), who said that if two independent judges agree equally on more than 10 percent of the ratings, the scale is too coarse and precision is being lost.

Rater Training

In most cases, supervisors or preceptors are simply sent the rating scale and asked to fill it out. On occasion, a written list of instructions is appended. Rarely, though, are the evaluators given any formal training in the use of the scale, the definition of terms, or the meaning of the various points along the continuum. This allows for a large degree of misinterpretation and idiosyncratic modes of responding. Most studies in industrial psychology have shown increases in reliability (e.g., Borman and Dunnette, 1975) and decreases in the halo effect (Borman, 1975) with rater training. While little research has been done in the clinical competence area, some authors have noted in passing (e.g., Gough et al., 1964; Printen et al., 1973) that the reliabilities of the evaluations have tended to improve during the second year that the scale was used, as the raters grew more familiar with it. Training should be formalized, rather than allowed to happen serendipitously, and this is particularly true when the attributes are vague or poorly defined.

Pooling Ratings

The above five recommendations are all designed to improve the reliability of a scale through minimizing the effects of "halo." As much as it may be reduced, however, it can rarely be eliminated entirely, especially when abstract and vague characteristics are being evaluated. If the average of a number of raters is used, then one person's positive bias may be counteracted by another's negative one, leaving a more accurate picture of the student's actual performance. From a statistical point of view, as Ebel (1951) has shown, even if raters do not agree with each other, the reliability of the average rating increases sharply as more judges are used.

In conclusion, we would say that the full potential of rating scales has not been realized. If it were possible to improve their precision and validity, they could serve as an extremely valuable tool in the ongoing evaluation of students. Rating scales as they are currently used, however, leave much to be desired and raise the possibility that the feedback students receive from them is not an accurate reflection of their performance. Whether the recommendations improve the utility of the instrument sufficiently to make it a practical device is an empirical question; however, given the seriousness of what we are trying to accomplish, it is imperative that we try these or other suggestions to improve the technique.

References

Allport, G. W.: Personality: A psychological interpretation. New York: Holt & Co. (1937).

Bendig, A. W.: The reliability of self-ratings as a function of the amount of verbal anchoring and the number of categories on the scale. J Appl Psychol 37, 38-41 (1953).

Bendig, A. W.: Reliability and number of rating scale categories. J Appl Psychol 38, 38-40 (1954).

Borman, W. C., Vallon, W. R.: A view of what can happen when behavioral expectation scales are developed in one setting and used in another. J Appl Psychol 59, 197-201 (1974).

Borman, W. C.: Effects of instructions to avoid halo error on reliability and validity of performance ratings. J Appl Psychol 60, 556-560 (1975).

Borman, W. C., Dunnette, M. D.: Behavior-based versus trait-oriented ratings: An empirical study. J Appl Psychol 60, 561-565 (1975).

Brumback, G. B., Howell, M. A.: Rating the clinical effectiveness of employed physicians. J Appl Psychol 56, 241-244 (1972).

Burnaska, R. F., Hollmann, T. D.: An empirical comparison of the relative effects of rater response biases on three rating scale formats. J Appl Psychol 59, 307-312 (1974).

Campbell, J. P., Dunnette, M. D., Arvey, R. D., Hellervik, L. V.: The development and evaluation of behaviorally based rating scales. J Appl Psychol 57, 15-22 (1973).

Cowles, J. T., Kubany, A. J.: Improving the measurement of clinical performance in medical students. J Clin Psychol 15, 139-142 (1959).

Cowles, J. T.: A critical-comments approach to the rating of medical students' clinical performance. J Med Educ 40, 188-198 (1965).

Cronbach, L. J.: Essentials of psychological testing (3rd ed.). New York: Harper & Row, (1970).

De Nio, J. N., Holmes, F. F., Pierleoni, R. G., Greenberger, N. J.: Evaluation of internal medicine clerkship students. Proceedings, 14th Annual Conference on Research in Medical Education, Washington, D.C. (1975).

Dielman, T. E., Hull, A. L., Davis, W. K.: Inter-rater reliability of clinical performance ratings. Proceedings, 18th Annual Conference on Research in Medical Education, pp. 191-196, Washington, D.C. (1979).

Dielman, T. E., Hull, A. L., Davis, W. K.: Psychometric properties of clinical performance ratings. Evaluation and the Health Professions 3, 103-117 (1980).

Donnelly, M. B., Gallagher, R. E.: A study of the predictive validity of patient management problems, multiple choice tests and rating scales. Proceedings, 17th Annual Conference on Research in Medical Education, New Orleans, La. (1978).

Dowaliby, F. J., Andrews, B. J.: Relationships between clinical competence ratings and examination performance. J Med Educ 51, 181-188 (1976).

Ebel, R. L.: Estimation of the reliability of ratings. Psychometrika 16, 407-423 (1951).

Erviti, V., Fabrey, L. J., Bunce, J. V.: The development of rating scales to assess the clinical performance of medical students. Proceedings, 18th Annual Conference on Research in Medical Education, Washington, D.C. (1979).

Gallagher, R., Donnelly, M., Scalzi, P. M., Deighton, M.: Toward a comprehensive methodology for resident evaluation. Proceedings, 16th Annual Conference on Research in Medical Education 16, 323-328 (1977).

Gardner, B.: A multivariate computer analysis of students' performances as a predictor of performance as a surgical intern. J Surg Res 12, 216-219 (1972).

Gardner, B.: Over-all student performance as a measure of internship performance. Surgery 74, 80-83 (1973).

Geertsma, R. H., Chapman, J. E.: The evaluation of medical students. J Med Educ 42, 938-948 (1967).

Goldberg, L. R.: A note on the assessment of "clinical competence" in internal medicine: A novel application of the external strategy of scale construction. ORI Technical Report 12, No. 5. Eugene, Ore.: Oregon Research Institute (1972).

Gough, H. G., Hall, W. B.: Prediction of performance in medical school from the California Personality Inventory. J Appl Psychol 48, 218-226 (1964).

Gough, H. G., Hall, W. B., Harris, R. E.: Evaluation of performance in medical training. J Med Educ 39, 679-692 (1964).

Gough, H. G., Hall, W. B.: The prediction of academic and clinical perfor-
   mance in medical school. Res Higher Educ 3, 301-314 (1975).
Guilford, J. P.: Psychometric methods (2nd ed.). New York: McGraw-Hill
   (1954).
Guion, R. M.: Personnel testing, New York: McGraw-Hill (1965).
Hammond, K. R., Kern, F.: Teaching comprehensive medical care. Cam-
   bridge, Mass.: Harvard University Press (1959).
Holt, R. R.: Experimental methods in clinical psychology. In: B. B. Wolman
   (Ed.), Handbook of clinical psychology. New York: McGraw-Hill
   (1965).
Jackson, D. N.: A sequential system for personality scale development. In:
   C. D. Spielberger (Ed.), Current topics in clinical and community psy-
   chology. New York: Academic Press (1970).
Kegel-Flom, P.: Predicting supervisor, peer, and self-ratings of intern perfor-
   mance. J Med Educ 50, 812-815 (1975).
Korman, M., Stubblefield, R. L.: Medical school evaluation and internship
   performance. J Med Educ 46, 670-673 (1971).
Landy, F. J., Farr, J. L.: Performance rating. Psychol Bull 87, 72-107 (1980).
Levine, H. G., Gustavson, L. P., Emergy, J. L. R.: The effectiveness of various
   assessment methods used in a pediatric junior clerkship. Proceedings,
   14th Annual Conference on Research in Medical Education, Washing-
   ton, D.C. (1975).
Likert, R. A.: A technique for the measurements of attitudes. Arch Psychol
   140, (1932).
Linn, B. S., Arostegui, M., Zeppa, R.: Performance rating scale for peer and
   self assessment. Brit J Med Educ 9, 98-101 (1975).
Linn, L.: Interns' attitudes and values as antecedents of clinical performance.
   J Med Educ 54, 238-240 (1979).
Murstein, B. I.: Theory and research in projective techniques. New York:
   Wiley (1963).
Nerenberg, R. L., Noe, M. J., Juul, D. H., Martin, I. C., Levine, S. P.: Predic-
   tion of graduate clinical performance ratings from multi-component
   medical school examinations. Proceedings, 17th Annual Conference on
   Research in Medical Education, New Orleans, La. (1978).
Nunnally, J. C.: Psychometric theory. New York: McGraw-Hill (1967).
O'Donohue, W. J., Wergin, J. F.: Evaluation of medical students during a
   clinical clerkship in internal medicine. J Med Educ 53, 55-58 (1978).
Paterson, D. G.: The Scott Company graphic rating scale. J Personnel Res 1,
   361-376 (1922).
Pierleoni, R. G., Dudding, B. A., Clark, G. M.: An analysis of pediatric clerkship performance in multicomponent evaluation system. Proceedings,
   17th Annual Conference on Research in Medical Education, New Orleans, La. (1978).
Printen, K. J., Chappell, W.: Clinical performance evaluation of junior medical students. J Med Educ 48, 343-348 (1973).

Rugg, H.: Is the rating of human character practicable? J Educ Psychol 13, 30-42 (1922).
Skakun, E. N., Taylor, W. C., Wilson, D. R., Langley, G. R.: The In-training evaluation report—stability of structure and relationship to other certifying examinations. Ann R Coll Phys Surg Can 9, 315-317 (1976).
Smith, P. C., Kendall, L. M.: Retranslation of expectations: An approach to the construction of unambiguous anchors for rating scales. J Appl Psychol 47, 149-155 (1963).
Symonds, P. M.: On the loss of reliability in ratings due to coarseness of the scale. J Exp Psychol 7, 456-461 (1924).
Thorndike, E. L.: A constant error in psychological ratings. J Appl Psychol 4, 25-29 (1920).
Thurstone, L. I.: Theory of attitude measurement. Psychol Bull 36, 222-241 (1929).
Thurstone, L. I.: The measurement of social attitudes. J Abnorm Social Psychol 26, 249-269 (1931).
Tukey, J. W.: Discussion. J Clin Psychol 6, 61-74 (1950).
Turner, E. B., Helper, M. M., Kriska, S. D., Singer, S. A., Ruma, S. J.: Evaluating clinical skills of students in pediatrics. J Med Educ 47, 959-965 (1972).
Weissman, S. H., Berner, E. S., Bombeck, C. T.: Evaluation of systematic observation of data gathering skills in sophomore medical students. Proceedings, 14th Annual Conference on Research in Medical Education, Washington, D.C. (1975).
Wells, F. L.: A statistical study of literary merit. Arch Psychol 1 (No. 7) (1907).
Wingard, J. R., Williamson, J. W.: Grades as predictors of physicians' career and performance: An evaluative literature review. J Med Educ 48, 311-322 (1973).

CHAPTER **8**

Medical
Record Review

PETER TUGWELL
CAROLINE DOK

Introduction

Patient records have traditionally been used for providing documentation of a physician's assessment and management to serve as a reminder in the subsequent care of the patient. More recently, the medical record has been recognized as having substantial potential for a number of other uses, including communication between different health providers caring for the same patient, clinical research, legal purposes, and the evaluation of the clinical competence of health providers. One continuing limitation of record review, however, is that recording practices have evolved haphazardly with few attempts at standardization. A result is that there are wide variations in recording practices, which impose important constraints on some applications.

Record review has been used to assess clinical competence in undergraduates, residents in postgraduate training, and clinicians practicing in the community. Record review has been used for both "formative" assessment (i.e, to provide feedback on performance that will be used to stimulate learning) and for "summative" assessment (used for a pass/fail decision for graduation or certification). Table 8.1 summarizes the main features of some of the most widely cited studies.

In undergraduate education, record review is widely used on an informal basis by supervising residents and faculty for formative evaluation of students on clinical rotations, using the data from the student's write-up as a basis for discussion and feedback. The supervisor usually integrates this information with knowledge from other sources in his global evaluation of students.

The medical record has been implemented as the primary basis for evaluation in the clinical program of an English medical school on the premise that audit of problem-oriented records allows constant monitoring of learning objectives and immediate feedback. Initial assessments of this method of evaluation in this hospital are encouraging (Dearden and Laurillard, 1976; Lloyd and McIntyre, 1979; McIntyre, 1979, 1980).

Nelson (1976) also used the record to evaluate performance on an Obstetrics clerkship and to evaluate the effectiveness of the training program by change in student performance. Goetz et al. (1979) have suggested that the undergraduate student's ability to review charts of patients written by others is a useful measure of competence on the basis that in order to review a chart well, the student must be able to quickly and accurately separate relevant from irrelevant patient information.

The use of the record by supervisors as an important source of data for evaluation of residents must be more widespread than for students, yet there are few documented studies. Scott and Sniderman (1973) used record review to study the performance of house staff in a university teaching hospital. The method was shown to discriminate among educational levels. Templeton et al. (1978) reported the results of a pilot study sponsored by the U.S. National Board of Medical Examiners and the American Board of Pediatrics, in which the medical record was used for assessing physician trainees' day-to-day performance in five pediatric training program centers. Performance was assessed using explicit criteria to evaluate medical history, psychological history, and the physical exam on ambulatory records. Substantial deficiencies in compliance with these standards were demonstrated.

The medical record has also been used extensively for assessing the clinical competence of practicing physicians, both in hospitals and in ambulatory practice, with the advent of the widespread quality-of-care audit activities that are requirements of government accreditation bodies. Most of the published studies have identified substantial deficiencies in compliance with criteria designed to measure assessment and management of patients (e.g., Brook and Appel, 1973; Payne et al., 1978; Thompson and Osborne, 1976). More recently, record review has been considered

TABLE 8.1
Variation in the Range of Components in Clinical Competence in Different Studies

Components of Clinical Competence	Bentsen (1976)	Brook & Appel (1973)	Clute (1963)	Dickie & Bass (1980)	Dixon (1973)	Hammett et al. (1976)	Hastings & Sonneborn (1980)	Kane et al. (1977)	Kessner et al. (1973)	Lindsay et al. (1976)
Problem Identification	+			+	+	+	+			
Data Collection—History identifies data required			+		+		+	+	+	+
Data Collection—Physical Examination identifies data required			+		+		+	+	+	+
Data Interpretation—History significance of history accurately perceived with significant negatives included			+		+		+		+	
Data Interpretation—Physical Examination significance of physical data accurately perceived with significant negatives included			+		+		+		+	
Problem Formulation problem definition problem assessment			+	+	+	+	+		+	
Data Collection—Investigations orders appropriate investigations		+	+	+	+		+	+	+	+
Data Interpretation—Investigations significance of investigative procedures or tests		+	+		+		+		+	+

Lloyd & McIntyre (1979)	Margolis et al. (1973)	Merrill (1979)	Nelson et al. (1976)	Neufeld & Tugwell (1977)	Payne et al. (1978)	Rakel (1979)	Reed et al. (1973)	Sanazaro & Worth (1978)	Saywell (1979)	Scott & Sniderman (1973)	Sibley et al. (1975)	Starfield & Scheff (1972)	Starfield et al. (1977)	Thompson & Osborne (1976)	Voytovich (1973)	Voytovich & Rippey (1978)	Williamson et al. (1967)
+	+		+				+			+			+		+		
+	+		+	+	+	+	+	+	+	+	+			+	+		
+	+		+	+	+		+		+	+	+			+	+		
+	+		+	+	+		+			+	+			+	+		
+	+		+	+			+			+	+			+	+		
+	+		+	+			+	+		+	+	+		+			+
+			+	+	+		+			+	+	+	+	+			+

(*continued*)

TABLE 8.1 (cont.)

Components of Clinical Competence	Bentsen (1976)	Brook & Appel (1973)	Clute (1963)	Dickie & Bass (1980)	Dixon (1973)	Hammett et al. (1976)	Hastings & Sonneborn (1980)	Kane et al. (1977)	Kessner et al. (1973)	Lindsay et al. (1976)
Refinement of Problem integration of results of procedures and laboratory tests		+	+	+	+	+		+		
Management			+	+	+	+				
therapy	+	+	+			+		+	+	
consultation							+			
patient education							+			
follow-up	+	+				+		+	+	+
Emergency care										
Knowledge demonstration of appropriate knowledge										
Appropriate Documentation in Medical Records for communication of management issues to peers for evaluation			+	+	+		+			
Self-assessment										
Teaching and Evaluation of Peers										

	Lloyd & McIntyre (1979)	Margolis et al. (1973)	Merrill (1979)	Nelson et al. (1976)	Neufeld & Tugwell (1977)	Payne et al. (1978)	Rakel (1979)	Reed et al. (1973)	Sanazaro & Worth (1978)	Saywell (1979)	Scott & Sniderman (1973)	Sibley et al. (1975)	Starfield & Scheff (1972)	Starfield et al. (1977)	Thompson & Osborne (1976)	Voytovich (1973)	Voytovich & Rippey (1978)	Williamson et al. (1967)
	+			+	+	+			+		+	+				+		
	+	+	+	+	+													
	+				+	+	+	+	+		+	+	+		+	+		+
	+				+	+							+					
			+		+	+	+	+	+			+	+	+	+	+		
				+														
									+							+		
	+																	
	+				+													

147

for recertification. The American Board of Family Practice administered its first mandatory recertification procedure in 1976, designed primarily as a physician self-audit (Rakel, 1979). At the time of writing this chapter, chart review is also used by the American Board of Obstetrics and Gynecology for recertification purposes (Merrill et al., 1979).

Record review has also been used to compare the competence of foreign medical graduates (Saywell et al., 1979) and physician assistants and nurse practitioners (Kane et al., 1978; Spitzer et al., 1974; Sox, 1979). Most of these studies showed little or no difference between the groups. A large study was reported by Sanazaro and Worth (1978), designed to determine the feasibility of a record review program that could be used for granting formal recognition of competence to practicing internists.

Formats of Medical Records

The two common formats of medical records are the traditional source-oriented record (SOR) and the problem-oriented medical record (POR) developed by Weed (1969). These two formats will be frequently referred to throughout this chapter, so it seems worthwhile to briefly describe here how they differ. In the source-oriented record the presenting complaint is usually recorded first, followed by a review of systems and then the physical examination; these are followed by a statement of the most likely provisional diagnosis, often accompanied by one or more differential diagnoses; the investigations and management are commonly listed together below the diagnosis or diagnoses. Progress notes follow the same format with no standardized approach for recording. The problem-oriented record uses a more standardized format with the following components: (1) A problem list that identifies all relevant clinical problems; the definition of these problems must fulfill certain specified requirements. (2) A defined data base that consists of (a) problem-specific information and (b) routine information that might be relevant to the patient's management. (3) Plans specified separately for each problem, including investigations, therapy, and patient education. (4) Progress notes specified separately for each problem and broken down into data base, assessment, and plan.

Using this introduction as a background to identify examples of different studies that use record review to assess competence, we will now consider the extent to which such studies meet methodologic criteria described in the introduction to this section.

Credibility

Clinical credibility is an important criterion that determines to a large extent the degree to which the results of record review are acceptable to those being assessed.

One of the basic issues relevant to the credibility and acceptance of the results is the extent to which predetermined criteria are formulated in a reproducible fashion and are clinically credible. It is generally felt that "explicit criteria" reflecting designated assessment and management activities need to be formulated and applied consistently if the results are to be acceptable. The majority of studies of physicians in practice and some studies including residents (Fessel and Van Brunt, 1972; Kane et al., 1977) use this approach.

Most of the record review studies of clinical competence in undergraduate and residency settings use the "implicit judgment" approach—i.e., subjective evaluation by physician assessors based upon the individual clinical judgment of the assessor (Margolis et al., 1973; McIntyre, 1980; Nelson et al., 1976; Scott and Sniderman, 1973; Voytovich and Rippey, 1978; Weed, 1969). The method is still employed for assessment of clinical competence of practicing clinicians in a few studies (Dawes, 1972; McAuley, 1980; Morehead and Donaldson, 1974; Therien, 1982). Fletcher (1974) in a study including implicit assessment of PORs compared with SORs found that inaccuracies were infrequently detected and concluded that this was due to the fact that the auditor was not using explicit criteria to look for specific information. It is probably reasonable for implicit record review to be used for identifying problems and providing the focus for day-to-day teaching, but this approach has serious methodologic limitations if used for making major decisions about clinical competence.

Brook and Appel (1973) compared five different methods for assessing the quality of care provided to patients with urinary tract infection, hypertension, or peptic ulcers: implicit process, implicit outcome, implicit process and outcome, explicit process, and explicit outcome. The proportion of cases judged to have acceptable care varied substantially according to the method employed, ranging from only 1.4 percent of cases using explicit criteria to a high of 63.2 percent when implicit outcome criteria were used. In addition, results using implicit criteria varied according to the condition under study.

Credibility is also related to the extent to which the actions of interest are known to influence the health of patients. Thus all criteria should be clearly relevant to therapeutic or prognostic decisions. If the "so-what" challenge from critics of the exhaustive lists of criteria of dubious relevance used in many audits in the past is to be avoided, criteria describing the assessment of the patient (history, physical examination, and laboratory investigations) should be clearly linked to a therapeutic decision. Ideally, therapeutic criteria should be based upon evidence from controlled trials, and diagnostic critera should be justified by evidence that the assessment criteria chosen influence the accuracy or the diagnosis of the monitoring of the patient's therapy. Sibley et al. (1975) emphasized the importance of these criteria in his selection of "indicator" conditions in which outcomes could be influenced by management. Sanazaro and Worth (1978) utilized "essential criteria," which are defined as process criteria derived from sound clinical research, adherence to which would be predictive of the desired end results of care. The opinion of a consensus of a group of respected clinicians, which is perhaps the commonest approach to ensuring credibility, does not always clearly address this issue.

Criterion lists consisting of a small number of therapeutic or follow-up items combined with large numbers of items of history, physical examination, and investigation also reduce the clinical credibility of results of process assessment. Therapeutic and follow-up criteria contributed only 4 out of 26 items in the myocardial infarction criteria list of Fessel and Van Brunt (1972), and 18 of 89 in the hypertension criteria list of Nobrega et al. (1977). When the level of competence is then determined by adding up all the items complied with, most of the score originates from the history and physical examination criteria, and an inappropriately small proportion of the score is based on the few management criteria. Thus a high score may reflect care that is good in most parts but disastrously inadequate due to one vital error (e.g., if a superb workup for hypertension was carried out but the patient was not treated correctly and died, the score would appear to be excellent).

Unreasonable expectation of performance can also occur due to lack of attention to the frequency of the event or complication of interest; for example, inclusion of items that are known to be relevant in less than one percent of cases are difficult to justify. Two examples will illustrate this point; first, in a study of hypertension, it was required that the presence or absence of a history of trauma to the flanks be recorded (Nobrega et al., 1977); and second, in all patients with acute myocardial infarction, a Venereal Disease Research Laboratory Test for syphilis should have been performed (Fessel and Van Brunt, 1972).

The emphasis of the topic chosen for assessment should be on problem/patient complaints rather than diseases or final diagnoses, since the latter method of selecting cases misses those patients who are misdiagnosed. Although it is technically a little more difficult to construct criteria, the studies of Sibley et al. (1975), Spasoff et al. (1977), and Greenfield et al. (1977) have demonstrated the feasibility of assessing problems and patient complaints in both ambulatory and hospital settings.

In situations other than acute emergencies, record review should allow assessment of episodes of care that may involve several visits where appropriate, since it may be inappropriate to insist on criteria even for the initial diagnostic workup being fulfilled at one visit—especially where the psychological aspects are important. Furthermore, the potential for assessing continuity of care including follow-up and monitoring of therapy is one of the major assets of record review.

Adjustment for disease severity and presence of complications also increases the acceptability of the results of record review; this entails incorporation of appropriate options to accommodate the differing criteria that are relevant depending upon the severity of the disease and/or complications. Sibley et al. (1975) established different criteria sets for different levels of severity for conditions such as hypertension; Greenfield et al. (1977) used a "criteria mapping approach" to handle this problem in conditions such as chest pain; this technique uses branching criteria that allow for the assessment of only those criteria relevant to the patient, thus differentiating different levels of clinical competence among homogeneous subsets of patients. Gonnella and Goran (1975) have developed another approach to this problem that they term "the staging concept." This is, in essence, a working system that operates by focusing on the cases with complications or who fare badly. When the frequency of these cases rises above arbitrarily defined acceptable levels, record review is then carried out.

Comprehensiveness

Comprehensiveness refers to the proportion of all of the components of clinical competence that can be or are assessed by record review. A number of different conceptual approaches for defining and measuring clinical competence have been employed depending on the purpose of the medical audit. Table 8.1 provides a comparison of the components of competence included in a sample of published record review studies using a standardized classification.

Assessment should include all of the clinically important dimensions of physician performance unless high correlations exist between them, in which case measurement of one dimension can be used to predict the other (Donabedian, 1969; Rhee et al., 1978). As can be seen from Table 8.1, the range of dimensions in reported studies varies considerably. Some studies have confined themselves to a specific focus; for example, Bentsen (1976) concentrated on the assessment of completeness of problem identification. The tracer concept (Kessner et al., 1973) addresses this issue of comprehensiveness by purposely sampling the different dimensions; this assumes that performance in specific dimensions is consistent across patients whether the clinical problem be similar or different, an assumption which is not borne out by two other studies. Lyons and Payne (1977) reported correlation coefficients of 0.80 or greater between only three pairs of diagnoses out of 80 pairs analyzed in ten diagnostic categories. Osborne (1975) found no correlation coefficients of 0.80 or greater in seven health care areas (four health supervision areas and three diseases). In the absence of data showing close correlations among the different components of clinical competence, it continues to be necessary to evaluate all components about which information is desired. Similarly, in view of the absence of evidence that performance by a physician is consistent for different diagnoses, it continues to be necessary to evaluate a variety of different conditions; nevertheless, a reasonable proportion of patients are represented by relatively few health problems so that by focusing on these, a reasonable sample of an individual's practice can be obtained.

Precision

Precision or reliability refers to the reproducibility of assessments of clinical competence using record review. As noted above, review of the literature in this area is complicated by the fact that different terminology and indices of competence are used in different studies.

Studies that rely upon the implicit clinical judgment of the observer tend to have lower reliability than those that rely upon predetermined explicit criteria (Brook and Appel, 1973; Dershewitz et al., 1979; Morehead and Donaldson, 1964; Peterson et al., 1965; Richardson, 1972). For example, Richardson (1972) found that as many as 16 to 28 physicians (depending on the case) were needed to read and judge each record to be 95 percent certain that care for a specific patient was or was not adequate. Morehead and Donaldson (1964) found that observers agreed on only 50 percent of cases, the level to be expected by chance alone, if physicians were not specifically trained in record review. Dershewitz et al., (1969) cited a level of 70 percent agreement if record review was performed by multiple physicians.

In Bentsen's (1976) study of completeness of problem identification, there was a total of 59 consultations by first-, second-, and third-year residents. They were observed by pairs of faculty physicians. The observers agreed on the main problem in only 48 of the 59 encounters (85 percent). By contrast, Voytovich and Rippey (1978) developed a scorable problem list for evaluating a student's problem identification. Three raters (a physician, a Ph.D, and a secretary) independently assessed the problem lists. The method was tested on a group of 88 medical students and faculty, who wrote problem lists based on a written standardized data base of a single patient. The method of scoring was pretested using the three raters and minor revisions were made upon noting discrepancies. Interobserver reliability ranged from 0.62 to 0.94 and 66 percent of the correlations were greater than 0.85.

Use of explicit predetermined criteria allows high levels of interobserver agreement in abstracting information from source-oriented records of practicing physicians. Sibley et al. (1975), using trained nurse abstractors, achieved an interobserver agreement of 88 percent, and of the abstracts about which they agreed, 94 percent agreed with an independent review by two physicians, providing a check on accuracy. Also in an ambulatory setting, Thompson and Osborne (1976) reported that medical record administrators were successfully trained to achieve a "high level of intra- and inter-observer reliability" although the exact level was not defined. Saywell et al. (1979), in a study comparing the performance of U.S. medical graduates with foreign medical graduates through record review, found that the agreement across all diagnoses and combinations of team abstractors was 90 percent. Payne et al. (1976, 1978) found that interobserver reliability was acceptable (88-95 percent) in studies of both hospital and ambulatory care using trained nonmedical abstractors.

Hastings and Sonneborn (1980) reported on the use of a 35-item checklist for peer review of ambulatory medical records. Interobserver variation was determined by having five pairs of reviewers rate the same ten records. They were consistent with one another, item by item, 72 percent of the time with Kappa = 0.35 ($p < 0.05$). Intraobserver variation was also determined by having ten physicians review the same ten records six weeks later. They were consistent with themselves, item by item, 74 percent of the time with Kappa = 0.53 ($p < 0.05$).

The American Board of Family Practice (ABFP) has developed self-assessment questionnaries for 20 diagnoses or problems common to family practice for use in the recertification program of its diplomates. Rakel (1979) discussed the assessment of the reliability of this method. Interobserver variation was determined by having a nurse and an auditor fill out a "self-assessment" questionnaire from the photocopied medical record submitted by the diplomate along with the accompanying self-assessment questionnaire. The mean agreement was expressed for each disease/problem category and ranged from 70.5 percent to 88.4 percent.

Payne et al. (1978) have used abstracts of medical records to assess individual physician performance in specified diagnostic categories. Criteria for optimal performance were weighted according to importance of the various items. This weighting of items allowed the development of a Physician Performance Index (PPI). Interobserver reliability ratings in their ambulatory study using the PPI averaged 90 percent with a range from 87 percent in gynecologic examination to 94 percent in use of drugs. Across pairs, interobserver reliability ranged from 88 percent to 92 percent. This high level of agreement was achieved through four weeks of training the four nonmedical abstractors in the ten study diagnoses.

Hermann et al. (1980) found that even with trained nurses there is considerable variability in the reliability of data abstraction. To improve the reliability of abstracted data they suggest standardized or structured forms and continuous monitoring and retraining of abstractors during the data-collection period. These findings led the authors to conclude that the quality and complexity of the medical record could affect observer variation.

The consistency of assessments of style of recording rather than the appropriateness of actions of care has also been examined. Margolis et al. (1973) developed a checklist from an outline of a POMR for use with pediatric patients. The Problem Oriented Medical Record (POMR) was divided into eight major sections each of which could be graded for structure and completeness for a maximum total of 162 points. Interobserver agreement was assessed by having seven faculty members and a teaching resident grade a single workup using the graded problem-oriented record (GPOR). The mean score was 114 (range 106 to 119) with a standard deviation of +3.2, signifying a high degree of agreement between observers; however, the reliability of the method was not stated.

Hammett et al. (1976) described a method to review certain indicators in the medical record as a basis for assessing whether the POMR format was adhered to. The Problem List and Progress Notes were the key components examined; the Initial Data Base was not reviewed since it was not problem oriented. Reliability of the format review procedure was assessed by having five individuals review the same 22 medical records. An analysis of variance technique established a reliability of 0.83 based on pattern scores.

Concurrent Validity

This addresses the issue of whether a substantial association with another available validated external measure has been demonstrated. When evaluating clinical competence using a measure such a record review, three dimensions will be addressed: (1) completeness of recording: the extent to which record review accurately reflects the action of interest of the health professional; (2) relationship to patient outcomes: the demonstration that patients who receive care from physicians judged more competent on the basis of evidence from the medical record have better outcomes; and (3) relationship to physician judgments.

Completeness of Recording

A major limitation of the medical record as the source of data for assessing clinical competence is the fact that individual physicians often fail to record all their clinical actions; as a result it is difficult to distinguish between actions not performed and actions performed but not recorded (Fessel and Van Brunt, 1972; Kroeger et al., 1965; Lembcke, 1956; Osborne and Thompson, 1975; Payne, 1979; Peterson et al., 1965). The problem-oriented record does have the theoretical advantage that the "SOAP" format, if complied with, results in pertinent information from history, physical, and investigations being clearly linked to the conclusions, whereas with the traditional source-oriented record it is often less clear which items of information were used in formulating diagnosis or management. Tufo et al. (1973) note that physicians in practice can achieve high levels of compliance with requirements for chart completeness using the POR. Checklists achieve the same end in situations where sufficiently large numbers of patients with the same problem are cared for (Frazier and Brand, 1979; Grover and Greenberg, 1976).

Few studies have addressed this issue directly. Lembcke found in 1949 that some surgeons postponed making a written record of their preoperative observations, including history and physical, until after the operation, potentially falsely inflating the accuracy of this information (Lembcke, 1956). Wiener and Nathanson (1976) observed the interview and examination of 145 patient encounters with residents and interns; the assessment included a chart audit. Although details are not provided, the authors state that recording inaccuracies were found due to: (1) forgetting a finding and not recording it (which they claim can be avoided by recording abnormalities on a card at the bedside); (2) illegible handwriting, obscure abbreviations, improper terminology, poor grammar, and incomplete recording of findings; and (3) recording a diagnosis and not the sign detected. Zuckerman et al. (1975) tape recorded 51 pediatric patient encounters involving three university staff physicians in an inner-city medical center; it is not clear whether the problems were confined to new complaints or whether repeat visits were included. Information from the tape recording was compared with the medical record. The frequency of recording of items present on the tape recording was as follows: diagnosis and problem—100 percent of 67 named diagnoses present on tape; historical items—56 percent of 297 items; drug name—100 percent of 28 names present on tape; drug dosage—54 percent of 68 dosages on tape; drug actions (purpose or intended pharmacologic effects)—95 percent of 55 actions present on tape; drug side-effects—0 percent of 8 named side-effects discussed on tape; specified follow-up appointments for the specific illness—100 percent of 39 items present on tape; diagnostic studies—100 percent of 24 investigations mentioned on tape. Physical examination was not possible to assess.

Norman et al. (1980) used videotaped interviews with simulated patients to compare the completeness of recording of items in the history and physical examination by medical students, residents, and practicing family physicians and internists; they were asked to interview and examine the patient and to complete the medical record as they would routinely do in the outpatient clinic or physician's office. The data base was classified into "essential" and "nonessential" by independent criterion groups of three family physicians and three general internists. Despite the fact that the participants knew they were being assessed, over 15 percent of physician actions judged "essential" by one criterion group which was elicited were not recorded.

The importance of individual items upon the completeness of recording has been commented on in the context of postoperative surgical care by Collopy (1979); in an audit of surgical procedures he found that the accuracy of the registrar's recordings was directly related to the seriousness of the complication. The recording of phlebitis at an intravenous infusion site (a relatively less serious complication), was rarely documented by the registrar but more accurately recorded by nurses; the recording of the more serious complication of wound infection had better than 80 percent accuracy when compared with records searched by a medical record administrator; the documentation of mortality was 100 percent accurate. The completeness of the nurses' recording and of the records searched by the medical record administrators themselves was not addressed in this paper, so the results should be accepted with caution. Stewart and Buck (1977) pretested the completeness of recording of management by family physicians by comparison with audio tapes. The number of encounters and detailed results were not given, but the authors state that there was virtually no underreporting of physicians' responses to patient discomfort and disturbance to daily living, but as much as 30 percent underreporting of responses for worries and social problems. These results are probably not generalizable since the physicians were chosen because of their interest in keeping good records.

A number of studies have addressed this issue indirectly. Peterson et al. (1965), Clute (1963), and Jungfer and Last (1965) all comment in their studies (based on implicit physician judgment) that recorded information was felt to provide an incomplete picture of clinical competence and quality of care. Kroeger et al. (1965), in a study of quality of care provided by internists in their office practice, found that only two-thirds of a random sample of 91 patient records were sufficiently complete and legible to allow nonphysicians to abstract information. Dawes (1972) examined 1,628 records of eight English general practitioners and found that symptoms were recorded in less than half of what were termed "disease episodes," recording of any physical signs in less than one-third, any diagnosis recorded in 60 percent of episodes, drugs prescribed in 70 percent of episodes, but the amount prescribed in the dosage in only one-quarter of these. Starfield et al. (1973) audited the medical records of 15 community practice pediatricians and found wide variations in the recording of preventive procedures (12-86 percent), throat cultures for suspected pharyngitis (2-100 percent), and urine cultures for suspected urinary tract infection on 11 of 12 occasions. There were insufficient numbers to assess each practice. These latter two studies assume that much of this variation reflects incomplete recording rather than incomplete performance, but there was no validation of this conclusion.

Thompson and Osborne (1976) asked 166 physicians in community practice whether they felt that the results of a record review accurately portrayed the care they were delivering, after they were told that only 52 percent of 10,500 charts fulfilled the predetermined explicit criteria satisfactorily. The majority of physicians felt that the records were incomplete due to the physicians performing but not recording many of their actions and that no documentation generally meant negative findings. This issue of negative findings being less often recorded than positive items indeed seems likely in most clinical situations, but apparently has not been studied. Again, confining the criteria to those essential for appropriate care is of course important in coming to reasonable expectations of completeness of recording; Greenfield suggests that the "criteria mapping" approach minimizes this problem of incompleteness by focusing on the essential items that influence management decisions. The presence of sufficient information to satisfy the criteria in over 60 percent of 118 episodes of care in a community primary care setting, using the indicator condition approach (Sibley et al., 1975), was probably at least partly attributable to realistic criteria sets and the use of predetermined special probes to obtain some types of pertinent information elsewhere in the record.

Do physicians record observations and actions that were not performed? Very little evidence exists to address this question. Fewer than 2 percent of items in pediatricians' records in the

study of Zuckerman et al. (1975) and 2 percent of items recorded by students, residents, and practicing physicians reported
by the McMaster group (Norman et al., 1980) were actually not
elicited. Margolis et al. (1973) comment that no data was recorded
that had not been elicited in the two observed encounters they
evaluated.

The question of whether the standard of record keeping pre-
dicts the overall competence of the individual physician is pertinent to the issue of completeness of recording. Peterson et al.
(1965) and Clute (1963) in their independent observational studies of general practitioners in North Carolina and Canada concluded that good recording was associated with better quality of patient care. Lyons and Payne (1974) found a mean correlation
coefficient of 0.2, which was statistically significant, between
good recording and good care for eight diagnoses (the correlation
coefficient ranged from -0.03 to +0.5) involving 1,239 charts;
on the basis of these figures and a review of other studies, they
concluded that good recording is related to good practice, but the
relationship is not strong. In any case, it appears that the assessment of style and completeness of recording have not yet been
demonstrated to predict the clinical competence of individuals
or groups at any level of training and experience to the extent
that it can be substituted for other measures of clinical competence.

Relationship to Patient Outcomes

The demonstration of a correlation between clinical competence
assessed by record-keeping behavior and patient outcomes would
provide the best evidence that the record review assessment
method is measuring an important component of clinical competence. Unfortunately, there are substantial methodologic problems in implementing such studies (Tugwell, 1979). Perhaps the
most important is the appropriate control of confounding factors
unrelated to physician actions, which can themselves substantially
influence patient outcomes. We will briefly review some of the
most relevant studies of the relationship of physician performance
to patient outcomes.

No studies appear to have been carried out with undergraduate medical students. The majority of studies involve only physicians in practice, although in some, resident staff were also involved. Brook (1973) compared process assessed by record review
with outcome in patients with hypertension, urinary tract infec-

tion, and peptic ulceration, using both implicit and explicit techniques. Outcomes were assessed on the basis of mortality and follow-up interview at five months for uncontrolled hypertension, positive urine cultures, and persisting peptic ulcer symptoms, activity, and mortality. The implicit process judgment was compared with the actual outcome and a few significant correlations between process and outcome were found. No adjustment was made, however, for external factors such as disease severity, and the outcome measure of persistent symptoms and decreased activity are questionable in a condition such as hypertension, which is usually asymptomatic.

Fessel and Van Brunt (1972) in their hospital study of residents and staff physicians found that neither quantity nor quality of recording process was related to outcomes of either acute appendicitis or myocardial infarction. However, the failure to standardize for confounding variables such as disease severity, the use of insensitive or inappropriate process measures, and the failure to use an inception cohort may have militated against finding a correlation between process and outcome measures.

Greenfield et al. (1977) studied the management of patients presenting with chest pain in an emergency department who were not admitted and assessed the relation between process and death or subsequent hospitalization for a condition related to chest pain. A sensitive method-assessing process from the medical record was used; this uses branching criteria to reflect sequential judgments and allows for assessment of only those criteria relevant to the patient. One hundred eleven patient charts fulfilled the process criteria and none of these had a poor outcome; 26 patient charts failed to fulfill the criteria, and 3 of these patients died within 3 weeks from cardiac causes. Although the relationship between process and outcome was statistically significant, one should be cautious in generalizing from such small numbers, and the outcomes were limited in scope. It is probable, however, that this method has advantages over the inflexible list of process criteria used in most studies.

Kane et al. (1977) have studied the relationship between the performance of residents, faculty, and physician assistants and the functional outcomes of a series of 410 acute episodes from two family practice centers. Explicit criteria developed by the Utah Professional Review Organization were used for 251 episodes and implicit criteria by faculty physicians for 159 episodes. In both the explicit and implicit approaches a positive relationship was demonstrated between process and outcome; with the explicit approach, patients with a good outcome had a 25 percent higher mean score for the appropriateness of management than those with a poor outcome: this relationship was positive in 5 of 7 conditions assessed. With the implicit approach using aggregated data of all types of patient problems, patients with a poor outcome had a 10 percent lower mean score (this was also statistically significant) for appropriateness of management than those patients with a good outcome. It is not clear whether the outcome assessors were blind to the process scores nor whether confounding variables such as severity of disease were comparable.

Lindsay et al. (1976) have studied the relationship between process and outcome in acute bacterial cystitis in women. Forty-two cases were reviewed by analysis of patients' records for process items; outcome measures included a positive urine culture six months later (two patients) and recurrent urinary symptoms (15 patients) obtained by a follow-up questionnaire. No correlation was found. As the authors state, this study was unlikely to have shown a relationship because of the infrequency of adverse outcomes with a sample this small.

In a second study, Lindsay et al. (1977) used the same approach with outpatient medical care of patients following hospital discharge after myocardial infarction, in which process was weighted and combined into an index and compared with mortality. A significant association between ten process items performed at the first post-hospital visit and mortality at two years was found, but later process did not show a correlation. Points of methodologic concern with this study include: (1) the insensitivity of mortality as an outcome with this sample size when the bulk of mortality occurs before and during hospitalization; (2) the fact that weighting was arbitrary when more sensitive approaches, such as discriminant function analysis, could have been used; (3) the absence of a baseline measure to avoid the contaminating effect of the differing process interventions such as patient education and medications that took place during hospitalization; (4) the fact that compliance may be important when assessing the association of process items such as antiarrhythmic drugs with the outcomes.

Nobrega et al. (1977) studied patients with hypertension in which process variables were compared to outcomes assessed by home interview and blood pressure determination. The failure to find an association between process and outcome could be a result of using insensitive methods of analysis that failed to make allowance for disease severity, compliance and vigor of therapy, and inappropriate process measures. As mentioned previously in the Credibility section, their criteria for audit overemphasized investigation of the etiology of the disease with exhaustive items of history and physical examination and minimized items on therapy and follow-up.

Payne et al. (1978) developed a Physician Performance Index (PPI) to provide an objective basis for evaluating individual physician performance in specific diagnostic categories. For six of the seven diagnoses studied, a significant relationship was found between the PPI and objective patient outcomes; however, patient compliance was a prerequisite for the demonstration of a relationship in three conditions (urinary tract infection, hypertension, iron-deficiency anemia). This adjustment for patient compliance is a particular strength of this study in comparison to most other studies.

Romm et al. (1976) studied patients with heart failure for correlations of process with the outcomes of activity and symptoms after six months; a significant association between physician awareness of patient concerns and the outcome of symptomatic cardiac failure was found only in a group of patients who were minimally symptomatic initially. Methodologic concerns here include: (1) the likelihood of significant process correlations with outcome being masked by initial disease severity, in view of the finding that disease severity had the strongest association with outcome; (2) the insensitivity of the management process criteria, and the method of index construction chosen; (3) the use of a checklist for instructions which will tend to change physicians' behavior and increase homogeneity, thereby reducing the correlation; (4) the importance of compliance for such process items as instructions on diet.

Sanazaro and Worth (1978) examined the effects of incorporating Concurrent Quality Assurance (CQA) into the mandatory utilization reviews of Professional Standards Review Organizations (PSROs) in five areas with randomly allocated experimental (24) and control (26) hospitals. The sets of criteria developed for the seven diagnoses audited were stated to be derived from clinical research which, when adhered to, would result in desirable outcomes (no details or citations were provided). The criteria comprised three categories: (1) diagnostic criteria which pertained to objective data required to substantiate the diagnosis; (2) documentation criteria which included data on comorbidity, risk factors, disease severity, and complications; (3) treatment criteria which indicated efficacious treatment or contraindicated treatment. The overall effect of CQA on adherence to essential process criteria was small. A slightly higher adherence of 1.5 percent to treatment criteria was seen in the experimental hospitals ($p < 0.03$). No association was found between the documentation or treatment criteria and patient outcomes if all diagnoses were pooled. However, failure to adhere to essential treatment criteria was associated with unsatisfactory outcomes in bacterial pneumonia ($p < 0.01$) and acute myocardial infarction ($p < 0.02$), suggesting that associations present for particular diagnoses may be masked or diluted when all patient diagnoses are pooled, though it is not clear from the report that the likelihood of spurious statistical associations due to multiple comparisons or adjustment for confounding variables was taken into account.

Starfield and Scheff (1972) compared process with outcome in the quality of care provided by residents and fellows to children with iron-deficiency anemia. For those patients given appropriate therapy and follow-up, the outcome hemoglobin level was >10 grams more often than in patients whose care did not satisfy these process criteria. This article does not allow the magnitude of the impact of the physician's action to be accurately assessed.

The above studies reflect the increasing awareness of the importance of the validation of measures of clinical competence against patient outcomes. The methodologic issues mentioned in connection with these studies place limitations on the application of the results. However, it should now be possible to avoid these pitfalls and such studies are indicated for the validation of record review if it is to be used on a large scale for the evaluation of clinical competence.

Relationship to Physician Judgments

Measures of clinical competence have been compared with the judgment of experienced clinicians based on the premise or construct that they should be expected to show agreement. Hastings and Sonneborn (1980) developed a 35-item checklist for peer review of ambulatory medical records. Competence-of-care estimates obtained using the checklist were compared with quality-of-care estimates obtained by physician reexamination of the patients. For 89 records of inmates of a Florida jail over a three-year period, a total of ten peer reviewers assessed the checklist, and using their implicit clinical judgment, three other physicians reexamined the patient within eight hours to assign a numerical value from 1 to 100 for each of nine areas of concern. The two measures correlated fairly highly with r = 0.44 ($p < 0.05$). In addition, a nurse practitioner reviewed 204 records using disease-specific review protocols with explicit criteria for diabetes, external otitis, gonorrheal urethritis, hypertension, sore throat, and urinary tract infection. Each record was also reviewed by a board-qualified internist using the checklist. Correlation coefficients between the overall scores obtained from these two measures ranged from r = 0.63 for hypertension to 0.28 for sore throat.

Dickie and Bass (1980) carried out a before-after study to assess the value of self-audit using a standardized 14-item form for improving medical record keeping in a Family Medicine Unit. The areas of concern applied to features that should be incorporated in POMR. In a pretest, validity of the checklist was established by demonstrating that the rank order of scores obtained from a random sample of 20 charts was in agreement with the author's implicit judgment of the same charts. The actual level of agreement was not stated. However, this study was only concerned with record keeping and did not address patient outcomes.

Construct Validity

Goetz et al. (1979) tested the relationship between record review and educational level by administering the charts to Phase I surgical residents who were both more proficient (selected a greater percentage of pertinent items) and more efficient (a higher percentage of pertinent items out of all items selected) than third-year medical students ($p < 0.01$ with sign test) on all four charts. Kane et al. (1977), in their study of family practice residents in Utah, showed that faculty performed better than residents and physician assistants when assessed by Utah Professional Review Organization explicit criteria. Voytovich and Rippey (1978) demonstrated discrimination between students, interns, residents, and faculty with their method of auditing a "Structured Problem List." Scott and Sniderman (1973) found that fewer major errors, which had a potentially major deleterious influence on the patients' welfare, were present in the records of the trainees with more experience.

The demonstration that the results of record review show a clinically significant change in performance of students, residents, or practicing physicians following an intervention such as an educational program also contributes useful evidence for the construct validity of the method; these studies are reviewed in the section on educational effects.

Predictive Validity

The ability of record review to predict the subsequent performance of the clinician in the future would be immensely helpful in deciding on the utility of record review. Unfortunately, there appear to have been no studies of this.

Feasibility

Medical record abstraction is certainly a more feasible method than many of the alternatives for assessing clinical competence in hospital and, in some cases, in ambulatory-care settings. Direct observation has been used especially in ambulatory practice, but this technique involves a large amount of professional time and, in addition, increases the possibility that physician behavior may change as a result of being studied. Record review by comparison is unobtrusive. Thompson and Osborne (1976) found that of 166 pediatricians and family physicians audited by record review, 81 percent said it did not interfere with their standard office practice and 99 percent said that they would agree to be reviewed by this method.

For medical audit, a significant amount of time of health professionals is required for the initial criteria selection stage, so as to render all the results acceptable to those being reviewed; in addition, systems of audit based upon disease-specific explicit criteria need to be updated according to ongoing changes in medical practice as a result of new knowledge from research. The use of outcome measures for assessing quality of care is even more constrained by factors of feasibility and cost (Payne, 1979). Immediate outcomes, such as those at the time of hospital discharge, although readily available, are not always appropriate, and determination of later outcomes from follow-up information is not always possible from reviewing the medical record.

The feasibility of using the medical record is enhanced by a high level of completeness of recording, legibility of handwriting, and ready availability of records. The issue of completeness was reviewed in the section on validity. Legible handwriting is usually a legal requirement as well as being important for other reasons such as an *aide-de-memoire*, and as a means for communicating critical information on a patient to others who are involved with his care. On a sample of 16,153 records, Payne et al. (1978) found that 88 percent were rated as being moderately to clearly legible or typed and only 1.5 percent received a rating of indecipherable. Availability of records depends to a large extent on the system used. Misplaced laboratory tests can also be an important cause of missing data (Payne, 1979).

Fletcher (1974) compared the speed and accuracy of auditing PORs versus SORs by adapting the medical records of four hospitalized patients with complex general medical problems; these were presented to 36 medical staff from two teaching hospitals. The results showed that physicians did not audit PORs more rapidly or with greater accuracy and comprehensiveness than SORs. The study has been criticized on the grounds that the adaptation itself removed many of the differences between PORs and SORs (for which, for example, the problems are listed and the justification for each summarized under each problem), thus making the conclusions of limited generalizability.

Kroeger et al. (1965) noted that printed forms may assist in keeping good records. Sixty-one physicians out of 91 studied had records judged by physician reviewers to be adequate on the basis of legibility and completeness for nonphysicians to review. More than 75 percent of the physicians using printed forms had adequate records and half of those having adequate records used a printed form. Reviewers required, on an average, between 20 and 40 minutes to review a record and to record items on the printed survey form.

Payne (1979) similarly found that for the 39 individual diagnoses studied, the average abstracting time by trained nonphysician abstractors was 20 minutes for hospital records and 30 minutes for ambulatory records. Unless physicians are trained specifically in abstracting and evaluation, not only are the costs increased substantially, but the reliability is decreased (Payne, 1979). Therefore, the use of trained, nonmedical abstractors is preferred.

McSherry (1976) showed that process evaluation can be expensive; evaluation of 690 records in a New York teaching hospital cost $104 per record, not including physician time. By contrast, Holloway et al. (1975) estimated that the records of 7,200 discharges in a community hospital in California could be evaluated at only $2.10 per record using the PAS—MAP computerized system. The direct cost of concurrent data collection for CQA, including documentation of immediate outcomes, was estimated at $1.23 per case. This figure does not, however, include costs for data processing and analysis. With increasing numbers of cases, computerized systems become more cost-efficient while the manual procedures vary considerably in proportion to the number of cases evaluated. Similarly, physician time is extremely expensive, and so the increasing use of nonphysicians for audit purposes significantly reduces costs.

Educational Considerations

Record review has a number of advantages that make it suitable for both formative and summative evaluation; it is based on real clinical behavior; it is experience centered and relevant to the patient-care problems of the learner; the learner can have the opportunity to participate in the setting of the goals and the implementation of the program (for example, criteria setting is educational in itself as it requires the physicians involved to review and think through the evidence for what constitutes competent care); active participative learning is more effective than passive transmittal techniques and record review allows a problem-based approach' that encourages active participation; concurrent record review allows rapid feedback which facilitates reinforcement of appropriate behavior and alteration of inappropriate behavior; record review is feasible to apply in the educational setting.

Sanazaro (1976) reviewed the circumstances in which there is empirical evidence from studies that the technical quality of care improved substantially, and he grouped them into four types of approaches. The first involved simply asking surgeons to provide systematic, critical clinical data before deciding to operate (de Dombal et al., 1974), and resulted in the surgeons improving their diagnostic skills and clinical judgment with subsequent reduction in unnecessary surgery. However, the improvement was not sustained four months after the study ended.

The second factor identified as improving performance involved preparation of a protocol to guide clinical action (Grimm et al., 1975). The initial development of the essential process criteria and its continuing availability resulted in physicians improving their recording habits and their treatment patterns substantially. An extension of this idea is the computerized printouts of warnings regarding potential treatment errors and suggested appropriate responses as defined by the protocols (McDonald, 1976). As a higher proportion of indicated changes was made by those who received computer alerts, their use resulted in improvement in patient care by modifying treatment.

The third factor revolves around the need for a firm commitment from all the staff involved to improve the quality of care once an audit has identified deficiencies in specific areas (Lembcke, 1956). Sanazaro (1976) emphasized that it is this commitment (with or without continuing medical education) which must be present in order to progress from quality assessment to quality assurance.

The fourth factor recognized as being associated with better physician performance is a teaching environment (Ehrlich et al., 1962; Goss, 1970; Lipworth et al., 1963; Morehead and Donaldson, 1964; Stapleton and Zwerneman, 1965). One example given was the more frequent ordering of critical tests on the teaching wards compared to the nonteaching wards. Similarly, care has been found to be superior in hospitals affiliated with a medical school. The above situations illustrate that for those cases where improved care was achieved, acceptable monitoring techniques were employed that primarily motivated the physicians involved to apply the knowledge and skills that they already possessed.

Formative Applications

It is important to stress that record review is only the measurement method for assessing clinical competence; a frequent misconception is that record reviews or audits must be flawed, since studies using these methods do not consistently result in change in physician behavior (Nelson, 1976). This is, of course, inappropriate since record review only assesses the competence of the care being given and does not itself address the issue of how to change physician behavior.

Studies utilizing the POMR suggest that record review for medical students and residents has considerable potential. Nelson et al. (1976) found that an education program based upon faculty review of medical students' records was associated with improvement on a short-term basis; they evaluated 318 patient records of 39 students doing a 4-week gynecology rotation. During this period extensive feedback was employed in addition to audit measures. They found that, although there was a large degree of variation both within and between students, on the whole the class improved in terms of the behavioral traits of thoroughness, reliability, sound analytical sense, and efficiency in identification and management of patient problems as reflected in the POMR. Record review, utilizing the POMR, is now used as one of the principal stimuli to identify educational issues in the curriculum of a medical school, the Royal Free Hospital in London, England (Dearden and Laurillard, 1976; Lloyd and McIntyre, 1979; McIntyre, 1979); the student's own POMR of his or her findings and plans for a patient workup form the basis for assessing his or her performance and for helping him or her correct any deficiencies identified. The advantages cited over didactic teaching include the individualization of the learning/teaching experience and the relevance of both the information acquired and the context for the experience; in addition, feedback for self-assessment of performance is available. Although there has been some resistance by both students and faculty, the process has been made less threatening by careful explanation and by measures such as encouraging students to evaluate faculty members responsible for organizing the record review program. No formal evaluation results are yet available on this enterprising experiment.

This same approach has been developed for improving feedback to medical students and residents about their ability to identify and synthesize problems in a large urban teaching hospital in the United States (Voytovich, 1973); efforts were first made to improve the clarity and usefulness of the medical record. A daily record review session was used as a form of reinforcement of behavior to emphasize performance and deemphasize knowledge by focusing on precise problem definition and subsequent problem solving. It has been accepted as a nonthreatening teaching tool mainly because of the precautions taken to guard against it becoming punitive in nature. The auditors were staff and senior house officers active in primary care areas; privacy was maintained and comments were detailed and specific, to provide useful educational feedback rather than general criticism. Praise was provided to minimize discouragement, and feedback was expected from the student. The audits and their responses were retained and later reviewed so that recurrent deficiencies within an individual could be identified and corrected. General weaknesses in the group were identified and used as topics for the didactic sessions. The one-to-one relationship between student and teacher was maintained throughout the audit process and was felt by those concerned to be highly educational.

Martin et al. (1980) recently reported the results of an interesting controlled trial involving medical residents, comparing educational feedback (concurrent chart review of 25 percent of residents' admissions and discussions to reinforce efficient strategies) with financial incentives in reducing the ordering of laboratory and radiologic tests by first-year residents. The two interventions were randomly assigned to two groups of residents, with a third serving as a control group. At the beginning of the study all three groups of residents received a one-hour lecture on patterns of test overuse, testing strategies, and test costs. Although all groups showed a temporary reduction in test ordering during the intervention period, only the chart review group showed a clinically important persisting reduction in test ordering during the intervention and following periods (a 32 percent greater reduction than the control group—a statistically significant difference). This study demonstrated that chart review was effective in reducing excess ordering of tests, although the short-term reduction in the control group indicates that the effect of being studied combined with the lecture may have temporarily affected the physicians' approach to test ordering.

Dixon (1973) has reported on the use of chart reviews of interns by their peers for continuing house staff education. The POMR approach was used for chart recording. In a before-after study of over 100 charts, this activity was associated with a reduction in misinterpreted data, missed significant data, significant omissions from the problem list, poorly organized and poor follow-up of the therapeutic plan by the interns.

More recently Dickie and Bass (1980) have shown that in a family practice setting, a self-auditing program based upon the POMR resulted in an improvement of 12.4 percent in the recording of drugs prescribed and 30.4 percent in the linkage of progress notes to the problem list. Neufeld and Tugwell (1977) also found that repeated self-auditing by students and independent review by other students and their faculty supervisor appeared to be associated with improved performance.

For physicians once they have left training programs, growing pressures from the profession, governments, and society have combined to make continuing medical education (CME) a primary means of improving clinical competence and patient care. Mandatory CME programs are increasingly being employed as a condition for maintaining certification. However, standard programs of CME have seldom been shown to substantially change physician behavior and improve patient care (Brown and Uhl, 1970; Lewis and Hassanein, 1970).

The use of medical records provides a means of providing

continuing medical education that is directed at patient care rather than relying on the more common relatively untargeted, didactic CME programs. This approach has been adopted by the Joint Commission on the Accreditation of Hospitals, the Peer Scientific Review Organization, and the Canadian Council of Hospital Accreditation. There is general support for this view that postgraduate education should relate learning directly to patient care; approaches to this include the "cybernetic approach" suggested by Williamson et al. (1967) and the bicycle approach developed by Brown (1968), which tailors the education to deficiencies identified from studying the patient care provided by the physicians participating in the educational program. The focus placed on the physician-patient encounter maintains the relevance for the physician-learner with ongoing evaluation and feedback possible throughout the process.

Brown and Uhl (1970) have reported a number of examples where this approach appears to have been successful in changing physician behavior. They quote improvement in antibiotic use as an example: (1) the needs of the physicians involved in a study of antibiotic use were first identified by audit; (2) the physicians were involved in criteria setting; (3) four conferences and an examination were held based on actual case record; (4) extensive feedback was provided; (5) performance of physicians was remeasured. Those physicians whose practice met the preestablished criteria of 75 percent appropriate usage of antibiotics remained in the patient care cycle, whereas those who did not were directed into the education cycle where new programs were developed to assist them in achieving that standard. The first 50 cases analyzed showed the department at a 48 percent level of proper usage and at the time the paper was written at a 60 percent level; the baseline level was 30 percent. This approach has also been successfully employed in improving hysterectomy and appendectomy care.

Reed et al. (1973) described a combination of an audit and an education program on acute myocardial infarction in a community hospital, based on Williamson's cybernetic concept. The three phases included (1) a record audit of myocardial infarction management practices prior to having a Coronary Care Unit (CCU); (2) a training and educational package, based on deficiencies identified in the audit; and (3) two subsequent record audits to identify changes in patient management and outcomes. Large improvements were noted in a number of patient care practices, and a decrease was found in at least one category of clinical complications; however, it is difficult to attribute improved quality of care to the educational component alone, as a coronary care unit with specially trained nurses was opened at the same time as the educational program was implemented.

The incentives for changing behavior are often much less powerful for physicians in practice than for those in training (indeed there is often a financial disincentive). Education is not always sufficient and other methods sometimes have to be developed aimed at motivating physicians to change their behavior. Williamson et al. (1967) found that a specially designed workshop and repeated bulletins failed to improve the quality or quantity of physician response to unexpected abnormalities in routine screening. Attempts to modify physician behavior were successful only after using a noneducational approach, which involved a ten week period of obscuring all abnormal results with fluorescent tape. Some of this success may have been due to the arrival of residency house staff which occurred at the time of introducing the fluorescent tape.

Starfield et al. (1977) studied the effects of an administrative change on physician behavior. They found that altering the format of the medical record, whereby a computer printout or "mini-record" was automatically produced after an initial patient visit and placed at the front of the chart prior to the next scheduled visit, resulted in improved recognition of patient information in a series of visits. This evidence of facilitated coordination of care was restricted to improved recognition of problems and therapies at the time of follow-up; the results of this study should be accepted with caution as they were generated from a before-after study and the reactive effect of being studied may have contributed much to the improvement.

Use of the POMR format itself has been suggested as facilitating high-quality care (Weed, 1969). Evidence is lacking, however, except for a nonexperimental study by Simborg et al. (1976), who found that follow-up of patients was better in clinics where the POMR was used and attributed this to the usefulness of the problem list in reminding the clinician. Switz (1976), in a before-after study, evaluated the effect of intensively introducing the POMR on the quality of care provided to patients discharged with the diagnosis of anemia. Twenty-nine consecutive records were reviewed four months after the period during 1972 and compared with 31 consecutive records of the same time in 1971, eight months prior to the introduction of the POMR. Two different groups of interns were thus compared. No statistically or clinically significant difference was observed in therapy process, defined as days until identification of anemia, days until appropriate therapy was initiated, and days until best diagnosis or resolution. In addition, the thoroughness of the history, physical examination and laboratory evaluation data base were compared. No statistically significant difference was observed between the pre- and post-POMR scores. Although the compliance with the POMR format was assessed to be adequate in the post-POMR period, it is not apparent how widely used this format was in the pre-POMR period. It was noted that the POMR had been in use on some wards since 1968 and that it had been promoted since 1970. If use was substantial, this would tend to minimize the possibility of finding any differences, thus obscuring a real effect.

Dinsdale et al. (1975) evaluated the impact of the POMR on staff communication, attitude change, and decision making in a rehabilitation setting. The study was a cohort analytic design with six different centers. The POMR was initiated in two sites at the beginning of the study; two sites where the POMR was already in use served as one set of controls and the last two sites served as additional controls where the POMR was never incorporated into the system. During the test period there was no change in the staff judgments of the above concepts. Therefore, it was concluded that introduction of the POMR did not result in improved staff perception of the medical record, the health care team, or the health professionals. This study did suffer from methodological problems that could impinge on the results, however; the different participating settings were markedly different on potentially confounding variables such as age, hospital case mix, and educational qualifications and experience of the staff. In addition, responses were poor in two of the settings, which resulted in the investigators initially deleting two of the sites (one of each control type).

Brook and Appel (1973) and Morehead and Donaldson (1974) also found substantial rates of failure to follow through on identified abnormal laboratory and X-ray results, suggesting that logistic and administrative factors are sometimes more important than lack of knowledge.

These studies provide considerable evidence of the potential and appropriateness of record review for educational purposes, but also highlight the need for further studies of the best way of integrating educational interventions with record review, with special attention needed for providing the motivation for behavioral change by physicians.

Summative Evaluation

Formal record review has rarely been used as a major basis for the terminal evaluation of undergraduate medical students and residents; an exception is a new program at the Royal Free Hospital in London, England, which is pioneering the use of the medical record as a major component of the evaluation of the clinical training of medical undergraduate students.

Recently there has been increasing interest in the potential of this approach for summative evaluation of physicians in practice. The American Board of Family Practice (ABFP) recertification program includes a physician self-audit of office medical records in addition to a multiple-choice examination and simulated patient management problems. Although this technique of assessment is still being evaluated, Rakel (1979) noted that there has been a significant improvement in the quality of the office record, due to better organization and legibility, felt to be a result of the stimulus provided by the ABFP's support of the POMR. The purpose of the ABFP's office record review is to assist the family physician to provide improved medical care. It is hoped that physicians will be motivated to change their behavior as a result of receiving a feedback form that compares their performance with that of a national peer group, where the criteria used reflect the consensus of the physician's peers.

The American Board of Obstetrics and Gynecology also uses a written examination and a self-audit of medical records for purposes of recertification, but with the criteria for audit focusing on outcomes rather than the process of care (Merrill, 1979).

The performance of United States medical graduates was compared to that of foreign graduates through audit of their medical records using both the Physician Performance Index component of the Payne Process Audit and the Joint Commission on Accreditation of Hospitals' Performance Evaluation Program. The results of both audits indicated there was no significant overall difference in the performance by physician type (Saywell, 1979).

Two provinces in Canada (Quebec and Ontario) have instituted a record review program that is aimed at assuring the Canadian public that the government and profession are providing appropriate surveillance of the competence of physicians in the community; this involves designated physician teams examining a number of patient records (using their implicit judgment) of a sample of registered physicians (McAuley, 1980; Therien, 1982).

The precision and validity of the methods used for these summative uses has yet to be demonstrated, but these examples show that there is considerable interest in such applications.

Conclusions

The main strengths of record review can be summarized as follows:

1. The medical record is an established component of clinical practice.
2. Actual practice behavior can be assessed.
3. Complete episodes of care can be assessed.
4. It allows application of explicit criteria with high levels of consistency in abstracting the information.
5. It allows the reactive effect of being studied to be avoided if the clinicians are unaware that their charts are being reviewed; and where they are aware beforehand, this effect can still be minimized by keeping those being evaluated blind as to which conditions are to be selected.
6. Relatively large numbers of cases with the same problem or diagnosis can be assessed, thus reducing the sampling problem that may result from basing conclusions on very few cases such as in oral examinations.

The main weaknesses are:

1. The fact that records are used more as an *aide-de-mem-oire* rather than a documentation of the justification for management decisions, which continues to compromise the validity of the medical record.
2. The inconsistency with which actions are recorded.
3. The difficulty in deciding who made the recorded decisions where more than one health professional discusses the patient before the record is written.
4. The difficulty in maintaining blindness of the assessor to the clinician involved.
5. The logistical difficulties in identifying a homogeneous sample in ambulatory settings, where there is no incentive to implement methods for retrieving charts with similar problems and diagnoses.

6. The failure to emphasize the evidence for the efficacy of the patient care being assessed, which has reduced the credibility and meaningfulness of the results and conclusions.

If record review is to be used for evaluation, then the clinicians involved have to commit themselves to recording sufficient information to reflect the care given to patients; given current financial realities, incentives should be considered to encourage better recording systems.

The problem-oriented medical record, appropriately adapted to the situation, is probably better suited to record review than the traditional source-oriented record, but this needs to be formally evaluated. The inconsistency of recording has to be overcome in situations where record review is being used to evaluate clinical competence, if the results are to have any meaning or utility. The most important area for research is probably that of improving the medical record as an assessment method, so that the results obtained accurately reflect the care given to patients.

There is also a need to improve ways of allowing identification of all cases with the same clinical problems and diagnoses where no computerized system is available, such as in ambulatory clinics and physicians' private offices. Linkage to billing procedures and the use of "day sheets" (Sibley et al., 1975) are the most promising approaches; recent advances in computerization of these activities will make this increasingly feasible.

Record review has several potential advantages over other forms of evaluation and is probably underutilized at present. The experience in situations where there is a high level of interest and commitment is encouraging.

References

Bentsen, B. G.: The accuracy of recording patient problems in family practice. J Med Educ 51, 311–316 (1976).

Brook, R. H., Appel, F. A.: Quality of care assessment: choosing a method for peer review. N Engl J Med 288, 1323-1329 (1973).

Brook, R. H.: Quality of care assessment: A comparison of five methods of peer review. DHEW Publication HRA, Rockville, Md. (1973).

Brown, C. R.: Continuing education performance deficits. Read before a conference-workshop on Regional Medical Programs. Washington, D.C. Jan. (1968).

Brown, C. R., Uhl, H. S. M.: Mandatory continuing education: sense or nonsense? JAMA 213, 1660-1668 (1970).

Clute, K. F.: The general practitioner: Study of medical education and practice in Ontario and Nova Scotia. Toronto: University of Toronto Press (1963).

Collopy, B. T.: A surgical outcome audit. Med J Aust 2, 689-691 (1979).

Dawes, K. S.: Survey of general practice records. Brit Med J 3, 219-223 (1972).

Dearden, G., Laurillard, D.: In-course assessment of clinical performance: a trial scheme. An interim evaluation report to the Curriculum Committee Royal Free Hospital, London, England (1976).

de Dombal, F. T., Leaper, D. J., Horrochs, J. C.: Human and computer-aided diagnosis of abdominal pain: further report with emphasis on performance of clinicians. Brit Med J 1376-1380 (1974).

Dershewitz, R. A., Fross, R. A., Williamson, J. W.: Validating audit criteria and analytic approach illustrated by peptic ulcer disease. Quality Rev Bull 18-24, Oct. (1979).

Dickie, G. L., Bass, M. J.: Improving problem-oriented medical records through self-audit. J Fam Pract 10, 487-490 (1980).

Dinsdale, S. M., Gent, M., Kline, G., Milner, R.: Problem-oriented medical records: their impact on staff communication, attitudes and decision-making. Arch Phys Med Rehab 56, 269-274 (1975).

Dixon, R. H.: The educational value of an audit of the medical record. In: H. K. Walker, J. W. Hurst, M. F. Woody (Eds.), Applying the problem-oriented system, Chapter 31. New York: Medcom Press (1973).

Donabedian, A.: A guide to medical care administration (Vol 2): Medical care appraisal. New York: American Public Health Association (1969).

Ehrlich, J., Morehead, M., Trussell, R. E.: The quantity, quality and costs of medical and hospital care secured by a sample of teamster families in the New York area. New York: Columbia University School of Public Health and Administration (1962).

Fessel, W. J., Van Brunt, E. E.: Assessing quality of care from the medical record. N Engl J Med 286, 134-138 (1972).

Fletcher, R. H.: Auditing problem-oriented records and traditional records. A controlled comparison of speed, accuracy and identification of errors in medical care. N Engl J Med 290, 829-833 (1974).

Frazier, W. H., Brand, D. A.: Quality assessment and the art of medicine—the anatomy of lacerations care. Med Care 17, 480-490 (1979).

Goetz, A. A., Peters, M. J., Folse, R., Beck, A. D., Finch, W. T., Wavak, P.: Chart review skills: a dimension of clinical competence. J Med Educ 54, 788-796 (1979).

Gonnella, J., Goran, M. J.: Quality of patient care—a measurement of change: the staging concept. Med Care 13, 467-473 (1975).

Goss, M. E. W.: Organizational goals and quality of care. Evidence from comparative research on hospitals. J Health Soc Behav 11, 255-268 (1970).

Greenfield, S., Nadler, M. A., Morgan, M. T., Shine, K. I.: The clinical investigation and management of chest pain in an emergency department: quality assessment by criteria mapping. Med Care 15 898-905 (1977).

Grimm, R. H., Shimoni, K., Harlan, W. R.: Evaluation of patient care protocol use by various providers. N Engl J Med 292, 507-511 (1975).

Grover, M., Greenberg, T.: Quality of care given to first time birth control patients at a free clinic. Am J Public Health 66, 986-987 (1976).

Hammett, W. H., Sandlow, L. J., Bashook, P. G.: Format review: evaluating implementation of the problem-oriented medical record. Med Care 14, 857-865 (1976).

Hastings, G. E., Sonneborn, R.: Peer review checklist: reproducibility and validity of a method for evaluating the quality of ambulatory care. Am J Public Health 70, 222-228 (1980).

Hermann, N., Cayten, C. G., Senior, J., Staroscik, R., Walsh, S., Wall, M.: Interobserver and intra-observer reliability in the collection of emergency medical services data. Health Serv Res 15, 127-143 (1980).

Holloway, C. D., Wiczel, L. J., Carlson, E. T.: Evaluating an information system for medical care evaluation studies. Med Care 12, 329-340 (1975).

Isborne, C. E.: Interdiagnosis relationships of physician recording in ambulatory child health care. Med Care 15, 465-474 (1977).

Jungfer, C. C., Last, J. M.: Clinical performance in Australian general practice. Med Care 1, 71-83 (1965).

Kane, R. L., Gardner, J., Dryer, Wright D., Snell, G., Sundwall, D., Woolley, F. R.: Relationship between process and outcome in ambulatory care. Med Care 15, 961-965 (1977).

Kane, R. L., Gardner, J., Wright, D. D., Wooley, F. R., Snell, G. F., Sundwall, D. N.: Differences in the outcome of acute episodes of care provided by different types of family practitioners. J Fam Pract 6, 133-138 (1978).

Kessner, D. M., Kalk, C. B., Singer, J.: Assessing health quality: the case for tracers. N Engl J Med 288, 189-194 (1973).

Kroeger, H. H., Altman, I., Clark, D. A., Johnson, A. C., Sheps, C. G.: The office practice of internists: the feasibility of evaluating quality of care. JAMA 193, 371-376 (1965).

Lembcke, P. A.: Medical auditing by scientific methods, illustrated by major female pelvic surgery. JAMA 162, 646-655 (1956).

Lewis, C. E., Hassanein, R. S.: Continuing medical education—an epidemiologic evaluation. N Engl J Med 282, 254-259 (1970).

Lindsay, M. I., Hermans, P. E., Nobrega, F. T., Ilstrup, D. M.: Quality of care assessment. I. Outpatient management of acute bacterial cystitis as the model. Mayo Clin Proc 51, 307-312 (1976).

Lindsay, M. I., Nobrega, F. T., Offord, K. P., Carter, E. T., Rutherford, B. D.: Quality of care assessment. II. Outpatient medical care following hospital dismissal after myocardial infarction. Mayo Clin Proc 52, 220-227 (1977).

Lipworth, L., Lee, J. A. H., Morris, J. N.: Case-fatality in teaching and non-teaching hospitals 1956-59. Med Care 1, 71-76 (1963).

Lloyd, G., McIntyre, N.: Educational aspects of the problem-oriented medical record. In: J. C. Petrie and N. McIntrye (Eds.), The problem oriented medical record. New York: Churchill Livingstone (1979).

Lyons, T. F., Payne, B. C.: The relationship of physicians' medical recording performance to their medical care performance. Med Care 12, 463-469 (1974).

Lyons, T. F., Payne, B. C.: Interdiagnoses relationships of physician performance measures in hospitals. Med Care 15, 475-480 (1977).

Margolis, C. Z., Sheehaw, J., Stickley, W. T.: A graded problem-oriented record to evaluate clinical performance. Pediatrics 51, 980-985 (1973).

Martin, A. R., Wolf, M. A., Thibodeau, L. A., Dzau, V., Braunswald, E.: A trial of two strategies to modify the test ordering behavior of medical residents. N Engl J Med 303, 1330-1336 (1980).

McAuley, R. G.: Report of the Committee on Peer Assessment and Education presented at the Annual Meeting of the College of Physicians and Surgeons of Ontario. Annual Report of the College of Physicians and Surgeons (1980).

McDonald, C. J.: Use of a computer to detect and respond to clinical events: its effect on clinician behavior. Ann Intern Med 84, 162-167 (1976).

McIntyre, N.: The new clinical curriculum at the Royal Free Hospital School of Medicine. Med Teacher 1, 252-257 (1979).

McIntyre, N.: Medical record review form. Med Teacher 2, 40-43 (1980).

McSherry, C. K.: Quality assurance: the cost of utilization review and the educational value of medical audit in a university hospital. Surgery 80, 122-129 (1976).

Merrill, J. A., Studnicki, J., Bean, J. A., Ludke, R. L.: A performance comparison: USMG-FMG attending physicians. Am J Public health 69, 57-62 (1979).

Morehead, M. A., Donaldson, R.: Quality of clinical management of disease in comprehensive neighborhood health centers. Med Care 12, 201-215 (1974).

Morehead, M. A., Donaldson, R.: A study of the quality of hospital care: described by a sample of teamster family members in New York City. New York: Columbia University School Public Health and Administration (1964).

Nelson, A. R.: Orphan data and the unclosed loop: a dilemma in PSRO and medical audit. N Engl J Med 295, 617-619 (1976).

Nelson, G. E., Graves, S. M., Holland, R. E., Nelson, J. M., Ratner, J., Weed, L. L.: A performance-based method of student evaluation. Med Educ 10, 33-42 (1976).

Neufeld, V. R., Tugwell, P.: Unpublished data (1977).

Nobrega, F. T., Morrow, G. W., Smoldt, R. K., Offord, K. P.: Quality assessment in hypertension: analysis of process and outcome methods. N Engl J Med 296, 145-148 (1977).

Norman, G. R., Anchel, G., Tugwell, P., Feightner, J. W.: The validity of the medical record in assessment of quality of care. Unpublished (1980).

Osborne, C. E., Thompson, H. C.: Criteria for evaluation of ambulatory child health care by chart audit; development and testing of a methodology. Pediatrics 56, supplement (1975).

Payne, B. C., Lyons, T. F., Dwarshius, L., Kelton, M., Morris, W.: The quality of medical care: evaluation and improvement. Chicago: Hospital Research and Educational Trust (1976).

Payne, B. C., Lyons, T. F., Neuhaus, E., Kelton, M., Dwarshius, L.: Evaluation and improvement of ambulatory medical care. National Center for Health Services Research Grant, Hyattsville, Md. (1978).

Payne, B. C.: The medical record as a basis for assessing physician competence. Ann Intern Med 91, 623-629 (1979).

Peterson, O. L., Andrews, L. P., Spain, R. S., Greenberg, B. G.: An analytical study of North Carolina general practice: 1953-1954. J Med Educ 31, 1-165 (1965).

Rakel, R. E.: The medical record in practice evaluation: results of investigations in establishing the office record review as a component of re-certification. Given at the American Board of Medical Specialties Conference on Recertification, Chicago. American Board of Family Practice, 91-102 Sept. (1979).

Reed, D. E., Lapenas, C., Rogers, K. D.: Continuing education based on record audit in a community hospital. J Med Educ 48, 1152-1155 (1973).

Rhee, S. O., Lyons, T. F., Payne, B. C.: Inter-relationships of physician performances. Med Care 16, 496-501 (1978).

Richardson, F. M.: Peer review of medical care. Med Care 10, 29-39 (1972).

Romm, F. J., Hulka, B. S., Mayo, F.: Correlates of outcomes in patients with congestive heart failure. Med Care 14, 765-776 (1976).

Sanazaro, P.: Medical audit, continuing medical education and quality assurance. Western J Med 125, 241-252 (1976).

Sanazaro, P. J., Worth, R. M.: Concurrent quality assurance in hospital care. Report of a study by private initiative in PSRO. N Engl J Med 298, 1171-1177 (1978).

Saywell, R. M., Studnicki, J., Beam, G. A., Ludke, R. L.: A performance comparison: USMG-FMG attending physicians. Am J Public Health 69, 57-62 (1979).

Scott, H. M., Sniderman, A.: Evaluation of clinical competence through a study of patient records. J Med Educ 48, 832-839 (1973).

Sibley, J. C., Spitzer, W. O., Rudnick, K. V., Bell, J. D., Bethune, R. D., Sackett, D. L.: Quality of care appraisal in primary care: a quantitative method. Ann Intern Med 83, 46-52 (1975).

Simborg, D. W., Starfield, B. H., Horn, S. D., Yourtree, S. A.: Information factors affecting problem follow-up in ambulatory care. Med Care 14, 848-856 (1976).

Sox, H. O.: Quality of patient care by nurse practitioners and physician assistants: a ten year perspective. Ann Intern Med 91, 459-468 (1979).

Spasoff, R. A., Lane, P., Steele, R.: Quality of care in hospital emergency departments and family physicians' offices. Can Med Assoc J 117, 229-232 (1977).

Spitzer, W. O., Sackett, D. L., Sibley, J. C., Roberts, R. S., Gent, M., Kergin, D. J.: The Burlington randomized trial of the nurse practitioner. N Engl J Med 290, 251-256 (1974).

Stapleton, J. F., Zwerneman, J. A.: The influence of an intern-resident staff on the quality of private patient care. JAMA 194, 877-882 (1965).

Starfield, B., Scheff, D.: Effectiveness of pediatrics: the relationship between processes and outcome. Pediatrics 49, 547-552 (1972).

Starfield, B., Seidel, H., Carter, G., Garvin, W., Seddon, J.: Private pediatric practice: performance and problems. Pediatrics 52, 344-351 (1973).

Starfield, B., Simborg, D., Johns, C., Horn, S.: Co-ordination of care and its relationship to continuing and medical records. Med Care 15, 929-938 (1977).

Stewart, M. A., Buck, C. W.: Physician's knowledge of and response to patients' problems. Med Care 15, 578-585 (1977).

Switz, D. M.: The problem-oriented medical record: evaluation and management of anemia before and during use. Arch Intern Med 136, 1119-1123 (1976).

Templeton, B., Erviti, V. F., Bunc, J. V., Burg, F. D.: Use of a medical record audit in assessing pediatric resident performance. A preliminary report. American Board of Medical Specialties Conference on Research in Evaluation Procedures. Chicago, Ill., March (1978).

Therien, B.: Experience of the professional corporation of Quebec in the evaluation of medical practice. In: V. Neufeld (Ed.), Symposium on recent advances in quality assurance. Ann R Coll Phys Surg (1982).

Thompson, H. C., Osborne, C. E.: Office records in the evaluation of quality of care. Med Care 14, 294-314 (1976).

Tufo, H. M., Eddy, W. M., Van Buren, H. C., Bouchard, R. E., Twitchell, J. C., Bedard, L.: Audit in a practice group. In: H. K. Walker, J. W. Hurst, M. F. Woody (Eds.), Applying the problem-oriented system, New York: Medcom Press (1973).

Tugwell, P.: Methodological perspective on process measures of the quality of medical care. Clin Invest Med 2, 113-121 (1979).

Voytovich, A. E.: Evolution of a non-threatening audit system in a large teaching hospital. In: H. E. Walker, J. W. Hurst, M. F. Wood (Eds.), Applying the problem-oriented system, Chapter 29. New York: Medcom Press (1973).

Voytovich, A. E., Rippey, R. M.: Audit of the structured problem list as a measure of clinical judgment: reliability and validity. J Ir Med Assoc 71, 346-349 (1978).

Weed, L.: Medical records, medical education and patient care. Cleveland: Case Western Reserve University (1969).

Wiener, S., Nathanson, M.: Physical examination—frequently observed errors. JAMA 236, 852-855 (1976).

Williamson, J. W., Alexander, M., Miller, G. E.: Continuing education and patient care research: physician response to screening test results. JAMA 201, 118-122 (1967).

Zuckerman, A. E., Starfield, B., Hochreiter, C., Kovasznay, B.: Validating the content of pediatric outpatient medical records by means of tape-recording doctor-patient encounters. Pediatrics 56, 407-411 (1975).

CHAPTER 9

Patient Management Problems

JOHN W. FEIGHTNER

Introduction

Beginning in the early 1950s there was a move within education generally and medical education specifically to standardized and objective examinations. At the same time some educators were attempting to further understand the nature of competence and to develop methods to assess it. The process of solving problems was seen as one essential feature of this competence, and efforts were made to develop objective measures of this skill, for example, by Rimoldi (1961, 1963), who used a card deck simulation to probe and describe the process. The potential role of written simulations in the assessment of competence was further strengthened by definitions of clinical competence which were developed in the 1960s (Hubbard et al., 1965), arising from concerns of the National Board of Medical Examiners and some specialty boards. These activities led naturally to early versions of the written patient management problem.

In the 1970s patient management problems (PMPs) flourished. Both major forms, linear and branching, became widely used for certification of competence at the undergraduate and postgraduate levels. While some studies assessing the psychometric properties of these instruments emerged through this decade, the enthusiasm for PMPs, accompanied by widespread implementation, was not complemented by a coordinated effort to firmly establish their psychometric properties. During this time many alternate forms of written and computer simulations were also developed, including such instruments as the diagnostic management problem (Helfer and Slater, 1971; Robinson and Dinham, 1977), the sequential management problem (Martin, 1975), and patient card decks (Tamblyn et al., 1980). Written patient management problems are, however, by far the most widespread format of written simulations and will be the main focus of this chapter. A section at the end will address the existing evidence regarding the psychometric properties of the other forms of written simulations.

PMPs have considerable potential not only to fulfill many key principles of learning but also to meet several evaluation demands. From the educational perspective:

1. The experience for the learner can be nonthreatening and can provide an opportunity to learn from mistakes without potential harm to the patient.
2. There can be instant initial feedback to the learner and the potential for very specific comments when the case is reviewed.
3. Educational planners can be specific and selective in designing a learning experience and the learner can encounter a wide variety of problems at varying stages.

From the perspective of evaluation:

1. The assessment can be standardized and specific performance criteria can be defined.
2. Large numbers of learners can be evaluated simultaneously and economically with a broad sampling of performance in different content areas.
3. PMPs have the apparent ability to assess intellectual skills other than factual recall in a fashion that approaches some psychometric qualities of a multiple-choice test (McGuire, 1963).
4. The instrument is generally seen as being highly relevant to the learning setting.

Measurement Criteria

The literature on the measurement characteristics of PMPs contains work of variable quality. Many early articles focused on face and content validity. Reliability and quantitative expressions of validity began to receive attention in the late 1960s. However, many of the published papers referred to internal studies in support of reliability and validity but do not provide detailed information about the design and analysis of these studies. In the 1970s several published studies specifically assessed the reliability and validity of PMPs and other written simulations. To date, however, there is very little objective information on the educational benefits of the instrument.

Credibility

A principal feature of written simulations is implied in their name—they simulate an actual clinical experience. Moreover, it has been widely held that PMPs measure not only knowledge but also problem-solving skills. Thus, the PMP is seen as an objective instrument capable of evaluating components of competence that could not be assessed by multiple-choice questions or other conventional test instruments (McGuire, 1963). The elements of scoring are seen by some as also lending credibility to the PMP. With most approaches to scoring, the weightings of the options are provided by a panel of experts knowledgeable in a clinical area. Furthermore, the formulas for arriving at a summary score are seen as being consistent with high-quality clinical performance (Williamson, 1965). It should be noted, however, that the enthusiasm for scoring algorithms has not been universal. This will be discussed in more detail later.

Comprehensiveness

By its design, the PMP demands performance in the four traditional categories of clinical competence: history taking, physical examination, laboratory investigations, and management. It is presumed to demand cognitive or problem-solving processes similar to those occurring in the actual clinical setting. Experts who have reviewed PMPs and students and physicians who have worked through them report on systematic inquiry that the PMP closely approximates the clinical setting (McGuire et al., 1972). In a novel approach, one study (Sedlecek and Nattress, 1972) asked judges to identify which options they would select at certain decision points in a PMP after having been given the standard set of preceding decisions. The inter-judge correlation on which decisions should be made ranged from 0.71 to 0.85. This approach might be considered further for assessing more empirically the content validity of PMPs. Other findings (Elstein et al., 1978) would indicate that the overall processes used by subjects to solve written PMPs closely resemble those employed in live simulations, providing further evidence for content validity.

Precision

Linear PMPs. The major studies assessing the reliability of linear patient management problems have been undertaken by the National Board of Medical Examiners. While the studies themselves are not published, internal consistency reliability is reported to be at the level of 0.80 to 0.85 using the Kuder-Richardson Formula 20 (Hubbard, 1978). Because the linear format assures that each candidate receives essentially the same examination, this conventional split-halves approach to reliability can be used.

Branching PMPs. There is an important conceptual distinction between linear and branching PMPs, which is crucial to the assessment of reliability. In the branching PMP, a candidate can make his own unique selection of which sections of the problem to explore and which options to select within a section. This creates a situation in which each candidate has taken a different test. Hence, the traditional split-halves approach which relies on each candidate selecting from an identical set of questions is inappropriate. Lewy and McGuire (1966) suggest an alternate approach whereby performance on a test is viewed as a sample of a universe of behaviors. Reliability then reflects the ability to generalize about an individual's behavior based on the sample provided by that test. Applying this approach, a coefficient of reliability ranging from 0.75 to 0.85 has been reported (McGuire and Babbott, 1967) for a single but lengthy problem. For tests of two or three long problems in one particular content area, reliability estimates range from 0.80 to 0.90. Finally, for tests composed of 10 to 12 problems and covering several medical content areas, the estimates range from 0.85 to 0.94. Using a similar approach to assess PMPs used for certification of residents Levine and Noak (1968) found a reliability coefficient of 0.90.

In general, then, the reliability of linear and branching PMPs is fairly well established although the evidence would suggest that fairly lengthy tests with many PMPs are required to achieve reliabilities sufficiently high to distinguish between individuals.

Validity

As noted in the introduction to this section, validity is not a uni-dimensional concept. Each approach to establishing validity assesses a different property of the instrument. Hence, when using an instrument for decision-making purposes it is critical to ensure that the appropriate dimension of validity has been established. For example, construct validity established by comparing performance of two levels of undergraduate students would be insufficient support for an instrument intended to certify the competence of a candidate about to enter independent practice after a residency program.

Construct Validity. In assessing construct validity the strength of the argument depends not only on the study design but also on the credibility of the actual construct and its underlying assumptions. The construct validity of an evaluation instrument is generally addressed by comparing two groups which differ in a critical way (e.g., number of years of training), or comparing the same group at different points in time or in different clinical settings. An alternate approach involves factor analysis of a multiple-component examination or the components of a specific instrument to identify whether the factor loadings follow a hypothesized pattern. This approach often incorporates a good deal of faith in interpreting the results and is generally an unacceptable strategy.

Linear PMPs. Construct validity has been studied at the undergraduate and residency levels. Hubbard (1978) reports the consistent finding that the performance of students at the third-year level was significantly lower than performance at the level of internship. Schumacher (1978) compared the scores of first- and third-year trainees in internal medicine and showed a statistical difference in their performance on PMPs. The numbers in each group, however, are relatively large, and while statistical significance was achieved, the actual difference in standard scores was approximately 4 percent. The percentage change in standard scores was less than half that observed for performance on multiple-choice and true/false questions. The constructs for these studies are credible and the results tend to support construct validity. Some might question, however, whether the magnitude of the difference in scores at the residency level is of practical importance.

Branching PMPs. Three approaches to comparison of different groups prevail; studies subjecting fundamentally different groups to the same test, comparisons of performance of the same group in different areas, and comparisons of performance on PMPs with actual clinical performance. Data are most extensive on the same test-different levels comparison. A number of studies of undergraduate students have yielded consistent findings. In an internal report, McGuire (1967) has identified a performance difference between 200 fourth-year medical students and 200 third-year students at the University of Illinois. In this study, 52 percent of the third-year students as compared to 6 percent of the fourth-year students failed to achieve a minimum passing level. In another study of junior and senior medical students, Juul et al. (1979) showed a significant difference in performance between groups.

At the residency level, the evidence is not as straightforward. Two reports (Levine and Noak, 1968; Miller, 1968) show no difference in PMP scores for residents across all four years of training. Other studies (Levine, 1967a, 1967b) suggest that specific management subscores are positively related to increase in training level, but that overall scores are not.

Donnelly and Prevot (1978), comparing the performance of two groups of medical students on PMPs representing two different clinical situations, found some support for construct validity. As hypothesized, students asked fewer questions and had, in general, higher efficiency scores on the PMPs dealing with emergency situations. For proficiency scores, however, the results were less conclusive. The definition of emergency and nonemergency settings was not clearly delineated. Palva and Korhonen (1976), focusing on outcomes, compared the rate of drug-induced agranulocytosis on a simulated clinical problem done by medical students to that on the actual medical service. House staff on the service were graduates of the same school as the students who worked through the PMPs. Similar rates of agranulocytosis were found in both groups. The approach is novel but lacks other controls and uses a low-frequency outcome for comparison. Other reports (McGuire, 1967; McGuire et al., 1972) have analyzed the performance of practicing physicians grouped by age or experience. The overall scores decreased with increased experience, reflecting the fact that more experienced physicians gather less data. The authors suggest that this is consistent with data from observational studies of physician performance (Clute, 1963; Peterson et al., 1956). The conclusions draw heavily on the presumed comparability of the different groups of physicians studied. As such, the findings are a helpful contribution but provide limited evidence in establishing construct validity.

McGuire et al. (1972), reporting results from factor analytic studies of multiple component examinations, identified three factors from the analysis. Multiple-choice questions loaded most heavily on "recall of information," while PMPs loaded most heavily on two other factors. The PMP data-gathering scores loaded on "persistence of inductive inquiry," whereas the management score loaded on a factor labeled "decisiveness and efficiency." While specific data is not provided in this report, the authors offer their results as a support for the construct validity of PMPs. Donnelly (1976) found two factors emerging from a factor analysis of PMPs: one factor was strongly related to data gathering and correlated across cases; the second factor related to management and was case specific.

Based on rigor of study design and the strength of the assumptions or constructs, those studies involving large groups of learners at different levels provide the most convincing evidence. While the findings at the undergraduate level are clear-cut, those from studies of residents and practicing clinicians do not provide consistent support for construct validity.

Concurrent Validity. Studies assessing concurrent validity of PMPs have generally taken one of two approaches. The first is to compare the scores on PMPs with the scores of the same individuals on other tests presumed to measure something other than what PMPs are measuring. An example of an alternate test would be a multiple-choice test. (While this approach is included here as one of concurrent validity, it has been considered by some as an assessment of construct validity. The distinction is not critical in this context.) The second approach is to compare performance on PMPs with measures that are hoped to reflect more specifically the individual's performance in a clinical situation.

McGuire et al. (1972) reports on studies comparing performance on PMPs and multiple-choice questions at all levels—medical student, resident, and certification exam candidate. The findings demonstrate uniformly low correlations, ranging from 0.20 to 0.40, and do not exceed 0.50 even when the tests are deemed highly reliable because of their length. Hence, they conclude that the instruments are measuring different competencies. The difficulty with this approach is that specific competency cannot be directly determined. This leaves certain questions unanswered. How firmly has it been established that the instrument measures the specific competencies of interest? Moreover, in what way are the findings influenced by a difference in content areas being measured by each instrument?

Some authors (McGuire, 1967) argue for content specificity of problem solving based on low correlation between PMPs of different content areas. If low correlations between PMPs result from variations of content, to what degree does content confound the findings of validity studies comparing PMPs and multiple-choice questions when the two tests have not been based on the same content? Proper studies controlling for content in an effective manner would provide a valuable contribution.

Attempts to compare scores obtained by students on written simulations to supervisor ratings of the students are fraught with problems (McGuire et al., 1972). The low reliability of supervisor ratings and the failure to identify and compare specific competencies have led to frustrating results to date. Evidence from studies which have properly overcome these problems does not currently exist.

An alternate route for comparing clinical performance to that on PMPs involves chart audit. Williamson and McGuire (1968) studied 18 physicians by auditing charts on their patients with problems similar to PMPs completed by the study physicians. Initial comparisons based on a pool of essential diagnostic data abstracted from the records showed considerably less data was recorded in history and physical than was elicited on the PMPs. There was no difference in the information elicited by laboratory investigations. Recognizing that less data may be recorded than was elicited in real life encounters, the investigators then reduced the data pool to six items that were felt certain to be recorded if elicited from the patient. Subsequent comparisons using these six items showed no difference between PMPs and chart audit. Unfortunately, three of these items were lab investigations, an area in which no difference existed in the initial analysis. Hence, the support for validity is actually based on a comparison involving one item of history and two of physical examination. The power of this comparison is not persuasive.

In a similar study by Goran, Williamson, and Gonnella (1973), a clinical team's performance on PMPs was compared with clinical performance assessed by chart audit. While exact cases were not compared, the chart audit and PMPs assessed similar clinical problems. The basis for comparison was a list of ten items of history, six items of physical examination, and a laboratory test

for urine culture. The clinical importance of each item was established by a literature review. Although a recording bias may still
be present, the ten items of history were requested far more frequently on the PMPs than they were recorded on the chart. Moreover, the critical decision to order a urine culture was also requested
twice as frequently on the PMPs. Differences in each comparison
achieved statistical significance. The authors add that the subjects perform consistently better on the PMP than in the clinical
situation and that those performing best on the PMP did not
necessarily perform best in the real life setting. These findings
raise doubts regarding the concurrent validity of PMPs.

Early work by McCarthy (1966) contributed further to concerns about behavior on PMPs. Although studying the effect of
cueing rather than validity per se, he found a 25 percent increase
in the amount of information collected on the PMP format as well
as a 50 percent increase in scores when compared to an oral examination. Once again, there was no correlation between the ranking
of students on two formats.

Three studies have explored the issue of cueing in greater
depth, one using real patients but with no control for content, and
two applying tightly controlled designs but using high-fidelity,
live, simulated patients. Donnelly and Gallagher (1978) observed
family practice residents with two to three real patients, scored
their performance using PMP formulas, and compared those performances to the residents' performance on PMPs. While less information was elicited in the visits with patients, the authors
found a positive correlation of scores between the two formats.
The authors rely heavily on their earlier work (Donnelly et al.,
1974), however, suggesting global performance across content
areas. The fact that other studies (McGuire, 1967) claim that performance is content specific might bring some to challenge Donnelly and Gallagher's conclusions.

Norman and Feightner (1981) compared the performance
of two similar groups of clinical clerks on four cases, each in the
written PMP format and in a live clinical simulation format. Their
study found that students elicited up to twice as much information on history, physical, laboratory, and management in the
PMP format. These differences achieved statistical significance and
held up on an analysis of a subset of clinical items deemed critical
for each of the cases. A weakness of the study is that live, simulated patients were used instead of real patients and that the same
student did not do the same case in each format. The findings,

nonetheless, are consistent with others (Goran et al., 1973; McCarthy, 1966; Page and Fielding, 1980), that raise questions about performance or behavior on patient management problems.

Page and Fielding (1980) assessed the performance of community pharmacists in their own pharmacies versus their performance on PMPs. Live, simulated patients were trained to simulate the same conditions as the patients represented in the PMPs and were sent into the community pharmacy to request medications from the pharmacist. Prior to assessing concurrent validity, the four PMPs in the study were shown to possess content and construct validity. Again, in this study, more information was elicited in the PMP format than in the actual clinical situation. For behaviors or actions judged critical to the problem, 79 percent of the items were elicited on the PMPs compared to 48 percent in the live situation. Thus the PMPs were viewed as poor predictors of actions judged as critical. Moreover, they were also poor at predicting behaviors which were critical to avoid, which occurred twice as often in the live situation as they did in the PMPs. The authors suggest that PMPs were good predictors of what pharmacists did not do in practice but poor predictors of what they actually do. While the study used live simulated patients, the pharmacists were unaware and unable to identify them as separate from other customers. While the study subjects were pharmacists, the results are consistent with those of other studies in medicine.

Predictive Validity

Predictive validity is the most difficult to assess. Proven instruments are not readily available for assessing the components of clinical competence in a practice setting. Moreover, it is difficult to develop a design which adequately controls for the many confounding variables between training and practice. One study by Nerenberg et al. (1978) attempted to assess the contribution of a multiple-component examination to the prediction of performance in the internship year. While the study found that PMPs explained some of the variance in clinical performance, there were too many problems with the study to draw any conclusions about the predictive validity of PMPs. Pawluk et al. (1976) found moderate correlations between a candidate's PMP score on a family medicine certification examination and scores on a subsequent quality-of-care assessment in that individual's practice. Considerable methodological hurdles must be overcome before any conclusive studies of predictive validity can be undertaken.

Scoring

In general, the scoring of PMPs involves the weighting of options by a panel of experts and the application of a formula to calculate a score based on the options chosen by a candidate. Positive weights are assigned to appropriate or helpful options, negative weights to inappropriate or harmful options, and a zero weight to an option considered neither of these. Rarely do the developers of PMPs have a criterion group actually work through the PMP and incorporate this into the scoring.

The National Board (Hubbard, 1978) assigns each candidate a handicapping score equal in magnitude to the total number of items labeled as definitely incorrect in the problem. Points are added for all positive score options selected and subtracted for negative score options. McGuire et al. (1972) have suggested an alternate approach using three algorithms for combining the weights into scores of proficiency, efficiency, and overall competence. Errors of omission and errors of commission can be identified and optimal pathways and minimal passing levels can also be established. Despite early recognition of flaws in the scoring formulas (McGuire and Babbott, 1967), insufficient attention has been focused on the implications of using various weighting scales or scoring formulas. Since many studies addressing the validity of patient management problems use the scores as the measure of interest, ensuring the validity of these intuitive formulas is essential to establishing the validity of the PMP itself. Results from three studies addressing these issues reinforce the need to look more closely at scoring. Connelly et al. (1974) compared one weighting system with a wide range of weights on individual items to another system with a narrow range and found a high correlation between the two systems on six out of eight PMPs. He concluded that the simple system (-1, 0, +1) was as adequate as the more complex one for scoring PMPs. Bligh (1980) looked more closely at scoring systems by varying the magnitude of the weights assigned and the range of scores applied. He, too, identified a high correlation across most of the scoring systems. While there was a high correlation across scoring systems, the changes in the scoring did have a major effect on the level at which a minimum pass score was established. Thus while a high correlation between scoring system exists, the decisions of whether a candidate passed or failed would differ depending on which weighting system was used. His findings suggest that this issue needs to be explored further. Marshall (1977) found that the most efficient problem solvers on their certification examination were not scoring well on PMPs because the instrument rewarded thoroughness in history taking and physical examination. While two candidates might arrive at the same diagnosis, the one that collected more minor positive items would score higher. By modifying the scoring system to set maximum scores for each section and reducing the weights assigned to minor routine data, he found that the best results on PMPs were now achieved by the most efficient problem solvers. While several questions have been raised about this study, in particular the small number of subjects, the results raise significant issues about conventional scoring of PMPs.

Educational Effect

The potential of PMPs to assist in student learning appears to be considerable. Examples exist of their use at all levels of training. The Royal College of General Practice of Australia has used PMPs as part of their self-evaluation program for practicing physicians. Corley (1976) has had extensive experience using PMPs to provide feedback to family medicine residents. Modifications of branching PMPs have been used for formative evaluation in pediatric clerkships (Feinstein and Levine, 1977). In general, however, it is difficult to assess how extensively PMPs are used for formative evaluation in medical education. Published studies exploring their effect on student learning are virtually nonexistent.

In addition to the feedback for individual students, the results from PMPs can provide useful information to instructors and program planners (McGuire et al., 1972). The patterns of individual student and group performance data can identify weaknesses in the instruction program. PMPs may well be underused for this purpose.

Synthesis

The literature on PMPs and other written simulations is diverse and often the final conclusions of studies are reported without the accompanying evidence. But what of the overall picture?

Strengths

Patient management problems and other written simulations have evolved from sound concepts and important intents. Developers have responded to the need to measure in a reliable fashion components of clinical competence other than factual recall. There is reasonable evidence for reliability both in the linear and branching formats. In general, there is acceptable evidence for content validity. The evidence supporting construct validity is reasonable, although not entirely consistent.

As instructional tools, PMPs and other written simulations appear potentially quite valuable and may well be inadequately used. Studies do not exist, however, to demonstrate their impact on student learning. They may have a role in evaluation of competence, because the PMP has advantages of objectivity and low cost compared to alternate instruments and approaches.

Concerns

Firm, consistent evidence regarding the validity of PMPs is lacking. The assessment of predictive validity is difficult and remains an unresolved issue and a challenge for the future. Concurrent validity has been addressed by a number of studies, the findings of which are disquieting. While studies showing a low correlation between PMPs and multiple-choice tests lend indirect support for concurrent validity, direct comparisons of PMPs with other measures of clinical performance have shown consistent differences and these findings seriously challenge the validity of PMPs. These findings are of particular concern considering the widespread use of PMPs for certification decisions, and it is surprising and unfortunate to find a lack of coordinated effort to adequately assess all of the measurement properties of the instrument. It seems clear that while PMPs simulate and approximate the clinical encounter, one cannot be certain that they allow a valid measure of an individual's performance in an actual clinical setting. Perhaps too much has been expected. It may be that a more circumscribed role can be defined as part of a battery of objective tests designed to assess specific components of clinical competence rather than anticipating that PMPs will measure problem solving or clinical judgment. Based on studies reported to date, however, it seems inappropriate for certifying bodies to rely so heavily on patient management problems to make certification decisions about clinical competence.

Other Written Simulations

The majority of the literature on written simulations has focused on the two most common formats, the linear PMP used by the National Board of Medical Examiners and the branching PMP developed most extensively at the University of Illinois. Both of these basic formats have been altered by various centers, but there is little to suggest that they have any methodologic properties which differ significantly from those already discussed. A limited amount of data does exist on three other formats of written simulations, namely, the sequential management problem (SMP) (Martin, 1975), the portable patient problem pack (P4 Deck) (Tamblyn et al., 1980), and the diagnostic management problem (DMP) (Helfer and Slater, 1971; Robinson and Dinham, 1977). They will each be discussed briefly.

The SMP was developed at the University of Illinois (Martin, 1975) in an effort to reduce the impact of cueing. This model begins with a small opening vignette. The subject is then asked at a sequence of stages to request data which he feels are most pertinent. Subsequent to each request for data, the subject is provided with a complete data set for that section including the items considered most pertinent by a criterion panel involved in developing the instrument. Thus, requests are made for items of history and physical, and then all of the pertinent information is provided regardless of whether it was requested. A similar exercise occurs for the request of lab tests and subsequent results, as well as components of management. Finally, the subject is asked to write down what he feels is the patient's diagnosis, prognosis, and appropriate continuing management. When comparing performance of a group of physicians on SMPs with another groups doing PMPs, the authors found higher scores on PMPs in the history and physical sections and higher scores on the SMPs in lab and management sections. While the higher PMP scores in history and physical may be the result of cueing, it is more difficult to interpret a comparison of lab and management scores since at this point the SMP subjects had been provided with all of the pertinent history and physical data. The degree to which this influenced their selection of laboratory tests and items of management was not explored. No studies of reliability and validity have been published for this instrument.

The P4 Deck is an extension of the Rimoldi card deck concept. The items the student might wish to ask in history, examine on physical, and select for lab investigations, management, and consultation are all contained on the front of the card with the corresponding results typed on the reverse side. This format allows complete flexibility for the student in working through the patient problem because he can move freely from any of the sections to another and back again. In addition to the clinical questions the card has a number of other stimulating questions for the student to consider in making that selection. This is intended to provide a richer educational experience while working through the problem.

There is one published study which addresses certain measurement characteristics of P4 Decks. Tamblyn et al. (1980), using a modified crossover design, compared performance of both nursing and medical students on a P4 Deck with their performance on live, high-fidelity simulated patients. The behaviors of both groups were compared with regard to which options were selected on history and physical, as well as in the areas of lab investigations, management, and consultations. The results showed no difference in the options selected between the two formats on history and physical. Unfortunately, a procedural error in the use of the P4 format did not allow comparison of performance as initially intended in the areas of lab investigations, management, and consultations. These results would lend some support for the concurrent validity of P4 Decks.

The diagnostic management problem (DMP) is also based on Rimoldi's card selection concept. As with the P4 Deck, not only can the options selected be recorded but the sequence in which they are selected can be documented as well. A report by Helfer and Slater (1971) describes the instrument and addresses the issues of its reliability and validity. The authors found a correlation of 0.66 ($p < 0.01$) between scores of 19 senior medical students who solved two dissimilar DMPs. The validity of the instrument was assessed by comparing the scores of 42 senior medical students on a single DMP with three alternate measures: their grade on the pediatric national boards, their subjective pediatric grade (supervisor rating), and their score on a branching PMP. The corresponding correlation coefficients were 0.09, 0.40, and 0.60, respectively. The latter two correlations were statistically significant. While this might suggest some support for the validity of the instrument, others have not found supervisor rating scales as a satisfactory "gold standard." There is insufficient information on the measurement characteristics of the supervisor reports to assess whether they are appropriate comparisons. No additional data are provided with regard to the content area of the branching PMP. One would assume that its content area was very close to that of the DMP; otherwise these results would tend to contradict those which some have used to suggest content specificity of problem solving based on low correlations across PMPs with differing clinical content.

Robinson and Dinham (1977) studied 41 clinical clerks on rotations in internal medicine or pediatrics. The clerks had been randomly assigned to the available clinical settings. Each group received three prerotation diagnostic management problems and three postrotation tests. Within each package the three DMPs were arranged in differing orders. The two packages were also systematically alternated so that the package that served as a pretest for one half of the students served as the post-test for the other half and vice versa. Scores relating to the process and the selection of positively weighted items showed a high internal consistency. Three other subscores, a selection of negatively weighted items, efficiency, and a diagnostic score, showed low internal consistency. While there is some support for reliability, the mixed results create certain questions which were addressed by the authors. Construct validity was assessed by comparing the prerotation scores with postrotation scores as well as the scores of students early in the clerkship with students late in the clerkship. Significantly higher postrotation scores were found in all of the five subscores except that relating to the selection of negatively weighted items. The picture is not as clear-cut when comparing less experienced with more experienced students. Significant differences were found only for certain subgroups on a process score, a score related to a selection of positive items, and a diagnostic score. No differences existed between complete groups. This study provides some support for construct validity of the DMP.

References

Bligh, T. J.: Written simulation scoring: a comparison of nine systems. Presented at American Educational Research Association Annual Meeting, New York (1980).

Clute, K. F.: The general practitioner: a study of medical education and practice in Ontario and Nova Scotia. Toronto: University of Toronto Press (1963).

Corley, J. B.: Evaluating residency training—an operational prototype. Charleston, S.C.: Medical University Press (1976).

Donnelly, M. B., Gallagher, R. E., Hess, J. W., Hogan, M. J.: The dimensionality of measures derived from complex clinical simulations. Proceedings, 13th Annual Conference on Research in Medical Education, Chicago, Ill. (1974).

Donnelly, M. B.: Measuring performance on patient management problems. Proceedings, 15th Annual Conference on Research in Medical Education, San Francisco, Calif. (1976).

Donnelly, M. B., Prevot, E. L.: Construct validity of patient management problems: emergency vs. non-emergency contexts. Proceedings, 17th Annual Conference on Research in Medical Education, New Orleans, La. (1978).

Donnelly, M. B., Gallagher, R. E.: A study of the predictive validity of patient management problems, multiple choice tests and rating scales. Proceedings, 17th Annual Conference on Research in Medical Education, New Orleans, La. (1978).

Elstein, A. S., Shulman, L. S., Sprafka, S. A.: Medical problem-solving: an analysis of clinical reasoning. Cambridge, Mass.: Harvard University Press, (1978).

Feinstein, E., Levine, H. G.: Using patient management problems for teaching clinical problem-solving. Proceedings, 16th Annual Conference on Research in Medical Education, Washington, D.C. (1977).

Goran, M. J., Williamson, J. W., Gonnella, J. S.: The validity of patient management problems. J. Med Educ 48, 171-177 (1973).

Helfer, R. E., Slater, C. H.: Measuring the process of solving clinical diagnostic problems. Brit J Med Educ 5, 48-52 (1971).

Hubbard, J. P., Levitt, E. J., Schumacher, C. F.: An objective evaluation of clinical competence: new techniques used by the National Board of Medical Examiners. N Engl J Med 272, 1321-1328 (1965).

Hubbard, J. P.: Measuring medical education: the tests and the experience of the National Board of Medical Examiners (2nd ed.), Philadelphia: Lee & Febiger (1978).

Juul, D. H., Noe, M. J., Nerenberg, R. L.: A factor analytic study of branching patient management problems. Med Educ 13, 199-203 (1979).

Levine, H. G.: An analysis of the construct validity of two simulation techniques. Chicago: University of Illinois, (1967a).

Levine, H. G.: Report on the January 1966 orthopedic certification examination. Chicago: University of Illinois, (1967b).

Levine, H. G., Noak, J. R.: The evaluation of complex eduational outcomes. Washington, D.C.: U.S. Dept Health, Education, and Welfare, (1968).

Lewy, A., McGuire, C. H.: A study of alternative approaches in estimating the reliability of unconventional tests. American Educational Research Association Annual Meeting, Chicago (1966).

Marshall, J.: Assessment of problem-solving ability. Med Educ 11, 329-334 (1977).

Martin, I. C.: Empirical examination of the sequential management problem for measuring clinical competence. Proceedings, 14th Annual Conference on Research in Medical Education, Washington, D.C. (1975).

McCarthy, W. H.: An assessment of the influence of cueing items on objective examinations. J Med Educ 41, 263-266 (1966).

McGuire, C.: A process approach to the construction and analysis of medical examinations. J Med Educ 38, 556-563 (1963).

McGuire, C. H.: A summary of the evidence regarding the technical characteristics of patient management problems. Report to AAOS Examinations Committee, University of Illinois (1967).

McGuire, C. H., Babbott, D.: Simulation technique in the measurement of problem-solving skills. J Educ Meas 4, 1-10 (1967).

McGuire, C., Solomon, L. M., Bashook, P. G.: Handbook of written simulations: their construction and analysis. Center for Education Development, Chicago, Ill. (1972).

Miller, G. E.: The orthopedic training study. JAMA 206, 601-606 (1968).

Nerenberg, R. L., Noe, M. J., Juul, D. H., et al.: Prediction of graduate clinical performance ratings from multicomponent medical school examinations. Proceedings, 17th Annual Conference on Research in Medical Education, New Orleans, La. (1978).

Norman, G. R., Feightner, J. W.: A comparison of behavior on simulated patients and patient management problems. Med Educ 15, 26-32 (1981).

Page, G. G., Fielding, D. W.: Performance on PMPs and performance in practice: Are they related? J Med Educ 55, 529-537 (1980).

Palva, I. P., Korhonen, V.: Validity and use of written simulation tests of clinical performance. J Med Educ 51, 657-661 (1976).

Pawluk, W., Roberts, R., Neufeld, V. R.: Concurrent validity of the Canadian Certification Examination in Family Medicine. Proceedings, 15th Annual Conference on Research in Medical Education, San Francisco, Calif. (1976).

Peterson, O. L., Andrews, L. P., Spain, R. S., Greenburg, B. G.: An analytical study of North Carolina general practice 1953-1954. J Med Educ 31, 1-165, (1956).

Rimoldi, H. J. A.: The test of diagnostic skills. J Med Educ 36, 73-79 (1961).

Rimoldi, H. J. A.: Rationale and applications of the test of diagnostic skills. J Med Educ 38, 364-368 (1963).

Robinson, S. A., Dinham, S. M.: Reliability and validity of simulated problems as measures of change in problem-solving skills. Proceedings, 16th Annual Conference on Research in Medical Education, Washington, D.C. (1977).

Schumacher, C. F.: Validation of the American Board of Internal Medicine written examination: A study of the examination as a measure of achievement in graduate medical education. Ann Intern Med 78, 131-135 (1978).

Sedlecek, W. E., Nattress, L. W.: A technique for determining the validity of patient management problems. J Med Educ 47, 263-266 (1972).

Tamblyn, R. M., Barrows, H. S., Gliva, G.: Units to facilitate problem-solving in self-directed study (portable patient problem pack). Med Educ 14, 394-400 (1980).

Williamson, J. W.: Assessing clinical judgment. J Med Educ 40, 180-187 (1965).

Williamson, J. W., McGuire, C. H.: Consecutive case conference. J Med Educ 43, 1068-1074 (1968).

CHAPTER 10

Computer Simulations

GEOFFREY R. NORMAN
CATHERINE PAINVIN

Over the past two decades, computers have played an increasing role in all aspects of medicine, to the point where a patient can almost anticipate an interaction with computers from the time of initial history taking to the payment of his account. Techniques such as computerized history taking (Warner et al., 1972), Bayesian diagnosis, and decision analysis (Weinstein and Fineberg, 1980) have been perceived as, not just an aid, but as a threat to the conventional practice of medicine. Computers have also been increasingly used in the evaluation of competence, ranging from simulation of the physiological dynamics of the cardiorespiratory system (Dickinson, 1972; Dickinson et al., 1973) to the evaluation of technical skills in anesthesiology (Abrahamson et al., 1969). The technical accomplishments which have accompanied these developments are impressive. In one application (Harless et al., 1971), the clinician can communicate with the computer using ordinary English statements such as "How are you feeling today?" typed on the computer terminal and anticipate an appropriate response from the computer "patient" nearly all the time. The SIM-1 project (Abrahamson et al., 1969) uses a mannequin under computer control—the clinician can auscultate or percuss the mannequin, and the "patient's" heart rate, blood pressure, and breathing will respond to interventions by the clinician.

In view of the considerable resources which have been invested in these projects, it is somewhat paradoxical that few have proceeded beyond the demonstration project stage, and few have been subjected to rigorous evaluation of reliability and validity. Where computers have achieved more widespread application, the goals and methods are usually much more prosaic than those achieved by the demonstration projects. A critical review of computer applications to the measurement of clinical competence would be remiss if it did not deal with this paradox.

Computer Simulation, Computer-aided Instruction, and Computer-aided Diagnosis

The use of computers in education has its roots in programmed instruction (Brigham and Kamp, 1974). Most conventional computer-aided instruction (CAI) deals with materials that can be readily presented in a textbook. Although computer simulation is one type of computer-assisted instruction, it can be distinguished from conventional CAI in that it is used chiefly to develop reasoning, problem-solving, and decision-making skills. Zemper (1973) clearly indicates the differences between CAI and computer simulation:

> Other modes of CAI are concerned with application of standard situations. The student is mainly learning new information and concepts and his interactions with the computer are in response to its direct stimulus. In simulation, on the other hand, a problem is posed, but how the student gets to a solution is an extremely flexible affair. He not only responds, but can ask questions as well. . . . the beauty of simulation is that with just a little imagination it can duplicate the realistic aspects of a problem situation. Thus learning is enhanced by being removed from the artificiality of the classroom and taking place in an environment which can closely approximate real-life situations.

The distinction between computer simulation and computer-aided diagnosis is less distinct. The essential feature of computer simulation is that the computer is playing the role of patient, providing information in response to the requests of the clinician, whereas in computer-aided diagnosis, the computer acts in the role of clinician cooperating (or competing) with the physician to diagnose the problems of patients presented to both. Where the distinction becomes fuzzy is that in educational application, it is appropriate for a computer simulation to provide feedback to the student when he or she errs, and in formal evaluation situations, the candidate must be judged against a criterion of performance. In both instances, the methods of computer-aided diagnosis, such as Bayesian calculations, are commonly used to formulate the criterion. Perhaps the distinguishing feature remains that, in computer simulation, the "patient" resides in the memory of the computer; in CAD, patient information is entered by the clinician.

Computer simulations can vary widely in sophistication, but in most applications the student can gather patient data from the computer, arrive at a diagnosis, and implement actions through typing his choices at a keyboard and viewing the computer response at the terminal. Schneiderman and Muller (1972) have expressed the utopian view that:

> Computers are tireless drillmasters; they can require students to learn actively, they can provide immediate feedback, and can keep records of student performance for evaluation. . . . The student thus has the opportunity to develop problem-solving skills free of the constraints of the real world. He can test his ideas by discovering their consequences and learn from his mistakes without bankrupting or billing his "patients." [p. 333]

The rationale for using computer simulation, or any other sort of simulation, in medical education can be summarized in six points:

1. To make the learner a participant in a realistic learning experience. The word "learner" is used with reference to students in health professions or health professionals in continuing education. The learner may take the role of the physician and the simulation gives him data about the patient.
2. To provide access for certain problems not readily available to the learner.
3. To allow reproducibility of the same problem either for the same learner until mastery, or for different students, facilitating the evaluation process.
4. To allow compression of time: the status of the patient can be changed in a few minutes, although it may take years in real life.
5. To eliminate risk to the patients.
6. To provide feedback to the learner about his performance, in the learning and evaluation situations.

These advantages of simulations provide a strong rationale for the use of any simulation technique; however, rarely are all accommodated within a single simulation device. For example, live simulated patients and some computer simulations such as SIM-1, already described, provide a realistic learning environment, but the degree of realism present in some of the computerized PMP approaches may be less than is available from a written PMP with photographs or slides. Relatively few computer simulations deal effectively with the time variable. Although the course of an illness over days or week may be simulated, with rare exceptions, the evolution of the problem is fixed and will not respond to the interventions of the student physician.

   Does computer simulation offer any advantages not offered by other forms of simulation? One obvious advantage is related to the vast capacity of modern computers, which can be available 24 hours a day, to a virtually limitless number of users, an attractive feature for certification, recertification, or continuing education. It is therefore not surprising that one of the most extensive developments in computer simulation is the CBX project (Senior, 1976), developed by the American Board of Internal Medicine and National Board of Medical Examiners for licensure and certification purposes.

   A second feature of computer simulations which may be of potential advantage in testing situations is the ability to correctly interpret queries directed in ordinary English. In contrast to a written PMP, in which the subject must choose options from a printed list and may be "cued" to seek information he would not otherwise have recalled, computer simulations such as the CASE system (Harless et al., 1971) require the subject to directly request information in natural language. These queries are then processed through sophisticated text interpreter programs to yield an appropriate response. Because cueing is apparently a strong bias of written PMPs (Norman and Feightner, 1981; Page and Fielding, 1980), this advantage of computers should not be ignored. This advantage is not achieved without some cost, however. In addition to the tedious requirement of typing the entire request at the terminal, the programmes misinterpret from 5 percent to 10 percent of requests.

   Other advantages of computer simulations are less obvious. Although it is now relatively straightforward to develop a written simulation on a computer, such simulations, unless they incorporate the flexibility to branch based on the student's responses, do not fully exploit the capabilities of the machine. The computer has enormous potential to provide dynamic responses to the interventions of the student. Physiological systems can be accurately simulated using complex mathematical models, and the computer can rapidly calculate the effect on the whole system of the change in any variable. Thus, the computerized "patient" can change over time in direct response to the interventions of the subject.

Finally, the computer simulation has the potential to provide immediate feedback—either in the form of process feedback, in response to a choice of particular options, or as outcome feedback in the form of summary scores at the completion of the problem.

Although we are not aware of any review of the literature in computer simulations, two comprehensive surveys of computer applications in North American medical schools have been conducted. The first, by Brigham and Kamp (1974), included 95 medical schools and was directed at determining the extent of educational use of computers in these schools. Forty schools were using computers in instruction and 31 expected to use them in the future. A total of 184 programs were available: 110 (59.8 percent) were on clinical subjects as opposed to basic science subjects, and 51 (27.7 percent) were a clinical application of computers, but not necessarily a computer simulation of patient problems. Seventy-five percent of the programs originated from three institutions and Ohio State University generated 44 percent of the programs. In the mid-1970s, the Office of Medical Education at Michigan State University, in cooperation with the National Library of Medicine (Zemper, 1973), identified 52 computer projects. Thirty-three percent presented factual information, 27 percent were programs dealing with patient management problems, but over 40 percent did not provide enough data for classification.

The present review used these two surveys as sources, but the present discussion is confined to projects where the intent is a simulation of an actual patient problem for instruction or evaluation of clinical competence.

We were able to identify a total of 15 projects involving computer simulation. About half of these programs were intended for instructional purposes, and half were primarily intended for evaluation. The range of content areas covered was impressive, although there were no projects in psychiatry and obstetrics. The measurement properties of these projects are summarized in Table 10.1.

The diversity in content areas is matched by a diversity in approaches. There is little commonality in the programming languages used to develop the problems, in the goals of the simulations

TABLE 10.1
Summary of Measurement Properties of Computer Simulations

Author	Name	Purpose*	No. Cases	Credibility	Reliability	Validity	Educ. Value	Cost
Senior, 1976	INDEX (CBX)	E	5	anecdotal "good"	.86-.91	↑	NR	$36-$60
Harless et al., 1971	CASE (CBX)	E,I	10	anecdotal	.34-.68	↑↓	NR	NR
de Dombal, 1969 de Dombal et al., 1971, 1972 Leaper et al., 1973	ODSAL	I	18	+/-	NR	→	↑	.10-.20
Schneiderman & Muller, 1972		I	?	anecdotal	NR	NR	NR	NR
Hoffer, 1973		I	∞	anecdotal	NR	Content only	NR	NR
Dickinson & Shephard, 1971 Dickinson et al., 1973	MACPEE MACPUFF MACMAN	I	∞	–	NR	NR	NR	NR

Study	System	Type						
Friedman, 1973 Friedman et al., 1977, 1978		I,E	21/25	realistic anecdotal	NR	↑↓	use only	$51
Schumacher & Burg, 1975	CPMP	E	8	↑	>.50 (Int. Con.)	↑↓	NR	$151
Senior, 1976	CRISYS (CBX)	E		NR	NR	NR	NR	NR
Gorry & Barnett, 1968	MATRIX (CBX)	E		NR	NR	↑	NR	NR
Johnson & Muller, 1975		R		NR	NR	Based on expert	NR	NR
Diamond & Weiner, 1974		I,E	10	NR	NR	NR	NR	$10/S
Abrahamson et al., 1969	SIM-1	I		NR	NR	NR	↑	$75,000

*I = Instruction, E = Evaluation, R = Research

207

or their intended audiences, or the manner in which the simulations are constructed. However, many of the simulations do have some common features. The goal of the simulation is generally the diagnosis and management of an individual patient problem. Usually the user interacts with the computer by selecting items of history, physical investigations, and management from a predetermined list and entering a numerical code. Programs appear to vary in emphasis and subject area, but many appear to follow this basic approach.

There are few notable exceptions to this rule, however. SIM-1, the computerized mannequin developed at the University of Southern California (Abrahamson et al., 1969), involves no verbal exchange and focuses entirely on technical skills in the management of the "patient." The CASE system of Harless et al. (1971), as previously described, uses natural language communication between computer and user, avoiding the potential cueing resulting from selection from a given list. Friedman's (1973; Friedman et al., 1977) and several other simulations (Hoffer, 1973) permit the simulation to evolve over time. And one class of simulation (Dickinson and Shephard, 1971; Hoffer, 1973) is based on a mathematical model of a physiological system, permitting an infinite variation in the clinical features by changing the input parameters and linking the clinical manifestations to underlying physiological processes for learning purposes.

Measurement Properties

It is evident from reviewing the literature that the extensive investment in the development of these simulations has not been matched by an equal investment in determining the effectiveness of the various approaches. More than half the simulations were developed for instructional purposes, yet only two studies have reported the instructional effectiveness of the computer simulation against some alternative instructional strategy. Validity studies have been more frequently reported for simulations intended for evaluation, particularly those simulations developed under the CBX project of the American Board of Internal Medicine and the National Board of Medical Examiners (Senior, 1976), but the results are mixed. The results of these studies will be reviewed in detail below.

Credibility

Systematic studies of credibility were reported for many simulations. Perhaps not surprisingly, authors reported a high degree of acceptability—for example, in a study of computerized PMPs (Fincham et al., 1976), 87 percent of candidates in a certification examination rated the PMP as pertinent, 84 percent found it easy to use, 68 percent felt it to be a better test than multiple choice, although only 42 percent felt it superior to oral examinations. And 78 percent of students using Friedman et al. (1978) simulations found them "enjoyable to use." De Dombal (1969) found that junior clinical clerks perferred the computer simulation over a structured oral examination or card problem. In another study (de Dombal et al., 1972), however, he reported reverse findings—a sample of clinicians, residents, and students preferred both oral and card problems to the computer simulation. Similar documented or anectodal evidence is provided for a number of other simulations.

The achievement of credibility is a necessary prerequisite for implementation of any evaluation method. In the case of computer simulations it is a positive comment on the achievement of computer specialists in making the interaction between the subject and computer sufficiently easy and realistic to obtain positive ratings by most users. However, although users may find the computer simulations a believable representation of a clinical encounter with a patient, it remains to be demonstrated that performance on a computer simulation can be used as a reliable and valid measure of clinical competence, or can result in learning.

Precision

At first glance, a discussion of the reliability of computer simulation may seem irrelevant, since as the measurements obtained by computer-based simulation testing, if they are objectively scored, do not involve observer variability, they should thus be completely reliable. Although the scoring of a computer interaction is usually based on a predetermined algorithm, therefore eliminating the subjective judgment of an observer as a source of variation in scoring, the essential notion of reliability is one of consistency or stability on repeated administrations and the observer is only one source of variation in the repeated administration of a test. The reliability of a computer simulation could be assessed by, for example, repeated encounters by subjects with the same computer problem, separated by a sufficiently long time interval that specific responses on the first administration would not be remembered.

If the computer simulation is intended as a general measure of competence, however, the nature of the presenting problem may be a source of considerable variation, and reliability must be examined across several different problems from different content areas.

In light of these comments, it is surprising that very few studies have examined the reliability of computer simulations. Schumacher and Burg (1975) reported coefficients in the 0.5 to 0.7 range for computerized linear patient management problems used in a pediatric certifying examination. Although not explicitly stated in the paper, it appears that these coefficients are a form of "internal consistency" reliability and do not encompass the sources of variation outlined above. Similar or higher reliabilities were reported for CASE problems (Webster et al., 1979) and the INDEX problems, also associated with the CBX project (Senior, 1976). However, the reliability of the CASE scores dropped to 0.35 when assessed across different problems (Webster et al., 1979).

Thus, the objective scoring frequently applied to computer simulations is no guarantee of reliability, in its more general sense. If computer simulations are to have a role as a measure of clinical competence, considerable attention must be paid in future studies to the sources of variation contributing to the unreliability of such tests.

Validity

In contrast to the paucity of reliability studies, a number of studies of validity have been reported. The problem in assessing concurrent validity of measures of clinical competence remains— there is no clear criterion against which performance on the simulation can be judged. As a result, computer simulations have been compared to a variety of other measures—simulated patients, record audit of physician practice, oral examinations, multiple-choice tests, and global ratings.

Two studies have examined performance against level of training. Friedman et al. (1978) showed that medical students took longer to complete a case, spent the most "money" on workups, and hospitalized patients longer than did housestaff or senior staff. Senior staff performed more poorly on these measures than housestaff, however, and no statistical analysis was conducted. Schumacher and Burg (1975) compared performance on a computerized PMP with level of training and found significant correlations on four out of six subscores.

Performance on the same two computer simulations has been compared to performance on licensing and certification examinations. Taylor (1976) found a low positive relationship between performance on the computer PMP and performance on a multiple-choice certification examination ($r = 0.24$), but no significant correlation with an oral examination. Friedman et al. (1978) found no correlation between subscores on the simulation and National Board scores, final examinations, or ward performance. Similarly, Schumacher and Burg (1975) found only a low correlation with an oral examination score, and Skakun et al. (1977) showed no correlation between performance on the computer and global ratings of performance.

The uniformly low relationship between performance on computer simulations and these measures is difficult to interpret. To the extent that the computer simulation is assessing clinical problem-solving skills, it may be a better measure of such skills than the criterion against which it is compared. And regardless of how accurately the computer simulation represents a clinical encounter, the reliability of performance across problems is so low (e.g., Friedman et al., 1978) that any comparison based on a limited number of problems is severely constrained.

The question of validity reduces to the question of the extent to which an individual's interaction with the computer reflects his performance if he were presented with a similar problem in the actual clinical setting. Although many authors allude to such a comparison, in nearly all cases the comparison is made on the basis of face validity, that is, whether the available options look reasonable. Friedman et al. (1977) did compare performance to a chart review of 20 patients with the same diagnosis. Their conclusion was that "the comparison showed a definite similarity in tests ordered." Since no data were presented, it is left to the reader to guess how similar the similarity was.

De Dombal et al. (1971) compared performance on a computer simulation to an oral examination and a card problem. They found that the number of questions asked on the computer was slightly less than in the oral exam format. In another study (Leaper et al., 1973), the investigators reported a significant difference in the same direction between the computer simulation and actual ward performance. They substantiated these data with the comment: "... the clinician's behavior under simulated conditions was totally different from that in real life. Particularly noteworthy is the way in which clinicians who in real life conducted adaptive interviews ... showed none of these attributes when under simulated conditions" (p. 572). Feightner and Norman (1978) used a sample of residents completing two problems each—one in the CASE computer format and the second as a live simulated patient. They found substantial differences in history taking and physical examination, with residents asking nearly twice as many questions in the simulated patient format. This effect is the converse of what is observed in written patient management problems and remains to be explained. Diagnosis, investigations, and management were, however, comparable in the two groups.

No clear conclusions regarding the validity of computer simulations are possible. The evidence is sparse and contradictory and suffers from the chronic problem in clinical competence assessment of lack of an accepted criterion. In any case, because computer simulation can run the gamut from a simple presentation of a series of multiple-choice questions at a video terminal to a conversant "talking telephone" (Friedman et al., 1978) or a lifelike mannequin (Abrahamson et al., 1969), any generalization may be inappropriate. On the other hand, the validity of a particular computer simulation is not an unanswerable question. It is incumbent on the developers of any simulation, having expended considerable resources to develop and test the software, to allocate sufficient funds and human resources to address the reliability and validity issues. The developments in computer simulation in the past two decades represent a remarkable technical achievement, but this has not been adequately matched by sound empirical research on which to base decisions for implementation.

Feasibility

It may be a reflection on our abilities as reviewers that the majority of articles we have located were published between 1970 and 1976. Alternatively, the paucity of recent articles may be a reflection of the feasibility of many of these demonstration projects. Feasibility reduces to two issues—cost and acceptability. The issue of acceptability will be addressed later in this section, but for the moment, let us examine the cost of initiating and maintaining a bank of computer simulations.

Most cost estimates cited in the literature are based on cost per student interaction and range from a low of 10¢ per session (in 1972 dollars) to a more reasonable estimate of $36-$60 per candidate for recertification in 1976. These estimates, however, frequently do not include the cost of development, estimated for one simulation as $20,000 (Diamond and Weiner, 1974). Further, the estimates are strongly contingent on a number of students using the simulation. In the only detailed cost analysis we found, Senior (1976) cited a cost per candidate for a nationwide testing system ranging from $1,000, based on a usage of one full day per year, to $82 for a use of 100 full days per year, for a total of 50,000 candidates per year. Clearly, in the development and application of computer simulations, there is an economy of scale which has implications for further development. If simulations are to continue, greater efforts must be made to write programmes in general languages such as FORTRAN in order to allow portability to other institutions and, thereby, distribute development costs. Furthermore, the most straightforward way to reduce the cost per session is to increase the number of users, an objective which can be best achieved by overcoming some of the traditional limitations of acceptability.

Friedman and Gustafson (1977) enumerated several impediments to a more universal application of computers in medicine, four of which are relevant to the present subject. The first one is the failure to accomplish a successful interaction with the computer, and there are six main reasons for this:

1. Many computer terminals have been poorly engineered, resulting in mechanical breakdowns.
2. The computer terminals have often been placed in out-of-the-way places making them inconvenient to operate.
3. The computer response time often has been quite slow because of low-speed teletype output or excessive delay between responses.
4. In order to obtain information from the computer the physician has often been required to take part in a long and complicated technical dialogue.
5. The use of computers has often required knowledge of special passwords, codes, or computer language.
6. Computer terminals have been expensive, and this has made it difficult to develop accessible yet cost-effective applications.

Many of these difficulties have been overcome by recent developments in computer hardware, resulting in cheaper, easier communication with the computer. A second impediment, as we have indicated, is the absence of easy transfer from one institution to another. There is no standard language of medical computing. Third is the inability to prove a significant positive impact on patient care, and the lack of investigation on the cost effectiveness of computer systems. This may be explained by the relative isolation in which computer researchers function. Finally, Friedman concludes that we have not learned from pervious mistakes. As a result of the rush to publish, the majority of projects in the area of computer application to medicine subsequently prove to be impractical, too expensive, or unacceptable. He sent a questionnaire to 52 authors of computer programmes applied to medicine. For 51 percent the work had been abandoned or temporarily stalled. In only 19 percent of the projects was the programme now in routine use at their medical center. The authors of the majority of the projects (63 percent) felt the work had lived up to their initial expectations, yet over 41 percent of these projects are now unfunded and only 18 percent were funded out of patients' fees or hospital funds. In almost every case where the project had been abandoned, the researchers indicated that this had occurred because the project never became cost effective.

Educational Considerations

As we have pointed out, some of the computer simulations surveyed in the present chapter are intended for use in a learning setting at the undergraduate, residency, or continuing education level. In view of this intent, it is surprising that very few researchers have attempted to determine whether the computer simulation is an effective device for learning. Abrahamson et al. (1969) evaluated the SIM-1 mannequin for anesthesiology skills using a randomized trial with proficiency in the clinical setting assessed by chart review as the measure of learning gain. Residents using the simulator achieved proficiency in significantly less time than control residents. However, the study can be faulted on two grounds—the sample size was very small (five per group) and no conventional training was given to the control residents.

De Dombal et al. (1971) used a before-after design to assess diagnostic accuracy following introduction of a Bayesian computer program in a gastroenterology clinic. They found a significant increase in accuracy following introduction of the computer. The learning gain was not sustained, however, and three months after the computer programme experiment was terminated, accuracy had returned to baseline levels. These authors (de Dombal et al., 1972) also examined the learning of students in an experimental design comparing simulation with instruction to a traditional course of instruction. Two forms of simulation exercise were used—computer simulation and card problems. Short-term retention of knowledge was equal in all groups; however, diagnostic ability was enhanced in the two experimental groups. No detectable difference was present between the two simulation groups who used computer and card problems.

To summarize, computer simulations have certain advantages for instructional purposes. Learning can be based on patient problems, and can be a result of active inquiry by the learner. Instruction can be highly individualized, yet large numbers of learners can be accommodated at little additional cost. Whether computer simulation can result in enhanced learning compared to other forms of simulation is, as yet, an unanswered question, although the de Dombal et al. (1972) results suggest that there may be no difference. The technology of computer simulation can be a double-edged sword, however. Although fascination with the hardware may provide a stimulus for learning, difficulties encountered in the course of a computer interaction, such as necessity for typing of responses, slow response times, inadequate or incorrect responses, and the necessity for at least some familiarity with the computer system, may ultimately "turn off" many students. Further, the cost of developing and maintaining hardware and software may become prohibitive, particularly if the computer possesses no advantages in learning gain over written or card problems.

In light of the complex issues surrounding the role of computer simulation in learning, and in face of an inevitable expansion of such projects as the hardware becomes more versatile and less expensive, it would be reassuring to have some clear indication that computer simulation has advantages over conventional instruction in learning effectiveness. At the present time, such evidence is lacking.

Conclusions

Whenever introduced a new technologic advance has been initially rejected or feared: rejected because of the belief that it could not work as well as existing devices; feared because of the suspicion that it might [Feinstein, 1967, p. 354].

The appearance of computer simulation of patient problems was a natural evolution of the teaching machines introduced in the 1950s. In medical education, computer simulations are an attempt to answer the needs for new methods of learning that are problem based, individualized, and adapted to the skills of the student and for new methods of evaluation of clinical competence. For many clinicians involved in teaching and evaluation, the computer is a luxurious toy that their faculty has not the financial resources to afford, and many of them are convinced that are problem based, individualized, and adapted to the skills evaluation. On the other side, with the growing dissemination of the computer, some think that they should use its potential and they pursue their efforts to develop a system that will be acceptable to clinicians and useful for teaching or evaluation purposes.

The area of computer simulation as a learning and evaluation tool is dependent on future developments which maximize the technical potential of the hardware and adequately investigate the measurement properties of the instrument. It is encouraging that most of the studies confirmed a positive attitude toward the computer, but much work needs to be done before computer simulations have a confirmed role in the evaluation of clinical competence.

References

Abrahamson, S., Denson, J. S., Wolf, R. M.: Effectiveness of a simulator in training anesthesiology residents. J Med Educ 44, 515-518 (1969).

Brigham, C. R., Kamp, M.: The current status of computer assisted intruction in the health sciences. J Med Educ 49, 270-279 (1974).

de Dombal, F. T.: A computer aided system for learning clinical diagnosis. Lancet 1, 145-148 (1969).

de Dombal, F. T., Horrocks, J. C., Stuniland, J. R., Gill, P. W.: Simulation of clinical diagnosis: a comparative study. Brit Med J 2, 575-577 (1971).

de Dombal, F. T., Smith, R. B., Modgil, V. K., Leaper, D. J.: Simulation of the diagnostic process: a further comparison. Brit J Med Educ 6, 238-245 (1972).

Diamond, H. S., Weiner, M.: A computer assisted instructional course in diagnosis and treatment of the rheumatic diseases. Arthritis Rheum 17, 1049-1054 (1974).

Dickinson, C. J.: A digital computer model to teach and study gas transport and exchange between lungs blood and tissue (MACPUFF). J Physiol 224, 7-9 (1972).

Dickinson, C. J. Shephard, P.: A digital computer model of the systemic circulation and kidney (MACPEE). J Physiol 216, 11-12 (1971).

Dickinson, C. J., Goldsmith, C. E., Sackett, D. L.: MACMAN: A digital computer model for teaching some basic principles of hemodynamics. J Clin Computing 2, 42-50 (1973).

Feightner, J. W., Norman, G. R.: Computer based problems as a measure of the problem-solving process—some concerns about validity. Proceedings, 17th Annual Conference on Research in Medical Education, New Orleans, La (1978).

Feinstein, A. R: Clinical judgment. Huntington, N.Y.: Williams & Wilkins (1967), pp. 354, 365.

Fincham, S. M., Grace, M., Taylor, W. C., Skakun, E. N., Davis, F. C.: Pediatrics candidates' attitudes to computerized patient management problems in a certifying examination. Med Educ 10, 404-407 (1976).

Friedman, R. B.: A computer program for simulating the patient-physician encounter. J Med Educ 48, 92 (1973).

Friedman, R. B., et al.: A simulated patient-physician encounter using a talking computer. JAMA 238, 1927-1929 (1977).

Friedman, R. B., Gustafson, D. H.: Computers in clinical medicine—a critical review. Comput Biomed Res 10, 199-204 (1977).

Freidman, R. B., et al.: Experience with the simulated patient-physician encounter. J Med Educ 53, 825-830 (1978).

Gorry, G. A., Barnett, G. O.: Experience with a model of sequential diagnosis. Comput Biomed Res 1, 490-507 (1968).

Harless, W. G., et al.: CASE: a computer-assisted simulation of the clinical encounter. J Med Educ 46, 443-448 (1971).

Hoffer, E. P.: Experience with the use of computer simulation models in medical education. Comput Biomed Res 3, 269-279 (1973).

Hoffer, E. P.: Computer aided instruction in community hospital emergency departments: a pilot project. J Med Educ 50, 84-86 (1975).

Johnson, P. E., Muller, J. H.: Analysis of expert diagnosis of a computer simulation of congenital heart disease. J Med Educ 50, 466-470 (1975).

Leaper, D. J., et al.: Clinical diagnostic process: an analysis. Brit Med J 3, 569-574 (1973).

Marshall, J.: Assessment of problem-solving ability. Med Educ 11, 329-334 (1977).

Norman, G. R., Feightner, J. W.: A comparison of behavior on simulated patients and patient management problems. Med Educ 15, 26-32 (1981).

Page, G. G., Fielding, D. W.: Performance on PMP's and performance in practice: Are they related? J Med Educ 55, 529-537 (1980).

Schneiderman, H., Muller, R. L.: The diagnosis game; a computer based exercise in clinical problem-solving. JAMA 219, 333-335 (1972).

Schumacher, C. F., Burg, F. D.: Computerization of a patient management problem to prevent retracing. Brit J Med Educ 9, 281-285 (1975).

Senior, J. R.: Toward the measurement of competence in medicine. Philadelphia: American Board of Internal Medicine (1976).

Skakun, E. N., Taylor, W. C., Wilson, D. R.: A follow-up study of the computerized patient management problem examination in pediatrics. Proceedings, Medinfo '77. Amsterdam, North-Holland (1977).

Taylor, W. C., Grace, M., Taylor, T. R., Finchman, S. M., Skakun, E. N.: The use of computerized patient management problems in a certifying examination. Med Educ 10, 179-182 (1976).

Warner, H. R., Rutherford, B. D., Houtchens, B.: A sequential Bayesian approach to history-taking and diagnosis. Comput Biomed Res 5, 256-262 (1972).

Webster, G. D., Langdon, L. O., Meskauskas, J. A., Narcini, J. J.: Results of a national study of a computer simulation and American Board of Internal Medicine's recertification examination: The MERIT project. Proceedings, 18th Annual Conference on Research in Medical Education, Washington, D.C. (1979).

Weinstein, M. C., Fineberg, H. Z.: Clinical decision analysis. Philadelphia: W. B. Saunders (1980).

Zemper, E. D.: Computer assisted instruction in medical education. East Lansing, Mich.: OMERAD Monograph (1973).

CHAPTER 11

Simulated Patients

GEOFFREY R. NORMAN
HOWARD S. BARROWS
GAYLE GLIVA
CHRISTEL WOODWARD

Simulation is a useful educational tool whenever a complex psychomotor task is to be learned and evaluated and the use of the real task setting is either not satisfactory from an educational standpoint, too expensive to use in teaching, or too risky. The playing of a musical instrument is a complex psychomotor task, yet simulators of musical instruments are rarely necessary. By contrast, aircraft cockpit, diesel locomotive, and space vehicle simulators are necessary to allow students to slowly develop mastery of the complex psychomotor tasks required for the operation of these vehicles in real life situations.

Similar considerations have led to increasing use of simulated patients in medical education for both teaching and evaluation (Barrows, 1968, 1971; Barrows and Tamblyn, 1980). "Simulated" patients is only one term used to describe individuals trained to portray the history, physical findings, and affect of an actual patient; they have also been called "programmed" patients, "pseudo" patients, "surrogate" patients, and "standardized" patients. Other methods have been labeled with similar terms; for example, patient management problems are often called "Clinical Simulations," and Maatsch (1980) has referred to a highly structured oral examination by the acronym SPE, for Simulated Patient Encounter.

The simulated patient technique has several potential advantages over the use of real patients: (1) the choice of an appropriate problem for teaching or evaluation is not dictated by the availability of such a patient in clinics or wards; (2) there are no ethical problems associated with the repeated examination of simulated patients or the examination of patients by junior students; (3) the interview and examination of the patient can be interrupted to maximize educational effect without problems of disclosure; (4) for evaluation, different students can be presented with an identical challenge, reducing one source of unreliability. Although some of these advantages are possessed by all forms of simulation, the simulated patient has perhaps the greatest face validity—i.e., is closest to the actual clinical setting.

In contrast to the other evaluation methods reviewed in this section, the simulated patient is not a method per se; rather, it is one component of a number of possible methods. For example, if evaluation is based on observation of the student with a simulated patient, the issues regarding reliability of direct observation methods are relevant. The simulated patient has been used to provide feedback on interpersonal skills (Maguire et al., 1978), for which some of the methods described in the next chapter are relevant. The simulated patient could be used in an attempt to standardize the traditional clinical oral examination by standardizing the stimulus situation presented to candidates, a method similar to those used by the College of Family Physicians of Canada (Lamont and Hennen, 1972). Finally, simulated patients have been introduced unknown into physicians' practices to assess quality of care by documentation, after the encounter, of which procedures were and were not done (Burri et al., 1976; Renaud et al., 1980).

As a result, the usual criteria of an evaluation method are relevant only in part to the use of simulated patients and, in part, to the evaluation method applied to the simulated patient encounter. The specific interpretation of the criteria will be discussed in later sections. For the moment, it is important to clarify what is meant by the term *simulated patient*.

Training of Simulated Patients

The training of a simulated patient is based on a case protocol developed from an actual patient. The clinician (physician, nurse, social worker, etc.) who worked with the actual patient being simulated either trains the simulated patient directly or acts as a resource to another trainer in the training sessions. The techniques employed in the training are aimed at helping the simulators actually take on the real patient problem as a believable self-role. They are encouraged, through a variety of techniques, to feel as if the patient's problems are their own.

Problems in a number of fields have been simulated: psychiatry, neurology, medicine, orthopedics, surgery, family medicine, psychosocial medicine, and so on, and an impressive array of physical findings have been simulated. Although it is not possible to simulate all physical findings (for example, wounds or fractures, heart sounds, edema, muscle wasting), a large number of physical findings have been accurately simulated. In addition, many medical conditions present with significant histories, which demand a careful or probing physical examination, although there may actually be no physical signs. Enough can be presented in the way of physical findings that a wide range of problems in many disciplines can be simulated.

Although the involvement of clinicians in training may appear expensive, experience indicates that it takes about three one-hour sessions to train a person who has never been a simulated patient for the first simulation. After this, the experienced simulator can take on additional patient roles in usually less than one hour. The training usually incorporates a few practice encounters in which the patient is examined by another clinician unfamiliar with the case, and errors or inconsistencies are eliminated.

Measurement Criteria

Credibility

Perhaps because the simulated patient possesses very high face validity or credibility, there is a paucity of studies of other measurement aspects of simulated patients. In contrast to many other methods, however, the high credibility of the simulated patient is supported by empirical evidence. In three studies (Burri et al., 1976; Reynaud et al., 1980; Owen and Winkler, 1974), simulated patients were introduced into primary physicians' offices unknown to the physician. None of the simulated patients was detected. Norman and Tugwell (1982), in a study designed specifically to assess the validity of simulated patients, asked residents to examine a total of eight patients, of which four were real patients and four were simulated patients programmed from the case histories of the real patients. Although residents performed better than chance in identifying real and simulated patients, 33 percent of the patients were incorrectly classified.

Comprehensiveness

Ostrow (1980) states that he believes "that surrogate [simulated] patients alone have the flexibility to be useful in the simulation and teaching of virtually all aspects of the doctor-patient encounter" (p. 84). In comparison to other types of simulations such as written or computer problems, the simulated patient has the potential to assess more areas, ranging from interpersonal skills to use of laboratory tests. There are some limits to the comprehensiveness of simulated patients, however, in addition to the limits already described, in the types of conditions that can be simulated.

There is also a limit to the range of skills capable of assessment by simulated patients. The simulated patient has been used to great advantage in two areas—the initial diagnostic workup of a new patient and the teaching of physical examination. It is clearly inappropriate to assess many invasive technical skills, from venipuncture to surgical skills, using simulated patients. Also, the long-term management of a hospitalized patient, although potentially suitable for simulation, is probably more appropriately assessed using observations in a clinical ward setting or perhaps computer simulations such as those developed by Friedman et al. (1978) that are specifically designed for these circumstances. Finally, those skills that are brought to bear after the initial encounter—laboratory use, management, follow-up—although capable of assessment using simulated patients, may be more efficiently assessed using some other approach, since the high fidelity of the patient encounter is not particularly relevant.

Precision

The precision of simulated patients is not amenable to the usual techniques for assessment of reliability, since precision, in this context, refers to the degree to which an individual trained to simulate a clinical problem presents a consistent picture from one encounter to the next. Although most users of simulated patients have the impression that the performances of well-trained simulated patients are consistent and periodic review is a necessary feature of maintaining a simulated patient, no studies have been reported that examine the consistency of performance. Because the clinical encounter is a human interaction, it would be unreasonable to expect, or strive for, complete consistency across encounters. Further, the question of precision involves a judgment of how much variability is a product of the different styles of the clinicians and how much represents real inconsistency in the performance of the patient. The occasion does arise in which a simulated patient will forget some feature of the problem or inaccurately simulate some physical finding, but it would appear that this is a relatively infrequent occurrence.

Validity

It is only recently that studies have been conducted to examine the concurrent validity of simulated patients. The early studies, indicating that physicians cannot reliably distinguish between simulated and real patients, provide some indication that they may well perform in a similar manner with the two types of patients. But only two studies have directly addressed this question of performance with real and simulated patients.

Sanson-Fisher and Poole (1980) used both simulated and real patients in a course on interpersonal skills, involving a total of 40 medical students. Each student conducted an interview with two patients; students were randomized into four groups. Group 1 saw both real patients; group 2, a simulated then a real patient; group 3, a real then a simulated patient; and group 4, both simulated. There was no control over the content of the patient problems and each patient (real or simulated) had a different problem. Students were aware that some patients were of each type, but they were not identified *a priori*. The dependent variable was a blind rating of level of empathy, using a validated rating scale with high reliability. Among several comparisons between real and simulated patients, no differences in the average empathy rating emerged. The results are encouraging, since the concern is frequently raised that students may not exhibit the same empathy to someone simulating a problem. However, the differing content of the problem may contribute some variability, which may decrease the power of the study to detect any differences.

Norman and Tugwell (1982) attempted to control for content in a study designed to assess the concurrent validity of simulated patients. Ten residents in family medicine and internal medicine each interviewed and examined eight patients in two half-day sessions. Four were real patients with chronic stable conditions and four were healthy individuals trained from the real patient protocols. No differences emerged in the number of questions asked, the number of physical examinations performed, the likelihood of arriving at the correct diagnosis and the number and type of laboratory tests ordered. The researchers did find that for one problem, residents elicited significantly more critical data from the simulated patient. On detailed examination, it emerged that the real patient suffered from a neurological condition, manifested in part by loss of memory and she repeatedly forgot to mention significant details of past medical history. The simulated patient was trained from a protocol containing the actual medical history rather than only the history recalled by the patient. This study, controlling for content, lends support to the concurrent validity of simulated patients, despite the one minor difference which emerged.

On the basis of these two studies, it can be concluded that the simulated patient is an accurate and valid representation of an actual patient, in circumstances in which the clinician is unaware that the condition is being simulated. But many situations in which simulated patients are used involve prior knowledge that the patient is simulated and frequently involve other intrusions on the normal setting, such as videotape, one-way glass, and observers. In these circumstances, the knowledge that the patient is simulated is one of many factors which may lead to "audience" or "reactivity" effects. The origin and magnitude of these effects are discussed in Chapter 4. It remains to be shown whether there is a measurable bias resulting from the known simulated patient which can be distinguished from the other potential sources of bias in this situation.

Educational Effect

In contrast to some of the other evaluation methods reviewed in this section, the educational effect of simulated patients has been extensively studied. Teaching by simulated patients has been compared to a variety of other educational techniques for interviewing skills and diagnostic thinking, interpersonal skills (de Dombal et al., 1972; Engel and Resnik, 1976; Helfer et al., 1975; Maguire et al., 1977), physical examination skills (Fraser and Miller, 1977; Tinning, 1975), and pelvic examination skills (Godkins, 1974; Johnson et al., 1975; Kerr, 1977; Livingstone and Ostrow, 1978). In particular, teaching using simulated patients has been contrasted to teaching with real patients in several studies (Helfer et al., 1975; Holzman et al., 1977; Johnson et al., 1975, 1976; Livingstone and Ostrow, 1978; Maguire et al., 1977; Tinning, 1975). A uniform finding has been that students taught with a simulated patient performed better on a variety of measures than students in the comparison groups. Measures used in these studies include student satisfaction with the course, student confidence, interviewing skills, general and specific (e.g., neurological examination, pelvic examination) physical examination skills, and patient satisfaction.

Based on these results, it is reasonable to conclude that simulated patients can have a significant role in clinical teaching. They can lead to a reduction in faculty teaching load because, as in many of the studies cited, the simulated patient can serve the three roles of instructor, subject, and evaluator, while improving the quality of instruction (Stillman et al., 1980).

Effect on Patients

One impetus for the use of simulated patients is the detrimental effect of repeated examinations on real patients. It is reasonable to question, however, whether the repeated demands of simulating a complex and personal role may have personal repercussions for individuals trained as simulated patients. One study (Naftulin and Andrew, 1975) addressed this question by comparing a sample of nine simulated patients and a sample of nine Hollywood actors, presumably selected on the basis that the actors were normal. Each subject was interviewed by one of the authors (presumably not blind) to elicit physical and/or emotional problems, and each subject completed an MMPI, which was interpreted blind by a clinical psychologist. No differences between the groups on either measure were detected, providing some reassurance that simulating does not have serious personal consequences. In view of the small sample size, however, the unusual comparison group, and the possible bias of the interviewer, these results cannot be viewed as definitive.

Applications of Simulated Patients

Simulated patients have been used in all areas of medical education, from teaching interviewing skills in the first undergraduate year to assessment of quality of care in the practice setting. They have been used in formative and summative evaluation in undergraduate medical education at McMaster University (Harper et al., 1983; Wakefield, et al., 1972). In the Harper study, all 100 students in a class were evaluated prior to entering the clinical clerkship, using a total of seven simulated patients all presenting the same problem. The Wakefield study was based on evaluation of all residents entering the residency programs at McMaster in a single year.

The College of Family Physicians of Canada have used simulated patients as a major component of the certification examination for more than a decade (Lamont and Hennen, 1972). Simulated patient encounters are observed by certified physicians and scored using evaluation forms incorporating features specific to each case as well as overall ratings.

Finally, two ambitious studies have used simulated patients, introduced incognito into physician practices, to assess quality of care. Renaud et al. (1980) have used a team of simulated patients (simulating a case of tension headache) to examine whether there are differences in medical management of physicians working in Quebec government health centers (CLSCs) and private group practice clinics in the Montreal area. The measure was not used to judge the general adequacy of a physician's care, but rather to ascertain whether adequacy of care for this problem (tension headache for three years with one-year history of daily diazepam usage) varied as a function of type of ambulatory care setting.

Owen and Winkler (1974) reported that simulated patients (portrayed by five women and five men) trained to portray a patient suffering from depression of psychosocial origin were entered into the practices of 25 randomly selected Australian general practitioners so that each doctor saw one woman and one man. In none of the 50 cases did the general practitioner recognize or suspect that the person was a normal person playing a role. Whether the physicians were told that the simulated patient would enter or had entered their practices is not clear, but it appears that the physicians remained unaware that they had participated in this study. All simulated patients were debriefed after each encounter and asked a series of standard questions about the length and content of the visit.

Conclusions

Since their invention over a decade ago, simulated patients have achieved a role in the armamentarium of educational evaluation. In contrast to the complexity of alternatives such as computer simulations or the austerity of multiple-choice tests, simulated patients possess high face validity; they are nearly indistinguishable from real patients. In addition, the cost of development of simulated patients is relatively low. A new simulated patient can be trained to high fidelity in one to three hours for less than the cost of developing a paper or computer simulation. Because of their capability to accurately portray nearly all aspects of a clinical encounter, along with their potential for educational intervention in the learning setting, simulated patients have found the most widespread application in instruction of various components of clinical skills and formative evaluation during training programs. Simulated patients, also because of their accurate representation of an actual patient, are unique in their capability to introduce a standardized, yet unobtrusive, stimulus into the actual practice setting for evaluation of quality of care.

In light of these apparent advantages, simulated patients have been relatively infrequently applied to routine clinical evaluation in the undergraduate and postgraduate years. One possible reason for this paradox may be that the major strength of simulated patients, their face validity, can also represent a liability. Student evaluation using simulated patients, because it is derived from the unstructured encounter between patient and physician, requires subjective judgments of competence and cannot be scored by machine. And these judgments are frequently made by a physician-observer, with a resulting heavy investment of faculty time. Such subjective ratings are also plagued by reliability problems, as described in Chapter 4.

Before the measurement problems inherent in subjective ratings can be resolved, more fundamental research to delineate the critical components of clinical competence will be needed. Assuming such variables can be identified and reliable measures of these dimensions developed, the use of simulated patients should be made more straightforward and economical. They remain virtually the only simulation device in medical education about which the substantive question of concurrent validity has been adequately addressed.

References

Barrows, H. S.: Simulated patients in medical teaching. Can Med Assoc J 98, 674-677 (1968).

Barrows, H. S.: Simulated patients (programmed patients). Springfield, Ill.: Charles C. Thomas (1971).

Barrows, H. S., Tamblyn, R. M.: Problem-based learning: an approach to medical education. New York: Springer Publishing (1980).

Burri, A., et al.: Using simulated patients to evaluate practicing physicians in a community. Proceedings, 15th Annual Conference on Research in Medical Education, San Francisco, Calif. (1976).

de Dombal, S. T., Smith, R. B., Woodgill, V. K., Leaper, D. J.: The simulation of the diagnostic process: a further comparison. Brit J Med Educ 6, 238-245 (1972).

Engel, I., Resnik, T. J.: The use of programmed patients and videotape in teaching medical students to take a sexual history. J Med Educ 51, 425-427 (1976).

Fraser, N. B., Miller, R. H.: Training practical instructors (programme patients) to teach basic physical examination. J Med Educ 52, 149-151 (1977).

Friedman, R., et al.: Experience with the simulated patient-physician encounter. J Med Educ 53, 825-830 (1978).

Godkins, T.: Utilization of simulated patients to teach the "routine" pelvic examination. J Med Educ 49, 1174-1178 (1974).

Harper, A. C., et al.: Methodological difficulties in clinical skills evaluation. Med Educ 17, 24-27 (1983).

Helfer, R. E., Black, M. A., Teitelbaum, H.: A comparison of pediatric interviewing skills using real and simulated mothers. Pediatrics 55, 397-400 (1975).

Holzman, G. B., Singleton, D., Holmes, T. F., Maatsch, J. L.: Initial pelvic examination instruction: the effectiveness of three contemporary approaches. Am J Obstet Gynecol 129, 124-129 (1977).

Johnson, C. F., Murchison, N., Reiter, S.: Sick infants versus simulated well-baby exam as an initial pediatric learning experience. J Med Educ 51, 1021-1023 (1976).

Johnson, G. H., Brown, T. C., Stenchever, M. A., Gabert, H. A., Poulson, A. M., Warenski, J. C.: Teaching pelvic examination to second year medical students using programmed patients. J Obstet Gynecol 121, 714-717 (1975).

Kerr, M.: Simulated patients as a learning resource in the study of reproductive medicine. Med Educ 11, 374-376 (1977).

Lamont, C. T., Hennen, B. K.: The use of simulated patients in a certification examination in family medicine. J Med Educ 47, 789 (1972).

Livingstone, R., Ostrow, D. N.: Professional patient-instructors in the teaching of the pelvic examination. Am J Obstet Gynecol 132, 54-57 (1978).

Maatsch, J.: Model for a criterion referenced medical specialty test. Final Report on Grant HS-02038-02. East Lansing, Michigan (1980).

Maguire, G. P., Clerke, D., Jolley, B.: An experimental comparison of three courses in history-taking skills for medical students. Med Educ 11, 175-182 (1977).

Maguire, G. P., et al.: The value of feedback in teaching interviewing skills to medical students. Psychol Med 8, 695 (1978).

Naftulin, D. H., Andrew, B. J.: The effects of patient simulations on actors. J Med Educ 50, 87-89 (1975).

Norman, G., Tugwell, P.: A comparison of resident performance on real and simulated patients. J Med Educ 57, 708-715 (1982).

Ostrow, D. N.: Surrogate patients in medical education. Programmed Learning Educ Tech 17, 82-89 (1980).

Owen, A., Winkler, R.: General practitioners and psychosocial problems: an evaluation using pseudopatients. Med J Aust 2, 393-398 (1974).

Renaud, M., et al.: Practice settings and prescribing profiles; the simulation of tension headaches to general practitioners working in different practice settings in the Montreal area. Am J Public Health 70, 1068-1073 (1980).

Sanson-Fisher, R. W., Poole, A. D.: Simulated patients and the assessment of medical students' interpersonal skills. Med Educ 14, 249-253 (1980).

Stillman, P., et al.: Patient instructors as teachers and evaluators. J Med Educ 55, 186-193 (1980).

Tinning, F. C.: Simulation in medical education. College of Osteopathic Medicine, Michigan State University (1975).

Wakefield, J. G., Pineo, G., Norman, G. R.: Experience with a single encounter assessment of clinical skills. Unpublished paper, Hamilton, Ontario (1972).

PART III

Applications

These three chapters are devoted to looking at the application of tools to special components of professional performance where it is likely that more than a single method is appropriate, or where major deficiencies in our present evaluation methods exist. These are the use of diagnostic tests, the assessment of technical proficiency, and the measurement of physician-patient interaction.

CHAPTER 12

Evaluation of the Doctor-Patient Relationship

CHRISTEL WOODWARD
BRIAN GERRARD

The doctor-patient relationship has been seen from antiquity as a crucial component of medicine that influences the quality of health care rendered (Engel, 1973; Hippocrates, 1923; Osler, 1904). The skill of maintaining rapport with a patient is an acknowledged prerequisite for the practice of clinical medicine and is a necessary component of patient management (Benjamin, 1969). Traditionally, the doctor-patient relationship was considered part of the "art of medicine" rather than the science of medicine. It was assumed that students could not be taught how to relate to patients and/or facilitate good doctor-patient relationships, and that these skills would be learned through role-modeling and experience. Similarly, since the quality of the doctor-patient relationship was seen as a consequence of the science of medicine, little attention was paid to measuring the quality of the relationship, which could be indirectly inferred by measuring the physician's diagnostic acumen and/or assessing the quality of the management plan or patient health outcomes.

Medicine has been increasingly criticized for the lack of attention physicians pay to the quality of the doctor-patient relationship (Mechanic, 1968; Reeder, 1972; Senate Report No. 94-887,

1976). Failure to ensure a good doctor-patient relationship has been implicated as a factor resulting in growing numbers of malpractice suits against physicians (Blum, 1960; Vaccarino, 1977). If the doctor-patient relationship is the keystone of medicine, why has it been neglected?

There is evidence that the trend toward impersonal treatment of patients was accelerated by the technical revolution in medicine (Wexler, 1976). Biomedical knowledge has expanded rapidly since the 1940s, and a vastly increased knowledge base is now needed to practice medicine. In our medical schools the educational program has primarily rewarded acquisition of this knowledge by students. Measurement of knowledge acquisition has outstripped assessment of other areas of clinical competence in the undergraduate curriculum. At the postgraduate level increased emphasis has been placed on developing excellence in using higher technology. The reward system within medicine has also given greater prestige and wealth to physicians who have mastered an impressive array of technical tools, helping to create large numbers of specialists and depleting the ranks of primary care physicians. It is alleged that the family doctor who knows his patients as individuals has become an endangered species in North America.

Conversely, the social reforms initiated in the 1960s have begun to reverse these trends in medical education (Benson, 1979; Cassell, 1976; Evans, 1964). The consumer movement has provided the impetus to greater accountability by the profession. In part because of an explosion of medical information in the media, physicians are facing better informed consumers than ever before. Concurrently, the population is aging, and more patients are suffering from chronic diseases that force them to take major responsibility for their own care by following special medical regimens, diets, and altered lifestyles. Medical schools have developed departments of Family Medicine and postgraduate training programs in this new discipline to meet perceived needs for greater continuity and caring in the delivery of medical services. Many have launched new programs to teach interpersonal skills to medical students (Kahn et al., 1979), and medical certifying boards are searching for better ways to evaluate candidates on those skills (Valberg and Firstbrook, 1977).

Empirical evidence is growing that the quality of the doctor-patient relationship may be related, not only to patient satisfaction, but also to compliance with medical regimens and health care outcomes (e.g., Hulka et al., 1976; Inui et al., 1970; Korsch, and Negrete, 1972; Liptak et al., 1977; Romm et al., 1976; Stone, 1979; Svarstad, 1976). Egbert et al. (1969) suggests that a positive doctor-patient relationship may decrease anxiety and promote recovery.

What constitutes the doctor-patient relationship? Sociologists, anthropologists, and psychiatrists have tried to describe the characteristics of the doctor-patient relationship in terms of the roles and responsibilities of the parties and various planes of interaction (Bloom, 1963; Ford et al., 1967; Fox, 1959; Freidson, 1961; King, 1962; Parsons, 1951). Yet these writers disagree about which role behaviors are appropriate, and measurement of these theoretical role constructs is difficult. Little is known regarding what kinds of role relationships occurring during an encounter are required to obtain desirable results (Stiles et al., 1979). Some writers have even suggested that the doctor's view of his role may be detrimental to a good doctor-patient relationship (e.g., Korsch and Negrete, 1972). The paucity of accumulated information on how this relationship operates is amazing, especially when compared with the information available on the biological aspects of disease.

Hess (1969) developed a working definition of skill in relating to patients by listing and classifying descriptions of the types of physician behaviors that are thought to be important to building patient understanding, trust, and compliance. The two major categories in this classification were (1) interpersonal skills (behaviors particularly important to patient acceptance of the doctor); and (2) communication skills (behaviors particularly important to information flow). Interpersonal skills is an umbrella term, however, comprising numerous quite separate skills. The teaching of facilitative skills such as empathy, warmth, and respect have been incorporated into teaching programs in medical schools (Kahn et al., 1979). Additional interpersonal skills important to effective doctor-patient relationships include concreteness—the ability to be specific in terms of the patient's level of understanding (Carkhuff et al., 1969); assertiveness skills such as refusal skills and constructive confrontation skills; and coping skills such as cognitive restructuring skills and stress management skills. These components of interpersonal skills have been carefully described and labeled only in the past 20 years (Carkhuff, 1969; Carkhuff and Berenson, 1967; Truax and Mitchel, 1971).

As Hess (1969) suggests, good communication is another hallmark of an effective doctor-patient relationship. The quality of communication may be examined in a variety of ways. The structure of communication (length of speech, silences, interruptions) can be dissected. The process of communication (style, clarity, content of language; attention paid to nonverbal cues) can be examined and, more importantly, the effects of communication can be assessed. The quality of communication between doctor and patient affects the degree to which the physician understands the patient's reasons for seeking medical care, the patient's expectations and perception of his illness (Korsch and Negrete, 1972), and the extent to which knowledge about his illness is imparted and understood by the patient. Communication also affects the patient's motivation and skills to adhere to the treatment regimen prescribed (Hulka et al., 1976), his willingness to return for subsequent visits (Korsch and Negrete, 1972), and his satisfaction with medical care (Aday and Anderson, 1975; Ware et al., 1978).

The doctor-patient relationship may also be influenced by physical arrangements. The availability of the physician as measured by length of waiting time and coverage received during "off" hours; his accessibility as measured by location of practice and cost of services; and the comfort afforded in his office, for example, by pleasant surroundings and privacy, may influence patient satisfaction with physician services.

Finally, the technical skills of the physician also impinge on the doctor-patient relationship. The physician's ability to accurately pinpoint the nature of the problem, to avoid unnecessary patient discomfort, to effect remission, stabilization, or cure of the medical condition, and to establish a regimen suited to the patient's lifestyle, all influence the patient's attitude vis-à-vis the doctor.

Assessment Methods

Numerous methods have been devised to assess aspects of the doctor-patient relationship. These assessment tools can be divided into five major categories: (1) measurement of specific physician attributes and attitudes seen as related to positive doctor-patient relationships; (2) assessment of the information base regarding skills and attitudes required for effective doctor-patient relationships; (3) measures of physician/student behavior in clinical encounters with patients or situations simulating patient encounters; (4) patient-based information regarding the doctor-patient relationship; and (5) measures of physician-patient agreement. No attempt is made to present an exhaustive review. Rather, measures were selected to illustrate the approaches currently taken. The measurement properties of these tests are summarized in Table 12.1.

Measurement of Physician/Student Attributes and Attitudes

Tests in this category assess general personality traits and attitudes, usually in the form of a pencil-and-paper self-report test. A number of personality tests have been used with medical students and physicians. Although the reliability and validity of these tests have been assessed for other populations, very little information is available on their use with medical students/physicians.

The Edwards Personal Preference Schedule (EPPS) is a self-report personality test containing 15 scales that measure the primary needs proposed by Henry Murray (Murray, 1938). Sullivan (1978) reported that the EPPS scales on which primary care physicians scored highest were achievement, dominance, and autonomy. An earlier study by Parker (1958) found that medical students scored high on endurance, nurturance, achievement, and deference. The EPPS scales that are theoretically most relevant to good physician-patient relationships are achievement, affiliation, intraception (understanding how others feel about problems), nurturance (treating others with kindness and sympathy), and endurance. The main advantages of the EPPS are that the majority of needs measured are interpersonal in nature, the needs are fairly low in social desirability (no obviously "correct" responses), and there is little overlap between scales.

The Personality Research Form (PRF) is a self-report personality test that also measures the needs identified by Murray (Jackson, 1967). It consists of fourteen scales, very similar to those on the EPPS. Parlow and Rothman (1974) found that compared to general arts students, first-year medical students scored high on achievement, endurance, order, nurturance, and understanding.

The Personal Orientation Inventory (POI) is a self-report that consists of 12 scales including inner-directedness, self-actualizing value, spontaneity, self-acceptance, feeling reactivity, self-regard, and capacity for intimate contact. The evidence for the construct validity of the POI with medical students is mixed. Robbins et al. (1979) found no differences in pre-to-post training scores on the POI for a group of medical students who received interpersonal skills training. Pascoe et al. (1976), however, found that medical

TABLE 12.1
A Comparison of Discrimination, Formulation, and Performance Tests on Selected Test Characteristics

Test	Empathy skills assessed	Warmth skills assessed	Initiating skills assessed	Assertiveness skills assessed	Reliability	Comprehensiveness	Concurrent validity	Construct validity
DISCRIMINATION TESTS								
Adler et al. (1968)			X			X		
Best et al. (1979)			X		X	X		X
Hopkins Interpersonal Skills Assessment (Grayson et al., 1977)	X		X			XX		X
Index of Facilitative Discrimination (Carkhuff, 1969)	X				XX			X
Physician-Patient Situation Test (Rasche et al., 1974)	X		X	X	XX	XX		X
Profile of Non-Verbal Sensitivity (Rosenthal et al., 1979)					X	XX	X	X
FORMULATION TESTS								
Affect Sensitivity Scale (Campbell et al., 1971)	X				X	X		X
Index of Communication (Carkhuff, 1969)	X				X		X	X
Response-to-Patient Inventory (Mathews, 1962)	X		X	X	XX	XX		X
Well's Empathic Communication Test (Pascoe et al., 1976)	X					XX		X
PERFORMANCE TESTS (RATING SCALES)								
Anderson et al., (1970)			X			X		
Brockway Medical Interview Checklist (Brockway, 1978)			X		X	X		X

TABLE 12.1 (cont.)

Test	Empathy skills assessed	Warmth skills assessed	Initiating skills assessed	Assertiveness skills assessed	Reliability	Comprehensiveness	Concurrent validity	Construct validity
PERFORMANCE TESTS (RATING SCALES) (*continued*)								
Carkhuff Rating Scale for Empathy (Carkhuff, 1969)	X				XX	X	X	X
Elements of Effective Communication (Kagan et al., 1967)	X	X	X		XX	XX		X
Interpersonal Relationship Rating Scale (Ryden, 1977)	X	X	X			XX	X	
Interview Evaluation Scale (Hollifield et al., 1957)			X		X	X		X
Queen's University Interviewer Rating Scale (Jarrett et al., 1972)			X		X	X		X
Truax Accurate Empathy Scale (Truax, 1961)	X				XX	X	X	X
PERFORMANCE TESTS (INTERACTION ANALYSIS)								
Behavioral Test of Interpersonal Skills for Health Professionals (Gerrard et al., 1980)	X	X	X	X	XX	XX	X	X
Helfer, 1970			X		XX	XX		
Hess, 1969	X	X	X	X	XX	XX	X	X
Interaction Process Analysis (Bales, 1950)		X	X	X	XX	X	X	X
Process Check Sheet (Hutter et al., 1977)	X		X		XX	X		X
Psychotherapy Interaction Scale (Adler & Enelow, 1966)		X	X	X	XX	XX		X
Verbal Response Mode Analysis (Stiles et al., 1979)			X		X	X		X

students who received interpersonal skills training scored significantly higher on existentiality, feeling reactivity, self-acceptance, and synergy than a control group. The main advantage of the POI is the theoretical relevance of most of its subscales to effective interpersonal relations. A concern is that the POI is subject to the effects of social desirability: the socially desirable response is obvious for most POI item pairs.

The Sixteen Personality Factor Test (16 PF) measures 16 personality dimensions (Cattell, 1965). Several dimensions are theoretically relevant to positive physician-patient relationships: outgoing, emotionally stable, assertive, trusting, placid, controlled, and relaxed. Stern et al. (1972) found that a composite profile on the 16 PF distinguished between medical and other types of students. Lipton et al. (1975) reports a number of significant correlations between medical students' scores on the 16 PF and both multiple-choice and essay examinations of clinical skills.

The Profile of Non-verbal Sensitivity (the PONS test) is a 45-minute 16-mm film test of a subject's ability to identify emotions communicated by actors in different nonverbal "channels": voice tone, facial expression, and body movement (Rosenthal et al., 1979). The PONS test has a reported average total test-retest reliability of 0.69 and an internal consistency reliability coefficient of 0.86 for the total test score. Test-retest reliabilities for subscores based on the different nonverbal channels, however, are all below 0.54. Evidence for concurrent validity comes from studies which have shown the PONS test to correlate significantly with other measures of sensitivity such as peer ratings. Construct validity has been examined by correlating PONS scores for physicians with patient satisfaction scores. DiMatteo and Taranta (1980) found a statistically significant correlation (r = 0.37, $p < 0.05$) between the PONS subscore for "body channel" and patient perception of the physician as a listening, caring, available person. In another study (Rosenthal et al., 1979) the authors found no significant difference in PONS scores between an experimental and a control group of physicians after the experimental group had received training in identifying nonverbal behavior. This may reflect the weakness of the experimental maneuver, however, rather than the absence of the construct validity of the PONS test.

The main advantage of attribute tests is their feasibility. They are usually paper-and-pencil tests that can be administered and scored with relative ease. Their main disadvantage is that there is little evidence for their validity with respect to positive physician-patient relationships.

*Assessment of the Information Base
Regarding Skills Required for an
Effective Doctor-Patient Relationship*

Tests in this category may be classified into two types: discrimination tests and formulation tests. The purpose of a discrimination test is to see whether the student can correctly identify the best response (out of several alternative responses that are provided) to a stimulus situation or correctly identify the most important behaviors, emotions, or dynamics involved in a stimulus situation. The purpose of a formulation test is to see whether the student can write down what he thinks is the best response to a patient statement. Discrimination tests and formulation tests consist of two parts: a standardized stimulus such as a film of a doctor interacting with a patient which is stopped at critical points, and a response format which is used to record the student's response to the stimulus materials.

Discrimination Tests. An example of a discrimination test is the Physician-Patient Situation Test (Rasche et al., 1974). This pencil-and-paper test presents 35 typical physician-patient incidents in which the stimulus is a typed comment made by the "patient." After each patient comment the student is asked to select one of five possible responses. The responses are divided into five categories (split-half reliabilities are shown in parentheses): evaluative (0.77), hostile (0.80), reassuring (0.74), probing (0.88), and understanding (0.92). The Physician-Patient Situation Test provides a comprehensive range of typical patient situations in the stimulus statements and assesses a variety of important interpersonal skills in the scoring system. Rasche et al. (1974) provide evidence for concurrent validity by comparing students' scores on the Physician-Patient Situation Test with scores (using the same five scoring categories) obtained by the students on actual patient interviews. This evidence is equivocal, however, because the authors failed to report any correlation coefficients and because the students assessed in actual interviews were a nonrandom subsample of the group administered the Physician-Patient Situation Test. Studies by Rasche et al. (1974) and Zisook et al. (1979) show that medical students' scores on the Physician-Patient Situation Test improve as a result of interpersonal skills training.

Jordan et al. (1980) have recently developed a discrimination test that consists of a series of typed doctor-patient vignettes. Subjects are asked to respond to each vignette by selecting the best response from several responses provided. This test has a reported internal consistency of 0.74. Construct validity was studied by correlating the discrimination test scores with scores on a number of cognitive, affective, and personality tests. Significant correlations were found between the discrimination test and the Personal Orientation Inventory, the Medical College Admissions Test, and Carkhuff ratings for Empathy and Congruence.

Formulation Tests. An example of a formulation test is Wells' Empathic Communication Test (WECT) (Pascoe et al., 1976). Ten brief videotaped excerpts from a woman role-playing a patient are used as the stimuli. After viewing each videotaped excerpt, the student writes down what he feels is a helpful response. The responses are later scored for empathy using the Carkhuff Rating Scale for Empathy (discussed below). A limitation of the WECT is that a limited range of stimulus statements are presented by only one person on the videotape. Pascoe et al. report 80 percent agreement between raters using the Carkhuff Empathy Scale with the WECT. Construct validity has been studied by examining the effects of empathy training on medical students' WECT scores as compared to WECT scores for a randomly selected control group. Pascoe et al. found that the experimental group was significantly more empathic than the control group after training.

An example of a multidimensional formulation test is the Response-to-Patient Inventory (Mathews, 1962). a pencil-and-paper test that consists of nine patient "statements." For three categories of patient statements (statements reflecting feelings of danger for one's survival, statements reflecting feelings of danger for one's self-esteem, and statements reflecting feelings of conflict over enforced dependency or submission), the student taking the test writes what he thinks is the most helpful response. Each response is classified as neutral, rule-centered, judgmental, threatening, person-positive, or person-centered (empathic). The test portrays a wide range of situations. An overall interrater agreement of 98 percent for the response categories is reported. Construct validity has been examined by correlating ratings of the administrative climate in hospitals with the person-centeredness scores of the nursing staff ($r = 0.94$). Although the Response-to-Patient Inventory was originally designed for use with nurses, the general nature of the stimulus situations make the test suitable for use with medical students and physicians.

The main advantage of the discrimination and formulation tests is feasibility. They can be administered and scored with relative ease and at low cost. Their main disadvantage is that although a student may have the ability to identify a correct response (discrimination test) or to formulate an effective response to use with a patient (formulation test), the student may not be able to actually *make* (e.g., say) the response in the actual situation (Carkhuff, 1969; Schwartz and Gottman, 1976). In fact Ware et al. (1971) showed an inverse relationship between knowledge of interviewing and performance. This potential discrepancy between knowledge of a correct response and ability to make a correct response is overcome by performance tests, which are discussed in the next section.

Measures of Physician/Student Behavior with Patients

Performance tests are tests that assess physician/student behavior (verbal and/or nonverbal responses) in actual patient interviews or in simulated patient interviews. Regardless of whether an actual patient or simulated patient is presented to the student, the student's actual *behavior* in response to the stimulus situation is measured. Performance tests are of two types: rating scales and interaction analysis.

The Truax Accurate Empathy Scale (Truax, 1961) is one of the most widely used rating scales for assessing empathy in clinical encounters. This nine-point rating scale can be used to rate interview segments (e.g., randomly selected one-minute segments on an audiotape of a physician-patient interview) or an overall interview. High interrater reliability in scoring has been reported (Sanson-Fisher and Poole, 1978, reporting an interrater agreement between 84 percent and 94 percent; Fine and Terrien, 1977, $r = 0.95$). Little validity research has been done on this scale with medical students or physicians. Fine and Terrien as well as Sanson-Fisher and Poole report that medical students show statistically significant gains in empathy scores following empathy training. In the counseling literature, the Carkhuff Rating Scale for Empathy (a five-point version of the Truax scale) is now the most widely used empathy rating scale.

Interaction analysis is a method for recording the frequency of accuracy of important interpersonal behaviors. One of the earliest and most widely used interaction analysis sytem has been Bales' Interaction Process Analysis or IPA (Bales, 1950). The IPA classification system is comprehensive and consists of four main categories, each of which is divided into three subcategories: (1) positive affect (friendliness, shows tension release, agreement);

(2) neutral statements (gives instructions, gives opinion, gives information); (3) neutral questions (asks for information, asks for opinion); (4) negative affect (disagrees, shows tension, shows antagonism). Each time a subject (physician or patient) demonstrates a behavior that fits into one of the 12 IPA categories, it is coded. At the end of the interview, physician and patient behaviors occurring in each behavior category are summed to obtain an interaction profile.

IPA reliability is quite good, with reported interrater agreement of 84 percent (Davis, 1971; Freeman et al., 1971). Freeman et al. (1971) and Davis (1971) have reported significant correlations among patient satisfaction, patient compliance, and several IPA categories.

Other researchers have modified Bales' IPA categories to make the interaction analysis systems more relevant to their particular populations. For example, the Psychotherapy Interaction (PIA) Scale was developed to assess psychotherapy interviews (Adler and Enelow, 1966). The PIA consists of 25 behavior categories grouped into three main areas: cognitive (e.g., confrontation, interpretation, agreement, disagreement); control (e.g., facilitation, question, counseling, suggestion); and affect expression (e.g, supportive, reassuring, happy, tense, anxious, depressed). Although the categories used in PIA are comprehensive, their focus tends to be psychiatric. Adler and Ware (1970) state that the PIA has high interrater reliability. They found that medical students who received programmed instruction in interviewing showed statistically significant changes in PIA categories in comparison with a group of medical students who received a traditional seminar-based interviewing course.

The Elements of Effective Communication rating scales developed by Kagan et al. (1967) are a part of a comprehensive "package" for the teaching and assessment of human relations skills. The scales assess four different dimensions of interpersonal behavior: affective vs. cognitive, exploratory vs. nonexploratory, listening vs. ignoring, and confronting vs. avoiding. A broad range of interpersonal skills are assessed. Interrater agreement is high (Robbins et al., 1979, $r = 0.77$; Werner and Schneider, 1974, interrater agreement = 80 percent). Robbins et al. found that training produced a statistically significant improvement on the affective scale, while Werner and Schneider found that training produced statistically significant changes on both the exploratory and the affective scales.

Verbal Response Mode Analysis is a method of interaction

analysis that classifies the verbal behavior of physicians and patients into eight categories (Stiles et al., 1979). Examples of the categories are question, interpretation, reflection, and advisement. An interrater agreement of 75 percent has been reported. Construct validity has been studied by correlating Verbal Response Mode Analysis scores of physicians with patient satisfaction ratings. Stiles et al. report correlations of 0.30 with patients' affective satisfaction and 0.31 with patients' cognitive satisfaction. A weakness of Verbal Response Mode Analysis is that it does not code nonverbal behavior.

The Behavioral Test of Interpersonal Skills for Health Professionals (BTIS) is a recently developed performance test that scores physician/student responses to a videotape of simulated patient and health professional vignettes (Gerrard and Buzzell, 1980). The test consists of 30 common patient and health professional situations that have been role-played by actors and recorded on videotape. There are 10 types of situations represented in the BTIS: commands, verbal attack, unreasonable request, crying, pain, anxiety, anger, happiness, affection, and performance evaluation. An important feature of the BTIS is the inclusion of health professional scenes which permit the assessment of team skills as well as interpersonal skills for dealing with patients. The subject whose skills are being assessed views each recorded problem situation on the videotape (e.g., a crying patient, a patient in pain, or an angry patient) and makes a verbal response as though he or she were interacting with a real person. Responses may be scored "live" or videotaped and scored later using rating scales for empathy, warmth, initiating, and assertiveness. The BTIS may also be scored for a corresponding set of 11 interaction analysis categories. Interrater reliabilities for these 11 categories range from 0.88 to 0.99. The effect of familiarity with the situations in the test on a second administration has been examined and none of the interaction scoring categories are influenced except the category Smile (i.e., subject responds with a warm smile). Concurrent validity was examined by comparing the BTIS scores for graduate nurses with peer and supervisor ratings. Significant correlations were found between 7 of 11 BTIS categories and relevant peer/supervisor ratings. Construct validity has also been examined. Differences in students at various levels of training have been shown as well as differences in students at the same level of training who have and have not received training in interpersonal skills (Gerrard, Boniface, and Love, 1980). The main advantage of the BTIS is that it is a stan-

dardized nonreactive performance test, especially suitable for pre-
and postassessment of interpersonal skills training.

Table 12.1 compares Discrimination, Formulation, and Performance Tests on the type of interpersonal skill assessed—empathy, warmth, initiating, and assertiveness (the rationale for regarding these four interpersonal skills as the most important ones
for health professionals is presented in Gerrard, Boniface, and
Love, 1980); reliability; comprehensiveness; concurrent validity
and construct validity. An "X" indicates the presence of the test
characteristic to an adequate degree. An "XX" indicates the test
characteristic is present to a superior degree.

Patient-based Information Regarding the Doctor-Patient Relationship

Assessment of the doctor-patient relationship through patient information has been gaining increased attention. Information is
sought through interviews and/or questionnaires about the quality
of the doctor-patient relationship and patient satisfaction with
the physician. Measures of agreement in perception between a
doctor and his or her patients have also been taken.

Information Provided by the Patient. Ware et al. (1978) have
suggested that the patient is the logical source of valuable data
on the health care he receives. Only patients experience all aspects
of the care provided and know how they react to it. These researchers published an interesting controlled study of the validity
of patients' reports on the art and technical quality of care. Four
videotaped doctor-patient encounters were constructed to ma-
nipulate two levels of technical quality (high, low) and two levels
of art of care (high, low). Over 100 volunteers viewed these tapes
and completed ratings of the encounter regarding the art of care,
technical quality and overall quality, using three ten-point rating
scales and ten items selected from the PSQ humaneness and technical quality rating scales. Questions regarding patient compliance,
willingness to return to the physician, and overall satisfaction
were also completed. In this study, "patients" could detect differences in the art and technical aspects of quality of care. These
differences had a substantial effect on patient satisfaction ratings
made, on stated intentions to comply with doctors' orders and to
return for another visit, and overall satisfaction with care. Ware
et al. concluded that the validity of patient satisfaction ratings as
reflections of real differences in the art and technical aspects of

quality of care was strongly supported by these findings. "Patient" ratings were more sensitive to differences in the art of care than to differences in technical quality, suggesting that patients are better able to discern differences in the affective component of the doctor-patient relationship than in a doctor's technical competence. The authors suggest replication of the study with a less educated population (mean educational attainment was college level for these volunteers) using direct observation of care and feedback in clinic settings. However, this study lends credibility to the use of patient-based information to evaluate the doctor-patient relationship.

A study of the doctor-patient relationship done by Korsch and her colleagues is considered a classic in the field. Korsch et al. (1968) used semistructured interviews of mothers of pediatric patients to elicit information regarding their perceptions of the doctor-patient relationship directly following a medical visit. These interviews were designed to obtain information concerning the patient's perceptions of her child's illness, her subjective experience with the illness, her expectations from the medical visit, her perceptions of the interaction with the physician, and the parent's satisfaction with the visit and the intent to follow through on medical advice. Korsch et al. found that mothers who saw their physicians as friendly, concerned and sympathetic, and willing to take the time and trouble to answer questions and explain the nature of the problem were much more likely to be satisfied with the services they received and comply with the medical regimen prescribed for their child.

Verbatim tape recording of the actual medical visit was used to allow later coding of this material and examination of its correspondence to interview data. The interview schedule used was pretested but no information regarding its reliability was available. (A shortened version of the interview schedule containing the questions that the authors found most informative and acceptable was presented in the literature: Korsch et al., 1968, p. 871). The interview schedule, constructed to meet the needs of this particular project, has not been adopted by other investigators, although the items employed have been useful models for others.

More recently Wolf et al. (1978) have reported development of a 26-item Likert-type scale to measure patients' evaluations of individual visits with physicians. The Medical Interview Satisfaction Scale (MISS) has three subscales (cognitive, affective, and behavioral). Included in the cognitive subscale are such items as "the doctor told me all I wanted to know about my illness." The affective subscale includes such items as "I felt really understood by my doctor"; "I felt free to talk to my doctor about private thoughts." Items from the behavioral subscale are "the doctor seemed rushed during his examination of me" and "this doctor was too rough when he examined me." Internal consistency of the scale, assessed using Cronbach's coefficient alpha, has been reported at 0.93 for the total scale and 0.87, 0.86, and 0.87 for the cognitive, affective, and behavioral subscales, respectively. Concurrent validity has been studied by correlating MISS subscale scores with indices of verbal interaction obtained by independently coding the interviews according to a detailed system of a discourse analysis (Stiles et al., 1979). This analysis suggests that patient satisfaction as measured by the affective and cognitive subscales of the MISS is specifically sensitive to the mutual exchange of information between the patient and the physician. The scale should have wide applicability. It is not directed toward a particular patient group and is seen as widely applicable across types of medical problem. The MISS is still an experimental scale that requires further field testing and validation studies before its properties can be fully assessed. However, evidence that the cognitive and affective subscales are significantly correlated with measures of clinically relevant patient and physician behaviors is encouraging.

At McMaster University, Wakefield, Norman, and Woodward, (1980) have been developing a patient feedback form (PFF) that is also designed to measure a patient's evaluation of an individual interview with his physician. The PFF is a 31-item Likert-type scale which is completed by the patient immediately after an interview. The item pool for this questionnaire was generated by reviewing the literature regarding investigations of the doctor-patient relationship, communication between doctor and patient, and patient satisfaction. Five clinical faculty involved in the teaching of interviewing skills to medical students were asked to critically examine this item pool for appropriateness, clarity, readability, redundancy, and comprehensiveness of coverage. Interrater reliability using patient/patient-observer pairs was calculated to be 0.70. The PFF has also been factor analyzed; six factors together account for 57 percent of the variance in scores. Fewer than ten separate patient encounter forms are needed to obtain a stable estimate of a given physician's performance ($r = 0.75$). Work is continuing in the development of this questionnaire. The item pool and structure of the PFF are highly similar to the MISS, developed independently by Stiles and his colleagues (1979).

A number of scales have appeared in the literature to measure patient satisfaction with health care services (see review by Ware, Snyder, and Wright, 1976a). Some of the questionnaires are concerned with how consumers feel in general regarding their health care. Others comprise many elements, including accessibility, convenience, availability of resources, continuity of care, efficacy/outcome of care, finances, humaneness, information gathering, information giving, pleasantness of surroundings, and quality/competence. The latter five dimensions appear to relate most closely to the doctor-patient relationship.

Such questionnaires can be used to evaluate the quality of the doctor-patient relationship perceived by patients who attend a particular physician's practice over time. They can also be modified to assess the doctor-patient relationship on a given occasion. Their major use to date, however, has been to evaluate health care services, to report on patients' general experience with the physicians, and/or to attempt to explain health and illness behaviors of patients.

The patient satisfaction questionnaire (PSQ) developed by Ware and his colleagues (1976b) is a good example of a questionnaire that could be used to examine a patient's perception of his relationship with a physician across a series of encounters. Doyle and Ware (1977) report that 41 percent of the variance in a global measure of patient satisfaction can be explained by the dimension of the PSQ they label "physician conduct." This dimension is represented by items pertaining to the humaneness of the physician and the technical quality and competence he exhibits as perceived by the patient. The PSQ has undergone extensive development and validation. Order effects, response sets, and even time needed to administer the questionnaire have been studied. The test-retest reliability to this questionnaire has been investigated not only for the entire questionnaire but for individual items of the questionnaire, and factor-analysis techniques have been used to allow scaling of the questionnaire. Concurrent validity of the PSQ has been studied by relating satisfaction ratings obtained with descriptions of health care experiences elicited by trained interviewers. There is good correspondence between PSQ scores and comments to open-ended questions on positive and negative physician conduct. Further, consumers' perceptions regarding what happened during the delivery of health care were clearly and consistently the most important factor in overall satisfaction with care as measured by the PSQ.

Another widely used patient satisfaction scale was developed by Hulka and her colleagues (Hulka et al., 1971; Zyzanski et al.,

1974). This scale has undergone two phases of development: (1) the initial construction of three Thurstone scales from 41 questionnaire items; and (2) the modification in the content, format, and scoring of these items in the revised 42-item questionnaire. In the latter version, a new method of scoring each item was devised so as to benefit from both the score resulting from response choice selected by each respondent on a five-point Likert-type scale and the Thurstone scale value associated with the item. The scale is divided into three content areas that have been labeled "professional competence," "personal qualities," and "cost/convenience." Internal consistency of 0.90 has been reported for the total scale and for the three-component 14-item subscales the values were 0.75 for professional competence; 0.86 for personal qualities; and 0.68 for cost/convenience. Test-retest reliability has not been reported. The measurement properties of the scale continue to be explored as it is used in numerous studies of health care services and correlates of satisfaction with medical care. Again, two subscales could be used to examine a patient's global perception of the quality of the doctor-patient relationship.

The effects of patient factors such as age, sex, educational level, and recency of care on responses to satisfaction questionnaires has been studied for some scales (e.g., Ware, Snyder, and Wright, 1976b). So far little attempt has been made to study potential sources of bias created by the type of presenting problem the patient exhibits. It is not clear whether patients with chronic or deteriorating health problems will find measured aspects of the doctor-patient relationship as satisfying as those who attend for health maintenance visits or acute illness episodes. Such data would be useful, especially if these scales are to be employed to measure a specific physician's performance with patients.

Measures of Doctor-Patient Agreement. Measures of physician-patient agreement have been developed which seem to have direct application to the measurement of the quality of the doctor-patient relationship. One measure quantifies the extent to which the patient has received the information the doctor thinks he conveyed. The second measure seeks to assess the extent to which the physician can describe the concerns of his patient regarding the medical condition for which he is treating the patient.

Communication. A measure of doctor-patient communication that evaluates the physician's success in communicating instructions and information to his patients has been described by Hulka and her colleagues (1971). For each medical condition studied, a series of items are identified to cover topics that are pertinent to the particular disease process and patient management for the condition. Given a condition-specific list of items, the physician indicates whether or not a particular patient has been instructed or informed in each area listed. The patient is subsequently presented with a corresponding series of questions to determine whether or not the information has been transmitted. A communication score is derived based on the proportion of information retained by the patient of the total amount provided by the physician. For example, to assess adequacy of communication between pregnant women and their physicians, information items such as taking vitamins or iron, weight control, consumption of nutritious food with limitation on fat and salt, and so on, were included. Hulka et al. (1976) have reported a significant relationship between communication scores and patient errors in taking medication for patients with congestive heart disease. Better communication scores were related to greater satisfaction with care among mothers with new babies (Liptak et al., 1977).

Physician awareness of patient concerns. Another measure of the physician-patient relationship developed by these researchers assesses the degree to which the physician is aware of his patients' attitudes and concerns (Hulka et al., 1971). This measure is built on the assumption that the physician's level of awareness should be a sensitive indicator of rapport developed in the doctor-patient relationship. A separate content-specific scale is constructed for each medical condition studied. Content relates to attitudes and concerns which have been expressed by patients and which a practicing physician can be expected to be aware of in his patients. For example, in pregnancy, the concerns scaled include the general emotional reaction to being pregnant; the desirability of having the baby; fear of an abnormal baby; concern over loss of physical attractiveness; and so on. The patient is asked to respond to each item along a continuum of 20 locations representing responses ranging from highly positive to highly negative. Questionnaires have been developed for four conditions: congestive heart disease, diabetes, pregnancy, and the first year of life. The questionnaires can be administered to patients by office staff. The physician is given an identical questionnaire to complete for his patient shortly after the patient's visit, and is asked to complete it as the patient would have filled it out without knowing the patient's responses. An awareness score is derived on the ability of the physician to predict patients'

responses. Some evidence for the construct validity of the awareness score has been reported. Hulka et al. (1976) indicate that a
decreasing number of office visits handled by a doctor is associated with an increasing awareness of his patients' concerns. Physician awareness of the concerns of new mothers is also positively
linked with a measure of mother-child adaptation (Liptak et al.,
1977).

Both measures of doctor-patient agreement appear to quantify important aspects of the doctor-patient relationship. The general methodology employed is straightforward. Since each scale
is tied to a specific medical condition, however, new scales must
be developed for each condition to be studied. This procedure
involves a lengthy period of item development, pretesting, and
refinement of each disease-specific scale. Further, to be used in a
physician's practice, a method is required for flagging eligible patients, arranging scale administration to patient and doctor independently near the time of the visit, and retrieval of the completed scales. These procedures are more cumbersome than simply
obtaining responses from all patients on a scale that is applicable
across medical conditions. Patient-based measures described
earlier are used more widely to assess the doctor-patient relationship than measures involving the responses of both doctor and patient because of these logistic problems.

Synthesis

As this review of the current literature indicates, aspects
of physician performance that correspond to good and bad doctor-patient relationships are not well defined. Interpersonal skills
and communications skills as judged by experts viewing the performance of a physician in real or simulated conditions and as
judged by patients are cardinal features of current evaluation
methods. However, the extent to which physical arrangements
and technical competence influence the doctor-patient relationship is largely unexplored. Several patient satisfaction questionnaires (e.g., by Ware et al., 1976b and Hulka et al., 1971) include
these dimensions in the assessment of patient satisfaction. They
report less relationship between patients' responses to these particular questions, however, than the relationship between patients'
responses to questions regarding communication and empathic
skills.

Tests developed to assess the doctor-patient relationship vary considerably in perspective adopted, comprehensiveness, and educational value. There is still no agreement on which perspective results in the best assessment of the doctor-patient relationship. Those investigators studying quality of care of physicians in practice have chosen the patient's perspective. Those investigating the effectiveness of a particular educational program to help develop skills tend to use professional ratings of the physician-patient interaction in a focus on process. Patient-based measures can measure a narrow spectrum of behavior (such as empathy) or provide feedback about many aspects of the encounter(s). Similarly, discrimination, formulation, and behavioral measures of physician/ students' communication and interpersonal skills can use a narrow range of stimuli or attempt to assess skill across a variety of patients. Although these measures can be comprehensive in the types of patient situations encountered, they tend to focus on one or two aspects of the doctor-patient relationship.

It would appear that patient-based information taps broader aspects of the doctor-patient relationship but does not have the kind of feedback value to the individual physician that direct observation assessment techniques offer. Brody (1980) reports that housestaff provided with feedback from patients regarding difficulties in listening well to the patient and understanding the patient's perceptions of his illness did not alter their behavior in dealing with subsequent patients. Patient feedback appears valuable in pointing out whether there is a problem or not, but it is not valuable in pinpointing exactly what the physician needs to learn or do to ensure that the problem does not recur with other patients.

Technological developments of the last 20 years have improved our ability to study the doctor-patient relationship. The availability of video technology allows an interaction to be captured for later review and rating by numerous assessors. This technology is not only useful for the teaching of doctor-patient relationship skills but may allow us to examine what the crucial factors are in this exchange. Further research is needed to better understand the doctor-patient relationship and its impact on patient outcomes, especially compliance. The availability of standardized tools that seem to have adequate reliability is also a recent development. We may be moving into an era in which established tools are used in a wide variety of situations so that their predictive validity is better understood and the relationship of the performance on these measures to other indicators of health outcome can be established. These developments suggest that we may be near an understanding of the art of care which can rival an understanding of the biological aspects of medicine.

It is quite obvious that a good doctor-patient relationship is an essential component of clinical competence. Studies of the quality of care rendered by a physician or groups of physicians that do not include this dimension omit documentation of an important area.

References

Aday, L. A., Anderson, R.: Development of indices of access to medical care. Ann Arbor, Mich.: Health Administration Press (1975).

Adler, L., Enelow, A.: An instrument to measure skill in diagnostic interviewing: a teaching and evaluation tool. J Med Educ 41, 281-288 (1966).

Adler, L., Ware, J.: Changes in medical interviewing style after instruction with two closed-circuit television techniques. J Med Educ 45, 21-28 (1970).

Adler, W., Ware, J., Enelow, A.: Evaluation of programmed instruction in medical interviewing. Los Angeles, University of Southern California Postgraduate Division (1968).

Anderson, J., Day, J., Dowling, M. Pettingale, K.: The definition and evaluation of the skills required to obtain a patient's history of illness: the use of videotape recordings. Postgrad Med J 46, 606-612 (1970).

Bales, R. F.: Interaction process analysis. Cambridge, Mass.: Addison-Wesley (1950).

Benjamin, A.: The helping interview. Boston, Mass.: Houghton Mifflin (1969).

Benson, H.: The mind-body effect. New York: Simon and Schuster (1979).

Best, A., Samph, T., Jordan, R., Moser, D., Templeton, B.: Two experimental examinations of medical student interpersonal skills. Paper presented at Eastern Educational Research Association in Kiawah, South Carolina (1979).

Bloom, S. W.: The doctor and his patient: A sociological interpretation. New York: Russel-Sage Foundation (1963).

Blum, R. H.: The management of the doctor patient relationship. New York: McGraw-Hill (1960).

Brockway, B.: Evaluating physician competency: what difference does it make? Eval. Program Planning 1, 211-220 (1978).

Brody, D. S.: Feedback from patients as a means of teaching nontechnical aspects of medical care. J Med Educ 55, 34-41 (1980).

Campbell, R., Kagan, J., Krathwohol, D.: The development of a scale to measure affective sensitivity (empathy). J of Counsel Psychol 18, 407-412 (1971).

Carkhuff, R. R.: Helping and human relations—a primer for lay and professional helpers. New York: Holt Rinehart Winston (1969).

Carkhuff, R. R., Berenson, B.: Beyond counseling and therapy. New York: Holt Rinehart Winston (1967).

Carkhuff, R. R., Collingwood, T., Renz, A.: The effects of didactic training in discrimination upon trainee level of discrimination and communication. J Clin Psychol 8, 104-107 (1969).

Cassell, E. J.: The healer's art. Philadelphia: Lippincott (1976).

Cattell, R. B.: The scientific analysis of personality. London: Penguin (1965).

Davis, M.: Variation in patients' compliance with doctors' orders: medical practice and doctor-patient interaction. Psychiatry Med 2, 31-54 (1971).

DiMatteo, R., Taranta, A.: Predicting patient satisfaction from physicians' non-verbal communication skills. Med Care XVI, 376-387 (1980).

Doyle, B. J., Ware, J. E.: Physician conduct and other factors that affect consumer satisfaction with medical care. J Med Educ 52, 793-801 (1977).

Egbert, L. D., et al.: Reduction of post operative pain by encouragement and instruction of patients: A study of doctor-patient rapport. N Engl J Med 270, 825-833 (1969).

Engel, G. L.: Enduring attributes of medicine relevant for the education of the physician. Ann Intern Med 78, 587-593 (1973).

Evans, L.: The crisis in medical education. Ann Arbor, Mich: University of Michigan Press (1964).

Fine, V., Terrien, M.: Empathy in the doctor-patient relationship: skill training for medical students. J Med Educ 52, 752-757 (1977).

Ford, A. B., et al.: The doctors' perspective: Physicians view their patients and practice. Cleveland: Case Western Reserve University Press (1967).

Fox, R. C.: Experiment perilous: Physicians and patients facing the unknown. Glencoe, Ill.: The Free Press (1959).

Freeman, B., Negrete, V., Davis, M., and Korsch, B.: Gaps in doctor-patient communication: doctor-patient interaction analysis. Pediatr Res 5, 298-311 (1971).

Freidson, E.: Patients' views of medical practice. New York: Russell-Sage Foundation (1961).

Gerrard, B., Boniface, W., Love, B.: Interpersonal skills for health professionals. Reston, Va.: Reston (1980).

Gerrard, B., Buzzell, M.: User's manual for the behavioral test of interpersonal skills for health professionals. Reston, Va.: Reston (1980).

Grayson, M., Nugent, C., Oken, S.: A systematic and comprehensive approach to teaching and evaluating interpersonal skills. J Med Educ 52, 906-913 (1977).

Helfer, Ray E.: An objective comparison of the pediatric interviewing skills of freshman and senior medical students. Pediatrics 45, 623-627 (1970).

Hess, J.: A comparison of methods for evaluating medical student skill in relating to patients. J Med Educ 44, 934-938 (1969).

Hippocrates: On decorum and the physician. London: William Heineman (1923).

Hollifield, G., Rousell, C., Bachrach, A., Pattishall, E.: A method for evaluating student-patient interviews. J Med Educ 32, 853-857 (1957).

Hulka, B. S., Kupper, L. L., Cassel, J. C.: Practice characteristics and quality of primary medical care: The doctor-patient relationship. Med Care 13, 808-820 (1975).

Hulka, B. S., et al.: A method for measuring physician awareness of patient concerns. HSMHA Health Rep 86, 741-751 (1971).

Hulka, B. S., et al.: Communication, compliance, and concordance between physicians and patients with prescribed medications. Am J Public Health 66, 847-853 (1976).

Hutter, M., Dungy, C., Zakus, G., Moore, V., Ott, J., Favret, A.: Interviewing skills: a comprehensive approach to teaching and evaluation. J Med Educ 52, 328-333 (1977).

Inui, T. S., Yourtec, E. L., Williamson, J. W.: Improved outcomes in hypertension after physician tutorials. Ann Intern Med 84, 646-651 (1970).

Jackson, D.: Personality research form manual. Goshun, N.Y.: Research Psychologists Press (1967).

Jarrett, F., Waldron, J., Barra, P., Handforth, J.: Measuring interviewing skill: the Queen's University interviewer rating scale (QUIRS). Canadian Psychiatric Association Journal 17, 183-188 (1972).

Jordan, A., Moser, D., Gleason, M., Samph, T., Best, A.: Psychological, cognitive and affective correlates of two experimental examinations of medical student interpersonal skills. Presented at the Eastern Educational Research Association Meeting (1980).

Kagan, H., Krathwohl, O., Goldberg, A., et al.: Studies in human interaction. Michigan State University, East Lansing: Education Publication (1967).

Kagan, N., et al.: Interpersonal process recall. J Nerv Ment Dis 148, 365-374 (1969).

Kahn, G. S., Cohen, B., Jason, H.: The teaching of interpersonal skills in U.S. medical schools. J Med Educ 54, 29-35 (1969).

King, S. H.: Perceptions of illness and medical practice. New York: Russell-Sage Foundation (1962).

Korsch, B. M., Gozzi, E. K., Francis, V.: Gaps in doctor-patient communication. I. Doctor-patient interaction and patient satisfaction. Pediatrics 42, 855-871 (1968).

Korsch, B. M., Negrete, V. F.: Doctor-patient communication. Sci Am 227, 66-74 (1972).

Liptak, G. S., Hulka, B. S., Cassel, J. C.: Effectiveness of physician-patient interaction during pregnancy. Pediatrics 60, 186-192 (1977).

Lipton, A., Huxhorn, G., Hamilton, D.: Influence of personality on achievement of medical students. Brit J Med Educ 9, 215-222 (1975).

Mathews, B.: Measurement of psychological aspects of the nurse-patient relationship. Nurs Res 11(3), 154-161 (1962).

Mechanic, P.: Medical sociology: A selective view. New York: Free Press (1968).

Murray, H. A.: Explorations in personality. New York: Oxford University Press (1938).

Osler, W.: The masterword in medicine. In W. Osler, Aequanimitas with other addresses to medical students, nurses and practitioners of medicine. Philadelphia, Penn.: Blackiston (1904).

Parker, S.: Personality factors among medical students as related to their predisposition to view the patient as a "whole man." J Med Educ 33, 736-744 (1958).

Parlow, J., Rothman, A.: Personality traits of first year medical students: Trends over six-year period 1967-1972. Brit J Med Educ 8-12 (1974).

Parsons, T.: The social system. Glencoe, Ill.: The Free Press (1951).

Pascoe, L., Naar, R., Guyett, I., Wells, R.: Training medical students in interpersonal relationship skills. J Med Educ 51, 743-750 (1976).

Rasche, L., Bernstein, L., Veenhuis, P.: Evaluation of a systematic approach to teaching interviewing. J Med Educ 49, 589-595 (1974).

Reeder, L.: The patient-client as consumer: some observations on the changing professional-client relationship. J Health Soc Behav 13, 406-412 (1972).

Robbins, A. S., et al.: Interpersonal skills training. Evaluation in an internal medicine residency program. J Med Educ 54, 885-894 (1979).

Romm, F. J., Hulka, B. S., Mayo, F.: Correlates of outcomes in patients with congestive heart failure. Med Care 14, 765-776 (1976).

Rosenthal, R., Hall, J., DiMatteo, M., Rogers, P., Archer, D.: Sensitivity to non-verbal communication: the PONS test. Baltimore, Md.: Johns Hopkins University Press (1979).

Ryden, M.: The predictive value of a clinical examination of interpersonal relationship skills. J Nurs Educ 16, 27-31 (1977).

Sanson-Fisher, R., Poole, A.: Training medical students to empathize: An experimental study. Med J Aust, May, 473-476 (1978).

Schwartz, R., Gottman, J.: Toward a task analysis of assertive behavior. J Consult Clin Psychol 44, 910-920 (1976).

Senate Report, No. 94-887. Washington, D.C.: Government Printing Office (1976).

Stern, M., Harris, F., Buckley-Sharp, M.: Personality factors in medical and other students. Brit J Med Educ 6, 268-276 (1972).

Stiles, W., Putnam, S., Wolf, M., James, S.: Interaction exchange structure and patient satisfaction with medical interviews. Med Care 17, 667-681 (1979).

Stone, G.: Compliance and the role of the expert. J Soc Issues 35, 1 (1979).

Sullivan, J.: Comparison of manifest needs of nurses and physicians in primary care practice. Nurs Res 27, 255-259 (1978).

Svarstad, B.: Physician-patient communication and patient conformity with medical advice. In D. Mechanic (Ed.), The growth of bureaucratic medicine. New York: Wiley (1976).

Truax, C.: A scale for the measurement of accurate empathy. Psychiatr Inst Bull 1, 1 (1961).

Truax, C. B., Mitchel, K.: Research on certain therapist interpersonal skills in relation to process and outcome. In: A. E. Bergin and S. L. Garfield (eds). Handbook of psychotherapy and behavioral change. New York: Wiley (1971).

Vaccarino, J. M.: Malpractice: The problem of perspective. JAMA 238, 861-863 (1977).

Valberg, L. S., Firstbrook, J. B.: A project to improve the measurement of professional competence for speciality certification in internal medicine. Ann R Coll Phys Surg (Can) 10, 278-282 (1977).

Wakefield, J. G., Norman, G. R., Woodward, C. A.: Development of in-training measures of physician-patient relationship. Final Report to the RS McLaughlin Centre, Edmonton, Alta (1980).

Ware, J.E., Kane, R. L., Daires-Avery, A.: Effects of differences in quality of care on patient satisfaction and other variables: An experimental simulation. Proceedings, 17th Annual Conference on Research in Medical Education, New Orleans, La. (1978).

Ware, J. E., Snyder, M. K., Wright, W. R.: Development and validation of scales to measure patient satisfaction with health services. Volume I of a Final Report. Part A: Review of Literature, Overview of Methods, and Results Regarding Construction of Scales. Carbondale, Ill.: Southern Illinois University School of Medicine (1976a).

Ware, J. E., Snyder, M. K., Wright, W. R.: Development and validation of scales to measure patient satisfaction with health services. Volume I of a Final Report. Part B: Results Regarding Scales Constructed from the Patient Satisfaction Questionnaire and Measures of Other Health Care Perceptions. Carbondale, Ill.: Southern Illinois University School of Medicine (1976b).

Ware, J. E., Strassman, H. D., Naftulin, D. H.: A negative relationship between understanding interviewing principles and interview performance. J Med Educ 46, 620-622 (1971).

Werner, A., Schneider, J.: Teaching medical students interactional skills: A research based course in the doctor-patient relationship. N Engl J Med, May, 1232-1237 (1974).

Wexler, M.: The behavioral sciences in medical education: A view from psychology. Amer Psychologist 31, 275-283 (1976).

Wolf, M. H., et al.: The medical interview satisfaction scale: Development of a scale to measure patient perceptions of physician behavior. J Behav Med 1, 391-401 (1978).

Zisook, S., Lloyd, C., Click, M.: Teaching and evaluating interviewing. J Med Educ 54, 117-119 (1979).

Zyzanski, S. J., Hulka, B. S., Cassell, J. C.: Scale for measurement of satisfaction with medical care: Modifications in content, format, and scoring. Med Care 12, 611-618 (1974).

CHAPTER 13

Assessment of Technical Skills

JOHN WATTS
WILLIAM B. FELDMAN

Introduction

Technical skills constitute an important component of clinical competence. However, exactly which technical skills should be taught during which stage of undergraduate and post-graduate medical education remains controversial. Weinburger (1976), in a survey of 300 primary care pediatricians in New York State, revealed that of 16 procedures acquired during residency training, only 8 were regularly performed by practitioners. The value of teaching a technical procedure which is unlikely to be used in practice is questionable since skill in performing such a procedure is likely to decay over time unless continually practiced; the value of evaluating such a skill, even more so. A first step in the evaluation of technical skills is obviously the choice of which skills to evaluate; unnecessary or rarely applied skills should be avoided and commonly used skills should be included, if necessary by extracting the common components of several complex procedures.

Unlike the situation regarding the assessment of knowledge and clinical skills, concerning which a body of literature is emerging, little has been written regarding objective measures of technical competence. Although it might be expected that research into measurement tools for technical skills would be best developed in those specialties in which technical competence is critical, e.g., the surgical specialties, this is not the case. Mueller (1981) has stated that surgeons rely heavily on "gut feelings" concerning the technical competence of their trainees; few attempts have been made to develop measurement tools for recording these technical skills or to assess the reliability and validity of these clinical impressions.

The few studies which have been conducted, reviewed later, have reported generally favorable results using a variety of methods. If it is indeed possible to critically evaluate technical skills, why has this apparently important area of evaluation received so little attention? The time-consuming nature of critical evaluation must be in part responsible, but one suspects this may be overemphasized. Possibly the fact that residency programs are in general the province of university teaching hospitals, which place greater emphasis on intellectual function and knowledge acquisition rather than on manual or technical dexterity, may also be important. The mere fact that technical incompetence or negligence weighs so heavily in medicolegal considerations, however, should be a stimulus to increasing the emphasis on appropriate evaluation of these areas during physician training.

Rationale for Technical Skills Evaluation

For the purpose of this discussion we will define technical skills as those diagnostic or therapeutic maneuvers which involve the use of instruments and/or manual dexterity; we have not included the use of instruments commonly regarded as part of the clinical examination of patients (such as ophthalmoscopes or auroscopes). Many of our conclusions about evaluation of technical skills, however, apply equally to the use of such instruments and indeed to the whole subject of physical examination of patients. We have, therefore, included in our discussion (1) diagnostic procedures such as lumbar puncture or arterial puncture and (2) major therapeutic maneuvers such as intubation, cardiopulmonary resuscitation, and operative surgery.

This broad description of the domains of technical skills does not, however, address the issue of which skills should be assessed in a particular specialty. The discussion in Chapter 2 is appropriate for such a decision—to what extent have these detailed specifications of technical competence been attempted by various specialties?

The American College of Emergency Physicians (Certification Task Force, 1976) has developed a detailed specification of technical skills. A similar list of items is contained in the instructional objectives of Canadian pediatrics residency programs, developed in 1974. However, the detailed objectives of the College of Family Physicians of Canada (1973) contain no references to technical skills. The American Board of Internal Medicine (1979), in defining clinical competence in internal medicine, explicitly considers "Motor and Technical Skills" as one prerequisite ability, but in its detailed specification of competence avoids the issue using statements such as "be technically proficient in the performance of those [diagnostic] procedures undertaken" and "be proficient in those therapeutic procedures requiring technical skills."

Thus, any attempt to evaluate technical skills in a specialty is likely to be handicapped at the outset by a lack of consensus regarding which skills are essential components of competence in the specialty.

Methods

The available forms of technical skills evaluation range from the informal "gut feelings" (unfortunately prevalent) all the way to sophisticated checklists of direct observation as described by Delaney et al. (1978) and Andrew (1977). If one excludes "gut feelings," methods of technical skills evaluation can be listed as follows: (1) procedure lists; (2) direct observation, without criteria; (3) direct observation using criteria checklist; (4) use of animals with direct observation and criteria checklist; (5) use of mechanical simulators with objective evaluation. The measurement properties of each approach are summarized in Table 13.1.

Procedural Lists

Listing of the procedures which should be conducted allows the trainee to log those procedures actually performed and allows the training institution some degree of certainty that the trainee has had experience in performing the desired procedures. This logging of procedures is the most common method and is the most easily measured. It is based on the assumption that the trainee, having performed that technical procedure sufficiently often, is competent in its performance. Although there is presumably some relationship between practice and competence, the simple listing

TABLE 13.1
Measurement Properties

Method	Credibility	Comprehensiveness	Precision	Validity	Feasibility
I. a) Procedure Lists with Logs	Merely tells us learner performed a procedure, not how well.	Doesn't tell us if all aspects of the procedure (preparation, etc.) were done.	Not applicable	No indication as to whether the learner has mastered the technique.	Cheap, easiest form of evaluation; this accounts for its wide use.
b) With prescribed minimum number	See (a); implies that "practice makes perfect."	See (a).	See (a).	See (a).	See (a).
II. Direct Observation with Patients without Criteria	More credible than I; at least someone with more experience has witnessed the learner performing the procedure.	The observer can assess comprehensiveness but without criteria; different observers may not agree as to "what comprehensiveness is."	Without criteria, there may be poor inter- or intra-rater reliability	More valid than I because the observer is comparing the learner to how he (the observer) feels it should be done; i.e., there is at least some gold standard.	More costly than I; logistics may be difficult, i.e., in real-life situation with patients, having the learner and the observer at the same place and the same time.

Method					
III. Direct Observation with Patients using Criteria Checklist	More credible than II; the successful learner will have met some previously established criteria of satisfactory performance.	Properly developed criteria will be very comprehensive from indications for the procedure to care of patient after the procedure.	This is the key feature of criteria checklist: very good interrater reliability.	If well-written criteria represent the "gold standard," then this method using criteria and real patients is the most valid.	Less feasible than II because criteria checklists have to be written; requires time and a motivated faculty; same logistic problems as with II.
IV. Direct Observation using Animals, Models, and Criteria Checklist	See III.	One element of comprehensiveness is "compassion." This is hard to measure anyway, but may be more so using an anesthetized animal.	See III.	The extent to which the animal or model approximates a human for whom the procedure will be performed constitutes the validity.	Very feasible; can be booked at convenient times for learner and observer; criteria checklists have to be written; cost of purchase and maintenance of animals and models.
V. Use of film and video-tape with real patients or animals	See III.	See III and IV.	Repeated viewing and training of observer may lead to increased precision.	See III and IV.	Extra cost of tape and equipment; cost of training faculty; can be viewed at observer convenience.

of procedures performed has no educational value and really in no way guarantees competence.

In some institutions, not only is there a listing of procedures to be performed but a specified number of each must be completed. There is not necessarily any requirement that supervision of these technical procedures be available, and the assumption is that "practice makes perfect." Although this method of evaluation of technical skills is commonly employed by training institutions, senior faculty have had the experience of trainees performing the same mistakes often enough to know that practice does not make perfect. Performing a number of lumbar punctures and obtaining bloody cerebrospinal fluid each time not only is of negligible educational value to the trainee but may submit patients to repeated risk.

Direct Observation without Criteria

At the next level of sophistication, a list of procedures is developed and assessed by a senior person (a more senior trainee or a member of faculty) who has been present at the performance of the procedure. This form of evaluation, where no explicit criteria are used, predictably suffers from low inter- and intra-observer reliability. The approach may be suitable for procedures in which outcome is more easily measured or assessed than process or technique. Certain laboratory procedures such as staining of microscopic slides may be particularly amenable to this approach; even so, too much emphasis on assessing outcome may result in the loss of an educational opportunity or even in an inappropriate evaluation (the materials may be more to blame than the trainee).

Direct observation without criteria checklists is more valuable than mere logs of procedures; however, the lack of explicit criteria results in a wide range of opinions as to what would constitute satisfactory performance. If one uses the lumbar puncture as an example, one observer may feel that a satisfactory performance merely constitutes the obtaining of a specimen of cerebrospinal fluid which can be used for diagnostic tests; on the other hand, another observer may feel, in addition, that an explanation to the patient and attention to aseptic technique are as important as getting usable cerebrospinal fluid.

Direct Observation with Checklists

Perhaps the most useful technique of assessment of technical skills is the criteria checklist approach. In this model, each step involved in the technical procedure is written down in advance by a group of experts and the trainee is then assessed with the checklist at hand to determine whether he or she goes through the appropriate steps in the appropriate sequence and in the appropriate manner.

Delaney et al. (1978), in a small pilot study, showed that when certain key aspects of surgical technique are systematically scored by pairs of faculty surgeons using explicit criteria, the interobserver reliability was higher for surgical skill assessment than for the knowledge and attitude components of their assessments. Andrew (1977) has shown that when clinicians design forms describing in behavioral terms the procedures associated with each physical examination skill, and when these check lists are used to assess physical examination skills, there is very high interrater reliability, ranging from 0.82 to 0.94. They also demonstrated construct validity, differentiating 150 physician's assistants who had graduated from a formal training program from the same number of PAs who had been trained on the job. The scores on the technical skills checklists correlated only 0.12-0.28 with scores on a concurrent written examination.

Although these checklists were devised for relatively simple physical examination procedures, similar reliabilities have been reported for more complex technical skills. Liu et al. (1980) have developed checklists for spinal anesthesia (49 items) and anesthesia setup and machine checkout (43 items) and had raters score videotaped performances of residents. The reliability for the spinal anesthesia checklist was 0.75 (using an intraclass correlation) and 0.83 for the machine setup checklist. This group has also developed a checklist for continuous epidural anesthesia and reported high reliabilities. These authors have found the checklists useful for formative evaluation as well, permitting identification of common errors and omissions in the performance of these procedures (Lane et al., 1979). A comment in their paper suggests a potential role for checklists in program evaluation. They state that many of the areas of error noted are especially relevant to the teaching situation where good habits must be inculcated.

We have used this approach for technical procedures in our pediatric residency program, including arterial puncture, exchange transfusion, lumbar puncture, and venipuncture. Some of the criteria for lumbar puncture are seen in Table 13.2. A similar check-

TABLE 13.2

Preset Criteria for Part of the Performance of Lumbar Puncture
on an Infant or Child. Used in Evaluation of Pediatric Residents
(the Criteria for Positioning, Preparation, Choice of Equipment,
Choice of Interspace, and Anesthesia are not shown).

Needling Procedure	*YES*	*NO*
1. Needle introduced		
(a) slowly and firmly	____	____
(b) in midline	____	____
(c) perpendicular to spinous processes	____	____
(d) pointing slightly cephalad	____	____
(e) puncture of anterior venous process avoided	____	____
2. (a) C.S.F. pressure measured (if appropriate)	____	____
(b) Rise and fall with respiration noted	____	____
(c) Queckenstedt's maneuver performed (if appropriate)	____	____
3. (a) Adequate volume collected	____	____
(b) Tubes appropriately labeled	____	____

list, used for the performance of cardiopulmonary resuscitation
by the Ontario Heart Foundation, is shown in Table 13.3.

One potential difficulty of the use of binary checklists for
summative evaluation is that the total score is a simple sum of
the individual items. Further, each item of behavior is usually
classified in two ways—adequate or inadequate. Fiel et al. (1979)
have devised a more sophisticated checklist approach and tested
it on blood pressure measurement skills. Each item on the 15-item
checklist was rated on four levels (a = did not do, 1 = poor, 2 =
satisfactory, 3 = good). The checklist also incorporated "outcome" criteria, scoring the student according to the difference
between his blood pressure reading and the patient's "true" blood
pressure assessed by the evaluator. Finally, each item on the
checklist was weighted on a 0-3 scale based on its importance to
the overall performance of the procedure. The authors quote reliabilities of 0.87-0.90, although these are based on assessments
of two students by nine evaluators so should be viewed with some
suspicion. They also demonstrated construct validity, showing
positive change in student performance as a result of a ten-week
clinic experience.

Harden et al. (1975) has used the checklist approach in developing an "Objective Structured Clinical Examination," aimed at overcoming many of the disadvantages of the traditional clinical oral as described in Chapter 5. In this examination students rotate through a series of "stations" where they may be asked to auscultate the chest, examine a microscope slide, or test a urine sample. The student is evaluated at many of the stations by a faculty observer or a trained simulated patient using a detailed checklist. After leaving the station, the student then completes a brief multiple-choice test containing questions relating to his interpretation of the findings he has elicited. The investigators did not report reliability data. They did, however, relate performance on the structured clinical examination (completed by 33 students) and on a traditional clinical examination (completed by 66 students) with their performance on a written final examination in medicine and surgery. There was no significant correlation between the traditional oral and the knowledge examination; however, the structured clinical correlated 0.63 with the multiple-choice test. The authors do not comment on this finding—whether the high correlation is a peculiarity of their structured clinical examination, which directly and objectively assesses knowledge related to the technical skills demonstrated or whether this high correlation suggests that performance of technical skills is strongly related to basic knowledge remains to be determined.

Use of Mechanical or Animal Models

The direct observation of procedures using checklists, as described in the previous section, has been conducted on real patients (e.g., spinal anesthesia), normal individuals (physical examination), and in a "laboratory" setting (interpretation of slides). There are a variety of situations where these alternatives are not appropriate and these have led to the use of various simulation devices—live simulated patients, mechanical simulations, animals, or computer-based simulations.

As a general strategy, simulation has a number of potential advantages, as described in the Chapters 10 and 11. For the instruction and evaluation of technical skills, there may be three reasons for the use of simulation devices:

1. Control over the presenting problems. An example would be the mechanical simulators for ophthalmoscopic examination.
2. Possibility of risk or lack of availability in the use of real

TABLE 13.3

Preset Criteria for the Performance of Cardiopulmonary Resuscitation Used in Ontario Heart Foundation Basic Life Support Program

Elapsed Time (Seconds) Min.	Max.	Activity and Time (Seconds)	Critical Performance	Pass	Fail
6	10	Establish unresponsiveness and call out for help Allow 6-10 sec. if face down and turning is required. Open Airway.	Shake shoulder, shout "Are you O.K.?" Call for HELP. Turn if necessary. Adequate time.		
10	15	Establish breathlessness (Look, Listen, and Feel). (4-5 sec.)	Kneels properly. Head tilt with one hand on forehead and neck lift or chin lift with other hand. Ear over mouth, observe chest.		
13	20	Four Ventilations. (3-5 sec.)	Ventilate properly 4 times and observe chest rise.		
20	30	Establish pulse and stimulate activation of EMS system. (7-10 sec.)	Fingers palpate for carotid pulse on near side (other hand on forehead maintains head tilt). Know local emergency number. Adequate time.		

Single-Rescuer — Heart Saver

74	96	Four cycles of 15 compressions 2 ventilations. (54-66 sec.)	Proper body position Landmark check each time. Position of hands. Vertical compression. Says mnemonic. Proper rate. Proper ratio. No bouncing. Ventilates properly.
81	106	Check for return of pulse and spontaneous breathing. (7-10 sec.) (Pupil check optional).	Check pulse and breathing. (Pupil check optional).
97	126	Minimum of *four* cycles of 5 compressions and 1 ventilation (16-20 sec.) Switch and repeat until examiner is satisfied.	Changes rate of compression. Says mnemonic. Interposes breath. No pause for ventilation. Call for switch Change after three next time. Switches. Switches back. Checks pulse (by ventilator). (Pupil check optional). Technique as above.

Two Rescuer
Heart Saver

For single rescuer, number of compressions is 60.
Number of ventilations is 12.

patients. Examples here would be the use of mechanical simulators for cardiopulmonary resuscitation or animals in teaching intubation.

3. Ethical problems. The use of live simulated patients or mechanical models instead of real patients in teaching pelvic examination exemplifies this area.

The use of live simulated patients has been adequately dealt with in a preceding chapter. An example of assessment of performance on an inanimate model may be found in the American Heart Association program, in which cardiopulmonary resuscitation is both taught and tested on a mannequin (Resusci-Ann). The assessment calls for the completion of a series of maneuvers, each of which is described in detail and should be completed within a given period of seconds (Table 13.3). Evaluation of technical skills on such a model has educational advantages in that models are available at any time and repetition, with or without evaluation, is simple; models are particularly useful in evaluating emergency procedures. Other models have been produced for teaching purposes (e.g., models for suturing and for endotracheal intubation) and would be suitable for evaluative use in a similar manner.

Animal models have been used for teaching and for practice as well as experimentation. Small animals such as rats are commonly used for teaching microtubular surgery. Somewhat akin to this is the use of human cadavers for education and practice; intubation is probably the commonest technical skill learned in this way. We have been evaluating the intubation skills of pediatric residents using a cat or kitten anesthetized with ketamine; the model closely approximates the difficulties of intubating an asphyxiated newborn infant (Jennings et al., 1974; Thompson, 1979). A set of criteria for intubation has been drawn up (Table 13.4) and performance is evaluated by an anesthetist or pediatrician. Direct feedback and criticism are possible and a criterion performance must be completed as part of residency training. This form of model overcomes the disadvantages of lack of realism while retaining the educational and availability advantages of the inanimate model.

Many of these simulation approaches still require the presence of an observer, and the advantages of detailed behavioral checklists apply equally well to the use of simulation methods. The mechanical simulations, in particular, however, can permit an additional assessment of "outcome" rather than "process," which does not require an observer. For example, in using an ophthalmo-

TABLE 13.4
Preset Criteria for the Performance of Laryngoscopy
and Intubation of Ketamine-anesthetised Cat, as Used
in Evaluation of Pediatric Residents

	YES	NO
1. Laryngoscopy		
(a) Handle held with fingers in position to stabilize chin/cricoid	___	___
(b) Laryngoscope held stable	___	___
(c) Absence of trauma	___	___
(d) Absence of excessive force	___	___
(e) Exposure—tongue not obscuring view	___	___
—cords visualized well	___	___
2. Intubation		
(a) Appropriate selection of tube size	___	___
(b) Tube introduced without obscuring view	___	___
(c) Position checked —bilateral auscultation	___	___
—gastric auscultation	___	___
(d) Absence of force/trauma	___	___
(e) Patient ventilated gently with chest movement checked	___	___
3. Response to Incidents		
(a) Accumulation of secretions—suctioned	___	___
(b) Vomitus—suctioned	___	___
(c) Patient cyanosed/bradycardia		
(1) rapid intubation completed	___	___
(2) procedure stopped and bag-mask used	___	___
(d) In case of prolonged procedure, recognizes problem and requests help	___	___

scopic simulator, the evaluation can be based on whether the candidate distinguished between normal and abnormal red reflex or recognized hemorrhages in the retina. The heart sound simulator permits programming and testing of a variety of heart sounds. The evaluation can then be based on the correctness of interpretation, using objective methods similar to those of Harden et al. (1975) and Penta and Kofman (1973), rather than detailed observation of process. The objectivity of such evaluation is not achieved without some potential cost, however; the mechanical simulator may not be a valid representation of real life and the opportunity for detailed feedback to the student is lost.

The ultimate in mechanical simulation is the computer-based simulation as exemplified by SIM-1 (Abrahamson et al., 1969) and HARVEY (Gordon, 1979). Unlike most computer simulations, these prototypes involve a lifelike mannequin under computer control which can be examined and will respond appropriately to the examiner. Both simulations can simulate a variety of conditions by simple instruction to the computer. HARVEY was designed for instruction in cardiac auscultation and focuses on accurate simulation of heart sounds and peripheral pulses for a variety of conditions. SIM-1 was designed to teach endotracheal intubation, including injector, oxygen administration, and so on. The simulations were designed primarily for instructional purposes; both have been showed to be more effective educationally than conventional instruction.

Performance on the cardiac simulator, however, has been used for evaluation with detailed checklists and reported inter-rater agreement of 95 percent. Although these computer simulations have demonstrated value for teaching, they are conceptually similar for evaluation purposes to more conventional methods such as mechanical heart-sound simulators or examination of real patients, and their cost-effectiveness in an evaluation setting remains to be demonstrated.

Conclusions

Observation, either direct (involving real patients, animals, or models) or indirect on film or tape, and employing criteria checklists, appears to be the method with the best measurement properties. Which form is used, direct or indirect, humans, models, or animals, will depend upon feasibility factors and the extent to which the animals or models approximate the "real thing."

Criteria checklists appear to enhance the credibility, comprehensiveness, precision, and validity of direct observations with patients, animals, or models. This is not meant to imply that absence of written criteria means there are not criteria; certainly the experienced observer has criteria of his own against which he is comparing the learner. But unless agreed-upon criteria as decided by a panel of experts are specified, satisfactory performance cannot be reliably assessed. The use of behavioral criteria allows everyone, including the learner, to have more confidence in the evaluation.

This chapter began by noting the necessity for credibility (face validity) and has demonstrated some approaches to the problem of validity and interobserver reliability. Although there is some evidence for construct validity, predictive validity remains to be demonstrated. The common thread running through all of these problems has been the issue of feasibility. From our considerations, two broad areas suggest themselves as foci for immediate concern and further study.

What to Evaluate

Given the already wide and still burgeoning field of technical or technologic medicine, how can we focus on areas that are important yet sufficiently few in number so that progress can realistically be achieved? We suggest that such areas should meet the following criteria: (1) the areas evaluated should be procedures that are frequently performed or that represent common components of infrequently performed maneuvers; (2) there should be areas where failure to perform adequately has major disadvantages or risks; (3) they should include any obvious life-saving or life-preserving maneuvers encountered in a specialty, even if these are uncommon.

How to Evaluate

The clear challenge is to develop evaluation techniques which combine feasibility with precision; it seems that the latter is most likely to be achieved with the use of predetermined criteria checklists and the former requires their use with simplified animate or inanimate models or with patient situations that can either be simplified or assessed in individual simplified components.

References

Abrahamson, S., Denson, J. S., Wolf, R. M.: Effectiveness of a simulator in training anesthesia residents. J Med Educ 44, 515-518 (1969).
American Board of Internal Medicine: Clinical competence in internal medicine. Ann Intern Med 90, 402-411 (1979).

Andrew, B. J.: The use of behavioral checklists to assess physical exam skills. J Med Educ 52, 589-590 (1977).

Certification Task Force. Emergency medicine condition/skills list. J Am Coll Emerg Phys 5, 599-604 (1976).

College of Family Physicians of Canada: Education objectives for certification in family medicine. Toronto, Ontario: Author (1973).

Delaney, P. V., Quill, R. D., Kalizser, M.: Assessment of operative surgical skills. J Ir Med Assoc 71, 13 (1978).

Fiel, N. J., et al.: A model for evaluating student clinical psychomotor skills. J Med Educ 54, 511-513 (1979).

Gordon, M.: HARVEY: The cardiology simulator. Proceedings of symposium on alternative mechanisms for assessing clinical competence. Ann Arbor, Mich. (1979).

Harden, R. M., et al.: Assessment of clinical competence using an objective structured examination. Brit Med J 1, 447-451 (1975).

Jennings, B. P., Alden, E. R., Brenz, R. W.: A teaching model for pediatric intubation utilizing ketamine-sedated kittens. Pediatrics 53, 283 (1974).

Lane, P. E., Savarjian, M., Miller, E., et al.: Common errors during resident performance of continuous lumbar epidural analgesia. Anesthesiology 51, 342 (1979).

Liu, P., et al.: Videotape reliability: a method of evaluation of a clinical performance examination. J Med Educ 55, 713-715 (1980).

Mueller, C. B.: Personal communication (1981).

Penta, F. B., Kofman, S.: The effectiveness of simulation devices in teaching selected skills of physical diagnosis. J Med Educ 48, 442-445 (1973).

Thompson, B.: Use of kittens in teaching neonatal resuscitation to family medicine residents. J Fam Pract 9, 128-129 (1979).

Weinburger, H. L.: An attempt to identify frequency of use of technical skills and procedures by the primary care physician. J Pediatr 88, 671-675 (1976).

CHAPTER 14

Assessment of the Use of Diagnostic Tests

R. BRIAN HAYNES
DAVID L. SACKETT
PETER TUGWELL

Introduction

The subject of this chapter is the use of diagnostic tests. Some of the measurement techniques described in earlier sections of the book are perhaps as capable of testing relevant concepts in using diagnostic information as they are for other aspects of clinical competence. As we demonstrate below, however, a review of the content of one type of examination shows that diagnostic test use is not evaluated comprehensively at present. This is hardly surprising, considering the lack of systematic teaching of the characteristics of diagnostic tests in medical schools and postgraduate training programs today. Thus the focus of this chapter is more on what concepts should be taught and tested than on how to test the concepts.

There has been an explosion in laboratory technology in recent years and a growing awareness of the importance of understanding the characteristics of diagnostic tests in order to interpret and apply them properly. Unfortunately, the increase in our ability to use diagnostic test results effectively has been a rather painful and slow process that has lagged behind the introduction of new tests into medical practice. As will be shown below, the saliency of laboratory technology in medical care has resulted in a considerable and even disproportionate emphasis on diagnostic test use in examinations, but the content of such evaluation is directed more at assessing the breadth of a student's inventory of diagnostic tests than at his or her depth of understanding of the information value of these tests. Indeed, recent studies have demonstrated that students and practicing physicians are woefully ignorant of even elementary concepts in test use such as predictive value (Casscells et al., 1978) and laboratory error (Skendzel, 1978). Such ignorance no doubt underlies other findings that physicians frequently persist in ordering tests even when they believe that the test will be of no value (Greenland et al., 1979) and yet fail to respond to unexpected abnormalities in test results (Olsen et al., 1976). Further, Dixon (1974) has reported that only 5 percent of the results of tests ordered by house officers were actually used in patient management. Under such circumstances it is hardly surprising that physicians and medical students have been frequently castigated by pathologists and other lab specialists for "underutilization, overutilization, and malutilization" of laboratory resources (Abrams, 1979; Martin, 1971; Murphy and Henry, 1978, p. 625). The fire in such condemnations is fanned by ever increasing demands on laboratories to do more tests at less cost while maintaining state-of-the-art facilities. Indeed, the growth in use of laboratory tests in medical care might be termed malignant: the doubling time in the volume of tests ordered has decreased from 10 years to 3.5 years in the last two decades, with no signs of abatement (Benson, 1978; Freeborn et al., 1972; Griner, 1979; Kralewski, 1980; Murphy and Henry, 1978; Reiser, 1980). At least some of this increase in test use has resulted in improved medical care, but it has been estimated that the use of laboratory tests could be reduced by 50 percent without any detriment to patients (Frazier, 1980).

It would also appear that the teaching of diagnostic test use is quite inconsistent from school to school and perhaps even within a medical school. Several studies of diagnostic test use among medical students, house officers, and practicing clinicians have documented extreme variability in the number and cost of tests ordered for patients (Eisenberg, 1977; Freeborn et al., 1972; Greenland et al., 1979; Schroeder et al., 1973). Schroeder et al., (1973), for example, found a 17-fold variation in the mean annual cost of tests ordered by general internists working at the same clinic. Interestingly, providing these physicians with the results of a cost audit produced a modest reduction in costs over the ensuing period but very little change in the relative ranking of the doctors and an increase in the variation between individual physicians.

Several studies (Freeborn et al., 1972; Greenland et al., 1979; Hardwick et al., 1975; Pineault, 1977; Schroeder and O'Leary, 1977) have shown that the variability in test use can be related to the physician's training and experience: more experienced physicians and those from "prestige" medical schools order fewer tests. Furthermore, while various interventions can modify physicans' uses of tests (Dixon, 1974; Eisenberg, 1977; Griner, 1979), the gains are likely to be small (Campbell and Makler, 1980; Schroeder et al., 1973) and transient (Eisenberg, 1977; Lawrence, 1979). It may be more expeditious to teach students good habits in test ordering early on in their training than to attempt to modify their use of tests later in their careers. As Griner (1980) has suggested, the educational needs of student physicians for the appropriate use of laboratory tests include "knowledge of the characteristics of disease; knowledge of both the tests and procedures available to confirm or exclude these diseases and their operating characteristics; the experience and perspective necessary to reasonably estimate the likelihood of disease prior to test use; and the correct interpretation of laboratory test results" (p. 3). It is from this perspective that current evaluation procedures for diagnostic test use are assessed and remedial activities in instruction and evaluation are proposed in this chapter.

Definition of Competence in the Use of Diagnostic Tests

The American Board of Internal Medicine (ABIM) (1979) has recently published guidelines for competency in internal medicine. The standards for competence in diagnostic test use appear in Table 14.1. This list was developed over several years with help from several other sources such as the American Board of Pediatrics (1974) and two "critical incident" studies (American Institute for Research, 1976; Price et al., 1971). The range of attitudes, knowledge, skills, and performance appear both credible and comprehensive and certainly constitute a worthy standard to be achieved in any area of clinical practice, not just internal medicine. These standards are idealistic, however. They are not described in sufficient detail to indicate

TABLE 14.1
Competence in Diagnostic Study as Defined by the
American Board of Internal Medicine*

In ordering or performing diagnostic procedures the internist should:

(Attitudes and habits)
1. Use the laboratory mainly to confirm or refute diagnostic hypotheses.
2. Accept responsibility for using most effective and least risky procedures that minimize cost of health care.
3. Be able to accept responsibility for ordering potentially risky or costly procedures that are essential for the solution of a patient's problem.

(Interpersonal skills)
4. Be able to explain to patients the purpose, possible complications, and factors necessary to make the procedures comfortable, safe, and interpretable.

(Motor and technical skills)
5. Be technically proficient in the performance of those procedures undertaken.

(Knowledge)
6. Know the range of biologic variation in test results.
7. Know the indicated procedures including special or unusual studies.
8. Know the diagnostic specificity and limitations of laboratory studies.
9. Know how to perform or order test procedures in a manner most likely to ensure interpretable results.
10. Recognize invalid test results.

(Pathophysiology)
11. Understand the underlying rationale of the indicated procedures.
12. Interpret the results of procedures in terms of alterations in underlying pathophysiology.
13. Recognize laboratory results that reflect homeostatic responses to disease in contrast to those that reflect the effect of disease.

(Organization)
14. Order laboratory studies in a logical sequence to avoid unnecessary procedures or costs and observe appropriate timing of procedures to avoid invalidating test results.
15. Record laboratory findings in a logical, organized fashion.

(Synthesis)
16. Accurately interpret test results.
17. Recognize patterns of diagnostic information.
18. Integrate data appropriately to confirm or refute diagnostic hypotheses.

TABLE 14.1 (cont.)

(Clinical judgment)

19. Select from alternatives those diagnostic procedures with the greatest likelihood of useful results, taking into account risk and cost.
20. Make appropriate judgments from conflicting laboratory results.
21. Adapt diagnostic procedures to meet the special requirements of the medical situation.
22. Discern when indicated procedures should be delayed, as in an emergency.
23. Judge the validity and reliability of laboratory studies in each clinical situation.

*From American Board of Internal Medicine (1979).

the level of performance expected nor how one might go about evaluating whether competence had been achieved.

For a practical definition of competence, it might be useful to turn to the evaluation procedures utilized by the ABIM, in order to compare the competencies actually tested against those included in Table 14.1. Unfortunately, the ABIM certifying examinations are not available for review. The American College of Physicians produces a very similar examination, however, for continuing education purposes, in cooperation with the National Board of Medical Examiners in the United States, entitled the Medical Knowledge Self-assessment Program (MKSAP). The latest version at the time of writing is MKSAP-V, published in 1980. Table 14.2 provides an analysis of all the responses provided for the first 260 questions of the examination. These questions cover the disciplines of allergy and immunology, infectious diseases, endocrinology and metabolism, and oncology. The complete examination has 768 questions and covers several other disciplines, but the remaining 508 questions were not analyzed, as a stable pattern appeared to emerge from the first 260 questions.

In the analysis, each *response* was categorized for the area of knowledge it appeared to examine. When a single response appeared to address more than one area of knowledge, it was tallied in all relevant categories. Thus 765 possible responses were offered for the 260 questions analyzed, resulting in 801 tallies because some responses tested more than one area of knowledge.

Review of Table 14.2 leads to several observations. First, diagnostic tests are the subject of 22 percent of all responses, and the synthesis of diagnostic test information with that from history and physical examination constitutes an additional 9 percent of

TABLE 14.2
Number and Distribution of Responses from the MKSAP-V Examination Related to Area of Knowledge Examined for Each Subject in Part I of the Exam

Area of Knowledge Examined	No. of Responses on Each of the Subjects of				Total No. of Responses	%
	Immunology	Infectious Disease	Endocrine/ Metabolism	Oncology		
1. History taking	2	0	0	1	3	0
2. Physical examination	0	0	3	1	4	0
3. Synthesis of 1 + 2	0	0	0	5	5	1
4. Diagnostic tests	36	47	69	22	174	22
5. Synthesis of 1 + 2 + 4	10	10	45	5	70	9
6. Mechanism/etiology	40	35	36	25	136	17
7. Pathology	16	24	16	19	75	9
8. Therapy	19	50	52	40	161	20
9. Toxicity of treatments	5	5	23	17	50	6
10. Basic science	51	13	7	16	87	11
11. Prognosis	0	3	0	9	12	2
12. Epidemiology	0	4	4	16	24	3
TOTALS	179	191	255	176	801	100

responses, making diagnostic test responses the most frequent of all those provided, exceeding even those relating to therapy. This pattern of frequency is present for all disciplines: diagnostic tests are within the top three in frequency for the four disciplines and in all but oncology exceed the frequency for therapy responses.

Skills relating to history taking, physical examination, the interpretation of findings from these activities, and the assessment of patient prognosis fare rather poorly in this analysis: they are tested in only 3 percent of responses. This is particularly surprising in view of Sandler's (1979) observation that most diagnoses and treatment plans can be made on the basis of history and physical examination alone and in view of the fact that the ABIM, for example, no longer conducts oral examinations to assess these skills.

With the relative emphasis placed on the use of diagnostic tests in the MKSAP-V examination, whether it be disproportionate or not, it would seem reasonable to surmise that a full range of knowledge of and competency in test use and interpretation could be accommodated in the examination. To ascertain whether this was so, the diagnostic test responses were categorized again, this time according to the measurement concept(s) they illustrated. Again, responses that could be classified under more than one category were so classified, so that the 174 diagnostic test replies led to 309 categorizations. The results are displayed in Table 14.3 and show that the majority of diagnostic test responses called for the examinee to make a judgment concerning the relevance or cogency of the test in a given clinical situation or to judge whether it should be combined with or was more appropriate than other tests for a given medical condition. A fourth most frequent response assessed the examinee's ability to reach a diagnosis, given a test result. A meager 3 percent of the responses concerned the method of performing a test, 2 percent the specificity of a test, 1 percent the sensitivity of the test, and 1 percent the predictive value of a test for a therapeutic response. The latter three concepts were addressed only in an indirect fashion. For example, the concept of sensitivity was approached with a response option such as "the serum level of carcinoembryonic antigen is commonly elevated in patients with teratocarcinoma." Finally, measurement concepts such as accuracy, reliability, bias, range of normal, referent values, positive and negative predictive value for diagnosis, cost, and cost-effectiveness were not assessed at all.

Because of the lack of detail in the ABIM standards of competence (Table 14.1), it is difficult to compare the concepts actu-

TABLE 14.3
Measurement Concepts Addressed by Diagnostic Test Responses
in Part I of the MKSAP-V Examination

Measurement Concept	No. of Responses	% of Responses
Relevance of test	118	38
Role of test in combination or comparison with other tests	90	29
Interpretation of test results	80	26
Method of performing test	9	3
Specificity	6	2
Sensitivity	3	1
Predictive value for therapeutic response	2	1
Adverse effects	1	0
Accuracy, precision, bias, range of normal, referent values, predictive value for diagnosis, predictive value for prognosis, cost, cost-effectiveness, efficacy	NOT TESTED	
TOTAL	309	100

ally evaluated in the MKSAP-V with those identified as important
by the ABIM. It is obvious, however, that most of the ABIM standards are not evaluated at all in the MKSAP-V examination. The
ABIM certification examination itself may be more comprehensive
in this respect, but unfortunately it is unavailable for review.

No doubt the major reason that current examination methods fall short of testing concepts and skills related to the use of
diagnostic tests is that these concepts and skills are not yet routinely taught in medical schools, despite their recognition by such
bodies as the American Board of Internal Medicine as expressed in
Table 14.1. We will now discuss some concepts of diagnostic tests,
then describe current approaches to teaching and some possibili-
ties for evaluation in the latter sections of this chapter.

Concepts Essential to the Effective Ordering and Interpretation of Diagnostic Tests

This section is offered as a brief primer, rather than an in-depth analysis, of some key characteristics of diagnostic tests. Although a considerable amount of technical jargon has been invented to label the various characteristics, the reader should not be deterred by this as it is the underlying concepts, rather than the labels, that are important and these concepts are relatively straightforward.

Observer Variation, Accuracy, Precision, and Bias

In Chapter 3 of this book, the concepts of observer variation, accuracy, precision, and bias are introduced. A thorough understanding of these concepts is crucial to the interpretation of diagnostic information, whether this be acquired at the bedside or derived from the laboratory.

Focusing on the latter, each lab employs quality-control techniques to ensure that its results are "accurate" or close to an accepted standard (concurrent or criterion validity) but accuracy is possible only within a range. The lab seldom provides this "range of error" to the clinician spontaneously. It is apparent from the study of Skendzel (1978) that clinicians can misinterpret changes in laboratory test results because of this.

The situation in the laboratory, however, is generally much better than that which occurs when clinicians attempt to interpret complex patterns such as those on radiographs, electrocardiograms, electroencephalograms and the like. For these, there is no "gold standard" or criterion by which to judge the accuracy of results and the problems in inter- and intra-observer variation are far greater than most clinicians realize (Dept. of Clinical Epidemiology & Biostatistics, 1980a, 1980b; Koran, 1975a, 1975b; Yerushalmy, 1969).

Sensitivity, Specificity, and Predictive Value of Qualitative Diagnostic Tests

The management of a patient's problems usually requires that the physician reach a definite decision concerning the presence or absence of disease so that an appropriate course of action can be undertaken. Frequently these decisions are based on cutoff points in test results. Since the tests are imperfect, biologic systems vary, and the cutoff points are arbitrary, it is not surprising that the wrong decision is made on occasion for individual patients. To make things more complicated, there are often tests with different characteristics which may enter into the same medical decision. Understanding, comparing, and controlling the errors made by these tests are essential to optimum medical care.

The relevant concepts which must be mastered by clinicians are illustrated by Tables 14.4a and b. In this example, blood pressure was assessed on 82 patients by direct arterial puncture, the most accurate method available. Patients whose average intra-arterial diastolic pressure was at least 90 mm Hg were termed hypertensive. The indirect blood pressures of these patients were then assessed by two methods, anaeroid and mercury sphygmomanometry, and the results were compared with the direct pressures. If the same cutoff point is used (a diastoic BP of 90 mm Hg or more) to define a person as hypertensive, it is seen from the table that both of the indirect methods will misclassify some hypertensive patients as normotensive and some normotensive patients as hypertensive. Furthermore, the anaeroid readings are somewhat different from the mercury ones, resulting in different types of misclassification. What are the error rates and their implications and how can these two indirect methods be compared?

In Table 14.4a, the correct and incorrect classifications provided by the anaeroid method are enumerated. The "sensitivity" of a test is its ability to identify correctly those people who actually have the disease. In this case, 34 people have hypertension and the anaeroid sphygmomanometer identifies 19 of them or 56 percent. The "specificity" of a test is its ability to correctly identify those people who do not have the disease. Here 45 of 48 normotensive people or 94 percent are correctly labeled. In most clinical settings, however, a physician would not have access to (or feel it warranted to obtain) intra-arterial readings. Therefore, the sensitivity and specificity of the indirect readings will be of less relevance than the "predictive value" of indirect readings above and below the cutoff point. The "positive predictive value" of a test is the likelihood that a person with a positive test actually has the disease in question. Here, a person with an anaeroid reading at or above 90 mm Hg has an (19/22 =) 86 percent chance of being found hypertensive by direct readings. If the indirect reading is below 90, the likelihood that the person will be found free of disease (i.e., normotensive on direct reading) is (45/60 =) 75 percent; this is the negative predictive value. Finally, the total number of correct tests (positive or negative) by the

TABLE 14.4a
Operating Characteristics of Anaeroid Sphygmomanometry at a Prevalence of Hypertension of 41 Percent Among 82 Subjects

Intra-arterial Pressure (mm Hg)

		≥ 90	< 90
Indirect	≥ 90	19 (a)	3 (b)
Anaeroid			
Pressure	< 90	15 (c)	45 (d)

Sensitivity = a/(a + c) = .56
Specificity = d/(b + d) = .94
Positive predictive value = a/(a + b) = .86
Negative predictive value = d/(c + d) = .75
Accuracy = (a + d)/(a + b + c + d) = .78

TABLE 14.4b
Operating Characteristics of Mercury Sphygmomanometry at a Prevalence of Hypertension of 41 Percent

Intra-arterial Pressure (mm Hg)

		≥ 90	< 90
Indirect	≥ 90	32 (a)	4 (b)
Mercury			
Pressure	< 90	2 (c)	44 (d)

Sensitivity = .94
Specificity = .92
Positive predictive value = .89
Negative predictive value = .96
Accuracy = .93

anaeroid method divided by the total number of tests done provides the "accuracy" of the indirect method, which in this example is [(19 + 45)/82 =] 78 percent.

The Range of Normal of Quantitative Diagnostic Tests

Technology permits the measurement of many biologic variables quantitatively rather than just qualitatively. Ideally, quantitative results would give the clinician an accurate statement about the nature and severity of a patient's disease and/or its prognosis or therapeutic responsiveness. Unfortunately, most test results are merely provided with a "range of normal" and, beyond that, the connection of the test result to various aspects of clinical care is left entirely to the clinician. As it happens, the range of normal is a very shaky base from which to make clinical decisions.

To begin with, the use of the term *normal* is ill-understood in medicine and Murphy (1976) has described no less than seven meanings of the word. In the laboratory setting, the range of normal of a test is often defined as "the mean plus or minus two standard deviations." That this definition is illogical is clear from its implications (Sackett, 1978). First, it means that all diseases have the same frequency (Sackett, 1973). Second, it implies that some patients must have negative values since the normal distribution has a limitless range. Finally, it guarantees that the only normal patient is the one who has not yet been worked up since the likelihood that a given patient will be defined as abnormal is 5 percent on each and every test he or she undergoes (see Table 14.5). The clinician who is unaware of these implications is ill-prepared to defend himself and his patient against multichannel analyses and "range of normal disease," let alone make appropriate interpretations of the laboratory tests he has selectively ordered.

Clinicians cannot depend on others to tell them what tests to use or how to interpret them because the use of diagnostic information must be adjusted to the clinical setting and tailored to the specific patient. Thus an understanding of the basic concepts of diagnostic test use and at least an appreciation of some of these concepts is crucial to the effective practice of medicine.

Those clinicians who have just read through this section will no doubt appreciate the gap between what they learned about the use of diagnostic tests in their medical training and what is currently known about such matters. As medical educators we must

TABLE 14.5
Relation Between Number of Independent
Laboratory Tests Performed (n) and
Proportion of Normal Patients called
"Normal" (0.95^n)*

n	0.95^n**
1	0.95
5	0.77
20	0.36
100	0.006

*From Sackett (1978)
**Normal range 95% of distribution

strive to narrow this gap so that future generations of physicians and their patients will not suffer under the same handicap.

Current Teaching and Learning of
Concepts Essential to Effective
Use of Diagnostic Tests

The evidence concerning teaching of appropriate principles in diagnostic test use is, unfortunately, only circumstantial and anecdotal. Most medical school courses that deal with laboratory tests are taught by pathologists or clinical chemists and dwell on the technical aspects of the tests and/or when, in conventional wisdom, they should be ordered. Epidemiology courses may deal with the predictive value of tests, but these are usually screening tests and such courses are seldom accorded much status or time in curricula by either medical schools or their students. It might be argued that diagnostic test principles should be taught as part of clinical skills programs in the wards and clinics rather than in pathology or epidemiology departments, if they are to be perceived by students as useful and to be effectively applied by graduates in clinical practice. It is unlikely that this occurs in many medical schools at the present time. In any event most of the concern about misuse of diagnostic tests has been expressed not by clinicians but by laboratory specialists (Benson, 1978; Freeborn et al., 1972; Galen and Gambino, 1975; Hardwick et al., 1975; Martin, 1971; Murphy and Henry, 1978; Pineault, 1977;

Skendzel, 1978; Ward et al., 1976), epidemiologists (Feinstein, 1974, 1975; Screening for Disease, 1974; Martin, 1971; Murphy, 1976; Sackett, 1973, 1978), and health care administrators (Eisenberg, 1977; Freeborn et al., 1972; Pineault, 1977). Studies by these groups and others have clearly documented that medical students, housestaff, and physicians frequently misuse or do not understand the rationale for and/or value of tests they order (Edwards et al., 1973). Surprisingly and rather distressingly, most reports of attempts to alter the test-ordering behavior of physicians appear to have emphasized cost containment and reduction in test volume rather than rational test use. To date, we have come across only one report of a formal instructional program for diagnostic test use that covers a broad range of appropriate issues, and this lacks systematic evaluation (Ward et al., 1976). Our efforts to discuss the extent of teaching of diagnostic test principles in medical schools hardly constitutes a survey, however, and readers will need to consider whether the teaching in their own schools is as devoid of relevant material on diagnostic test use as we have been led to believe is the general case.

If we are correct, then curriculum change is necessary before issues of evaluation can be assessed or addressed. The suggestion of curriculum change raises the inevitable question of how the systematic teaching of diagnostic test use can compete for time in an already crowded and expanding curriculum. While this question is beyond the scope of this chapter, we would like to offer those who must deal with it two beneficial consequences of diagnostic test concept application. First, when we apply these concepts in the everyday practice of clinical medicine, it simplifies rather than complicates clinical decision making by rendering some inferior tests unnecessary and clarifying the interpretation of others. Second, when confronted by claims concerning a new diagnostic test in our clinical reading, application of these concepts permits easy assessment of whether the test has been evaluated properly and, if so, whether or how we can use it in our own practices. Thus the concepts are not merely "academic" but are valuable for providing rational and efficient medical care and for sorting out the wheat from the chaff in new developments in medical diagnostics.

Future Teaching and Evaluation
of the Use of Diagnostic
Test Concepts

If the teaching of the effective use of diagnostic tests is inadequate, then it is difficult to imagine that evaluation can be in a much better state. Indeed, it would be unfair of examinations to test concepts that had not been taught. Thus it is difficult to criticize or praise our current approaches to evaluating diagnostic test use.

The future of evaluation of diagnostic test concepts similarly depends upon developments in the teaching of these concepts. If these are guided by the acquisition of competencies as outlined by the American Board of Internal Medicine (1979) (see Table 14.1) and other groups (American Institute for Research in the Behavioral Sciences, 1976; Price et al., 1971), then a fuller range of concepts will be taught and their appropriate application at the bedside and in other settings will follow.

The teaching of effective test use can be assisted by laboratory specialists and epidemiologists, particularly if these individuals have a clinical base. It is improbable, however, that students will achieve the level and range of competence expected by the ABIM unless clinical faculty are similarly qualified. Most clinical faculty do not possess these skills at present (Casscells et al., 1978).

Our response to this problem at McMaster University has been the evolution of teaching materials and methods designed to provide faculty, housestaff, and students with "critical assessment skills" applicable to diagnostic test use and a range of other pertinent matters including treatment efficacy, patient prognosis, quality of medical care, and errors in clinical assessment. The materials are provided in problem-oriented format including a series of self-contained instructional packages that present clinical problems, information on the methods that apply to such problems, and an exercise on the clinical problem that the student can tackle. The part of the course on diagnostic tests can be covered in about two hours of student preparation plus two hours of tutorial time; the complete course usually requires five tutorial sessions plus student assignment time and concludes with students applying the methodologic principles to an issue from their own clinical practice. Faculty and housestaff who have participated in these "critical appraisal" courses have been generally highly enthusiastic and at present demand for such courses greatly exceeds our capacity to offer them. To attempt to deal with this delightful problem we have asked graduates of previous courses to act as co-tutors so that they can subsequently provide such courses within their own discipline on a continuing basis. To assist in making the clinical problems relevant to the students, we have developed a "bank" of problems with examples from several clinical disciplines. In addition, students who work up relevant problems as part of their course work or after it are invited to contribute them to the bank.

For our own undergraduate medical students, diagnostic test concepts are introduced into the curriculum in a number of ways. First, the importance of the concepts is recognized in the objectives of the program. Second, each of the biomedical problems that form the basis of the curriculum is reviewed by a "discipline consultant" from clinical epidemiology and from laboratory medicine and, where appropriate, diagnostic test issues and resources are identified. Third, students can take electives in laboratory medicine or clinical epidemiology or both. Fourth, pathologists, laboratory medicine specialists, clinical epidemiologists, and biostatisticians act as tutors in the regular M.D. program. It is important to point out here that no time is set aside in the curriculum for formal teaching about diagnostic tests. Rather, diagnostic test issues are raised only when they arise naturally in discussing the management of a clinical problem.

Our most recent step to complete the integration of diagnostic test concepts into the acquisition of clinical skills has been to teach the tutors of clinical clerks (senior medical students) these skills. The training of tutors has been modeled on the apprenticeship principles of "see one, do one, teach one." We show tutors how the principles apply to a clinical problem ("see one"), invite the tutors to work through an example from their own practice ("do one"), and then offer tutors the opportunity to work through their example, in tutorial fashion, with one or more volunteer medical students ("teach one"). The tutors are then provided with self-learning packages on diagnostic tests (described above) for their clinical clerks and asked to introduce these at an appropriate opportunity in the workup and discussion of clinical cases. The concepts to which students are introduced in the fashion outlined above include the sensitivity, specificity, and predictive value of diagnostic tests.

We have recently completed a controlled trial to evaluate how well students can handle these concepts and how well our teaching approach improves students' handling of them (Tugwell et al., 1982). In this study, tutors were allocated to receive or not receive our "see one, do one, teach one" sessions on diagnostic test use. Those who were allocated to receive the sessions were provided afterwards with learning packages for their tutorial groups (usually comprising five students).

All students (with or without tutors who had special instruction) were given a pretest and posttest to assess their use of diagnostic test information. The format of these tests consists of a paper patient problem, some questions on the sensitivity, specificity, and predictive value of a diagnostic test ordered for the patient, and an article from the recent medical literature from which the appropriate diagnostic test information can be extracted. To test the concepts rather than the recollection of jargon, we avoided use of terms such as *sensitivity, specificity,* and *predictive value.* For example, students were asked, "What is the likelihood that this patient has a urinary tract infection?" rather than, "What is the positive predictive value of the test result?"

According to preset criteria of "clinically important" improvement, the ability of the students in the intervention group to handle scientific concepts applicable to the evaluation of both diagnostic tests and treatments was substantially and significantly improved in comparison with students in the control group.

Although the results of this study are encouraging, we consider it to be only one step along the path of evaluation of diagnostic test principles and practice. Other steps would comprise expanding the principles taught to include observer variation, accuracy, precision, bias, and the range of normal. Evaluation will ultimately have to test how well students use and interpret diagnostic tests for their own patients. Review of clinical records and direct observation will be more appropriate for these tasks than paper-and-pencil patient management problems.

Conclusion

Although the modern clinician has a multitude of highly sophisticated diagnostic tests at his or her fingertips, the clinician's ability to use these tests is limited sharply by lack of knowledge of their characteristics. This situation is tragic because information on test characteristics is readily available. To remedy this problem, medical educators must apprise themselves of the features of tests in common use, must develop curricula to describe these features to students, and must generate valid tools to evaluate student performance in the use of diagnostic tests. It is our view that all of this should be integrated with clinical teaching rather than added to the curriculum as yet another course, taught by yet another group of specialists. A start on this enterprise has been made here and elsewhere, and we believe that future generations of clinicians will be better able to use advancing diagnostic technology to the benefit of their patients. If this is so, we should be able to document the competency of these new clinicians by many of the methods described here and in other chapters in this book.

References

Abrams, H. L.: The "overutilization" of x-rays. N Engl J Med 300, 1213-1216 (1979).

American Board of Internal Medicine: Clinical competence in internal medicine. Ann Intern Med 90, 402-411 (1979).

American Board of Pediatrics: Foundations for evaluating the competency of pediatricians. Chicago: American Board of Pediatrics (1974).

American Institute for Research in the Behavioral Sciences: The definition of clinical competence in internal medicine; performance dimensions and rationales for clinical skill areas. Palo Alto, Calif.: American Institute for Research in Behavioral Sciences (1976).

Benson, E. S.: Research and educational initiatives in improving the use of the clinical laboratory. Ann Biol Clin 36, 159-161 (1978).

Campbell, J. A., Makler, M. T.: Cost awareness: the effect on laboratory use. Presented at the Conference on Clinical Decision Making and Laboratory Use. University of Minnesota, Minneapolis, Minn. (1980).

Casscells, W., Schoenberger, A., Graboys, T. B.: Interpretation by physicians of clinical laboratory results. N Engl J Med 299, 999-1001 (1978).

Department of Clinical Epidemiology and Biostatistics, Clinical Epidemiology Rounds: Clinical disagreement: how often it occurs and why. Can Med Assoc J 123, 613-617 (1980a).

Department of Clinical Epidemiology and Biostatistics, Clinical Epidemiology Rounds: How to read a journal. II: To learn about a diagnostic test. Can Med Assoc J 123, 499-504 (1980b).

Dixon, R. H.: Utilization of clinical chemistry services by medical house staff. Arch Intern Med 134, 1064-1067 (1974).

Edwards, L. D., Levin, S., Balagtas, R., Lowe, P., Landau, W., Lepper, M. H.: Ordering patterns and utilization of bacteriologic culture reports. Arch Intern Med 132, 678-682 (1973).

Eisenberg, J. M.: An educational program to modify laboratory use by house-staff. J Med Educ 52, 578-581 (1977).

Feinstein, A. P.: The derangements of the "range of normal." Clin Pharmacol Ther 15, 528-540 (1974).

Feinstein, A. P.: On the sensitivity, specificity, and discrimination of diagnostic tests. Clin Pharmacol Ther 17, 104-116 (1975).

Frazier, H. S.: Medical decisions and society. Presented at the Conference on Clinical Decision Making and Laboratory Use. University of Minnesota, Minneapolis, Minn. (1980).

Freeborn, D. K., Baer, D., Greenlick, M. R., Bailey, J. W.: Determinants of medical care utilization: physicians' use of laboratory services. Am J Public Health 62, 846-853 (1972).

Galen, P. S., Gambino, S. R.: Beyond normality: the predictive value and efficiency of medical diagnoses. New York: Wiley (1975).

Greenland, P., Mushlin, A. I., Griner, P. F.: Discrepancies between knowledge and use of diagnostic studies in asymptomatic patients. J Med Educ 54, 863-869 (1979).

Griner, P. F., Liptzin, B.: Use of the laboratory in a teaching hospital: implications for patient care, education and hospital costs. Ann Intern Med 75, 157-163 (1971).

Griner, P. F.: Use of laboratory tests in a teaching hospital: long-term trends. Reductions in use and relative costs. Ann Intern Med 90, 243-248 (1979).

Griner, P. F.: Training housestaff in effective laboratory use. Presented at the Conference on Clinical Decision Making and Laboratory Use. University of Minnesota, Minneapolis, Minn. (1980).

Hardwick, D. F., Vertinsky, P., Barth, R. T., Mitchell, V. E., Berstein, M., Vertinsky, I.: Clinical styles and motivation: a study of laboratory use. Med Care 13, 397-408 (1975).

Koran, L. M.: The reliability of clinical methods, data and judgments. Part I. N Engl J Med 293, 642-646 (1975a).

Koran, L. M.: The reliability of clinical methods, data and judgments. Part II. N Engl J Med 293, 695-701 (1975b).

Kralewski, J.: Medical decisions, technology and social need. Presented at the Conference on Clinical Decision Making and Laboratory Use. University of Minnesota, Minneapolis, Minn. (1980).

Lawrence, R. S.: The role of physician education in cost containment. J Med Educ 54, 841-847 (1979).

Martin, S. P.: The clinical laboratory: cost-benefit and effectiveness. Ann Intern Med 75, 309-310 (1971).

Murphy, E. A.: The logic of medicine. Baltimore: John Hopkins University Press (1976).

Murphy, J., Henry, J. B.: Effective utilization of clinical laboratories. Hum Pathol 9, 625-633 (1978).

Olsen, D. M., Kane, R. L., Procter, P. H.: A controlled trial of multiphasic screening. N Engl J Med 294, 925-930 (1976).

Pineault, R.: The effect of medical training factors on physician utilization behavior. Med Care 15, 51-67 (1977).

Price, P. B., Taylor, C. W., Nelson, D. E., Lewis, E. G., Laughmiller, G. C.: Measurement of predictors of physician performance. Two decades of intermittently sustained research. Salt Lake City, Utah: L.L.R. Press (1971).

Reiser, S. J.: Decision making and the evolution of modern medicine. Presented at the Conference on Clinical Decision Making and Laboratory Use. University of Minnesota, Minneapolis, Minn. (1980).

Sackett, D. L.: The usefulness of laboratory tests in health-screening programs. Clin Chem 19, 366-372 (1973).

Sackett, D. L.: Clinical diagnosis and the clinical laboratory. Clin Invest Med 1, 37-43 (1978).

Sandler, G.: Cost of unnecessary tests. Brit Med J 2, 21-24 (1979).

Schroeder, S. A., Kenders, K., Cooper, J. K., Piemone, T. E.: Use of laboratory tests and pharmaceuticals. Variation among physicians and effect of cost audit on subsequent use. JAMA 225, 969-973 (1973).

Schroeder, S. A., O'Leary, D. S.: Differences in laboratory use and length of stay between university and community hospitals. J Med Educ 52, 418-420 (1977).

Screening for Disease. A series from The Lancet. Reprinted from the Lancet October 5 to December 21 (1974).

Skendzel, L. P.: How physicians use laboratory tests. JAMA 239, 1077-1080 (1978).

Tugwell, P., Bennett, K. J., Haynes, R. B., Neufeld, V. R., Sackett, D. L.: A controlled trial of teaching critical appraisal to M.D. clinical clerks. Clin Res 30, 24/A (1982).

Ward, P. C., Harris, I. B., Burke, M. D., Horwitz, C.: Systematic instruction in interpretive aspects of laboratory medicine. J Med Educ 51, 548-656 (1976).

Yerushalmy, J.: The statistical assessment of the variability in observer perception and description of roentgenographic pulmonary shadows. Radiol Clin North Am 7, 381-392 (1969).

PART IV

Implications

This section considers the implications of present evaluation procedures and methods in various areas of medical education. The authors examine the role of evaluation of competence in three areas: education (undergraduate and postgraduate), licensure and certification, and the delivery of health care. One additional chapter is devoted to implications for further research.

CHAPTER 15

Implications
for Education

VICTOR R. NEUFELD

This book has led the persistent reader through a detailed review of research directed toward the definition of clinical competence to a consideration of the various methods used to assess components of competence and into some areas where these insights can be applied.

This chapter, by contrast, is a synthesis for the benefit of individuals directly responsible for the education of physicians in a clinical clerkship, a postgraduate residency program, or a program of continuing medical education. Three educational problems have been selected to provide a focus for this discussion. Each problem is derived from one of the three preceding sections of the book and is approached in a way that hopefully will be useful to clinician-educators.

The problems are:

1. The problem of categorization. Derived from the Part I, on the definition of clinical competence, this section proposes an approach to categorization which is intended to be simple, realistic, and adaptable.
2. The problem of selecting assessment methods. The reader may feel overwhelmed by the number of tools available and by the detailed critique of each in Part II. We offer a grid which displays the relative appropriateness of a particular assessment method for a specified ability.
3. The problem of educational differentiation. Insights on the definition and measurement of clinical competence

can be applied in a variety of educational situations. Out of this concern, we examine the question of how new ideas about clinical competence can be adjusted for the quantitative and qualitative differences in education programs.

The Problem of Categorization

This problem is not unique to medical education. Any complex activity is plagued by the search for satisfactory classifications or "typologies" of that activity. This problem presents itself to medical educators when they are faced with such tasks as writing (and clustering) educational objectives, preparing appropriate learning opportunities, and selecting methods of competence assessment.

There are several features of the categorization problem. First, there are different conceptual schemes upon which a proposed categorization is based. A simple scheme, borrowed from the general educational literature, divides competence into cognitive, affective, and psychomotor domains (in other words, knowledge, attitudes, and skills). Another scheme uses the components of the clinical encounter: history taking, physical examination, ordering tests, designing a plan of management, and following the patient. Some schemes go beyond those activities of the physician-patient encounter to include self-education, teaching, and managing activities (Gonnella and Storey, 1981).

An interesting variant was described in the recent report of an *ad hoc* committee of the Association of American Medical Colleges which reviewed external examinations (Clemente et al., 1981). This report categorizes components of competence into three groupings: cumulative, enduring, and inferred qualities. Again, while some may quarrel with the adjectives used, the ideas are of interest to educators. *Cumulative* qualities are those that are directly influenced by the educational process (knowledge, technical skills, efficiency under stress, effective use of time); *enduring* qualities are not usually modified by educational interventions (examples are sensitivity and ethical behavior); *inferred* qualities are those which become important in postgraduate education and in practice (supervising ability and teaching ability are examples).

Another feature of the categorization problem is complexity. Admittedly there is a danger in oversimplification, but excessively complex schemes may discourage potential users and force a relatively simple activity to fit a complicated scheme. An example of complexity is the three-dimensional framework developed by the American Board of Pediatrics for the construction of a certification examination (Burg et al., 1976). The three dimensions are subject matter, tasks, and ability. An example is given where appropriate behaviors are described for the management of an infant with clinical features of meningitis, which involves a total of 15 cells in a matrix. While some theoretical utility can be seen in this approach, its widespread application is doubtful because of its complexity. Another version of this matrix has recently been proposed by the National Board of Medical Examiners (NBME) for its proposed "comprehensive qualifying evaluation (CQE) program" (Levitt, 1979). The matrix consists of 5 abilities (similar to those in the American Board of Pediatrics project) and 10 activities resulting in 50 cells. The CQE, as proposed, is described in 12 of 50 cells.

For some activities performed by physicians, a classification may simply not fit. For example, when a physician performs a lumbar puncture, several components of competence are observable *concurrently*. These include clinical judgment (the decision that a lumbar puncture is required), knowledge (of the anatomical structures involved), technical skills (using the lumbar puncture needle and equipment correctly), and interpersonal attributes (explaining the procedure to the patient and giving the patient confidence that the physician knows what he is doing). Also in this example the classifier may have difficulty knowing whether this is a diagnostic test or a therapeutic intervention—it could be both or either.

What conclusions can be drawn from this discussion and what practical approaches can be taken? It should be apparent that no one categorization scheme will be suitable for all educational and assessment situations. Educators will have to adapt any schema to the requirements of a particular situation. It would seem reasonable to keep any proposed categorization scheme relatively simple and realistic; a simpler scheme is likely to be more widely used and more easily adapted.

An example of a simple categorization is found in Table 15.1, adapted from the list of "Abilities" in the NBME matrix. It differs in that it has no "task" dimension. "Clinical skills" is a separate category from "Technical skills" although acquiring clinical information by taking a history and performing a physical examination in real life tends to be a composite activity. It is

TABLE 15.1

A Categorization of Clinical Competence

The following abilities are required in encounters between a physician and individual patients:

1. Clinical Skills

   The ability to acquire clinical information by talking with and examining patients, and interpreting the significance of the information obtained.

2. Knowledge and Understanding

   The ability to remember relevant knowledge about clinical conditions in order to provide effective and efficient care for patients.

3. Interpersonal Attributes

   The expression of those aspects of a physician's personal and professional character that are observable in interactions with patients.

4. Problem Solving and Clinical Judgment

   The application of relevant knowledge, clinical skills, and interpersonal attributes to the diagnosis, investigation, and management of the clinical problems of a given patient.

5. Technical Skills

   The ability to use special procedures and techniques in the investigation and management of patients.

---

recognized that separating "clinical skills" from "technical skills" is an arbitrary decision.

It should be noted that the categories used in Table 15.1 are restricted to those abilities which are required in the clinical encounter between a physician and an individual patient, consistent with the focus in this book. There are, of course, a number of other abilities (behaviors, competencies) which are desirable in physicians and are usually expressed or observable in situations other than the direct clinical encounter between a physician and a patient, such as a physician's responsibility to himself, to his immediate colleagues, to the profession, and to the community or society at large. This wider perspective of physician competence is displayed in Table 15.2.

To summarize, the "categorization problem" will never be

TABLE 15.2
A Categorization of General Physician Competence

This can be expressed in terms of responsibilities of the physician:

1. To Patients (Clinical Competence)

   Those abilities required in the individual physician-patient encounter.

2. To self

   This includes recognition of personal strengths, weaknesses, and emotional reactions; and habits of effective and efficient continuing learning.

3. To Immediate Colleagues

   Behaviors expressed in useful working relationships with other physicians, nurses, and health care personnel.

4. To the Profession

   Participation in professional organizations and activities.

5. To the Community and Society

   Awareness of broader issues in health and health care, and participation in selected community activities to promote health.

fully resolved, but the very act of discussion and revision may improve our understanding of clinical competence. In the meantime, any proposed scheme should be simple and realistic. An educator using any proposed scheme should be prepared to adapt it for a given situation.

The Problem of Selecting Assessment Methods

Having read this book, the clinician-educator may be uncertain about which assessment method to use. Some, while appearing attractive at first, turn out to be weak when certain measurement criteria are applied. Others may be relatively reliable in their application but are of limited validity. Still others are both precise and valid but are impractical to develop or apply in a given setting. How can all this be sorted out?

To begin, it must be restated that clinical competence is a multidimensional entity. No single assessment method can adequately measure it. Given this reality, two basic approaches have been used in the selection of assessment methods. The first involves using some combination of several separate instruments. And second, some individual assessment exercises tap several components of competence. We will take a brief look at some examples of both of these approaches.

Multiple-Method Combinations

This approach has been used mostly by agencies and organizations responsible for specialty certification. An early description of such a "comprehensive" examination was the result of several years of intensive research and development with the American Board of Orthopedic Surgery (Miller, 1968). Another example is the certification examination of the Canadian College of Family Physicians (CCFP). This examination specifically identifies several components of physician competence, then combines a number of methods of obtaining data including a paper-and-pencil (multiple-choice question) examination, patient management problems, a structured oral examination, and direct observation of an encounter with a simulated patient.

Similar approaches have been used in undergraduate medical education (Newble et al., 1978) and in residency training (Corley, 1977). In this latter example, Corley describes an evaluation system in a family practice residency program which includes a comprehensive entry assessment using a personality inventory, a test of medical knowledge, and a standardized observation of a physician-patient encounter. Further ongoing assessment during the course of training includes data from several sources: direct observations of randomly selected patient encounters using a TV camera, global ratings by family practice faculty, nurses, and supervising physicians from hospital rotations, chart audits, and an annual intensive two-day in-training examination (consisting of multiple-choice, patient management problem, and oral examinations).

Single Events with Several Components

A second approach to the problem of selecting appropriate assessment methods involves the design of a single event which systematically incorporates several components of clinical competence.

A good example of this approach is the Objective Structured Clinical Examination (OSCE), first described by Harden and Gleeson (1979). This examination involves having students move individually through a sequence of "stations," typically 15 to 20, as described in Chapter 13. While this approach has some drawbacks in terms of feasibility and artificial discontinuity, it has considerable credibility and has now been adapted to a variety of settings.

Another example of a single exercise which incorporates several components of competence is the "triple jump exercise" used at McMaster University (Painvin et al., 1979; Powles et al., 1981), a three-step structured oral examination (nicknamed by the students) designed specifically to tap performance in several areas including clinical reasoning, application of relevant knowledge, self-directed learning, and self-assessment. In step one, a student "thinks aloud" through a clinical problem—with the examiner role-playing the patient—allowing an assessment of problem definition, hypothesis generation, application of existing knowledge, and ability to identify knowledge gaps. In the next stage, the student spends some time (usually two hours) in searching out relevant information and in further problem analysis. On returning to the examiner for step three, the student's efficiency and effectiveness of self-directed learning can be assessed. The student then presents a synthesis of the problem, using any new insights acquired during the information search stage. Finally, the student is given an opportunity for detailed self-assessment, which is compared with the assessment of the examiner.

What practical advice can be given to the clinician-educator faced with the task of selecting appropriate methods of assessment? A simple three-step approach is proposed. The first step is to think through the competencies (abilities, components) of interest and display these using the categories in Table 15.1 or in some similar categorization. Second, from among the many methods available, select one or more methods as appropriate for assessing the components of interest. To assist with this step, we have displayed on a grid (Table 15.3) the methods of assessment described in Part III. The ordinate on the grid lists the five general categories of clinical competence (from Table 15.1), and the cells indicate the degree of appropriateness of the assessment method for a given ability. This weighting, using a system of plusses, is somewhat arbitrary, but attempts to reflect the critique of each method in earlier chapters. For more details on a

TABLE 15.3
The Methods/Abilities Grid

Abilities \ Methods	Oral Examinations	Written Examinations	Direct Observation*	Written Simulations (PMPs)	Computer Simulations	Record Review	Global Rating Scales
Clinical skills	+ (indirect)		+++	++	+	++ (indirect)	+
Knowledge and Understanding	+	++	+	+	+	+	+
Interpersonal Attributes	+		+++				+
Problem Solving and Clinical Judgment	+++		+	++	++	++	+
Technical Skills			+++			+ (indirect)	+

*Using either actual or "standardized" patients.

given assessment method, one can refer back to the relevant chapter. The third step involves making a choice of methods. This can result in a combination of several different methods or in the preparation (or adoption) of a single event which incorporates several components of competence, as described earlier.

The Problem of Educational Differentiation

Studies cited earlier in this book exemplified the application of aspects of clinical competence to various educational areas including undergraduate medical education, residency (graduate or postgraduate) education, continuing education of practicing physicians, and the special problems of licensure and certification. A common theme in all these discussions is the concept of educational differentiation.

This terms refers to the observation that there are both qualitative and quantitative differences in various educational programs. Different *levels* of competence are expected when comparing undergraduate, postgraduate and continuing education. Within each of these areas (with the possible exception of continuing education) again various levels of competence from neophytes to senior students are expected, corresponding to a quantitative differentiation. Similarly, different *components* of competence are emphasized within and across these broad areas of educational activity, corresponding to qualitative differences in evaluation of competence. Several examples of both aspects will be discussed; then we will propose an approach to clarifying some of the confusion which exists.

Quantitative Aspects

One might assume that as medical students progress through their medical school education and then through a residency program, there is an incremental increase in their level of competence. This assumption, however, bears closer inspection. Some components of competence do not necessarily become enhanced—they may, in fact deteriorate with increasing training. The capacity of students to empathize with patients, for example, may decrease with time; that is, their "cynicism" increases (Becker et al., 1961; Diseker and Michielutte, 1981). Similar observations have been made in other areas. Interviewing skills acquired during the first year of medical school training may deteriorate by the final year, particularly if there have not been opportunities to practice these skills in intervening years.

When applying standard assessment measures (for example, measures of knowledge, clinical skills, and clinical judgment), it is usually possible to differentiate between undergraduate and postgraduate trainees. The same is not the case, however, when comparing postgraduate trainees and practicing clinicians. Residents, particularly in their more senior years, appear to know more than their teachers. In fact, there are few available measures which accurately reflect accumulated clinical experience, so that knowledgeable but relatively inexperienced postgraduate trainees consistently perform better than experienced clinicians. Carefully prepared and structured oral examinations may prove the exception to this trend (Maatsch, 1980) and other measures are still at a developmental stage (Norman et al., 1979).

Qualitative Aspects

Not only are there differences in levels of competence, there are also differences in the components of competence that are emphasized in various parts of the educational continuum.

The recently published AAMC report on external examinations, referred to earlier, provides a good example of this qualitative differentiation (Clemente et al., 1981). The report, to recapitulate, describes three types of competence: there are qualities that are assumed to increase systematically with increasing training (these are *cumulative* and include knowledge, technical skills, and efficiency under stress). Other *enduring* qualities, notably interpersonal attributes, are not expected to change with training. A third set of *inferred* qualities assumes importance in postgraduate training and practice; included are supervisory ability, teaching ability, and independent decision making. These categories illustrate the need to pay attention to qualitative differentiation in clinical education.

As another example, we can refer to the accumulating experience, particularly in the United States, with recertification. A major stumbling block to the routine application of recertification is the fact that practicing clinicians have become highly differentiated. For example, the Medical Knowledge Self-assessment Program (MKSAP) has items categorized under nine medical subspecialities. The consultant internist with a practice specializing in cardiology may have considerable difficulty with the sections on neurology or allergy. Some procedures to handle this dilemma have recently been described (American Board of Medical Specialties, 1978).

This same qualitative differentiation is at the heart of the "content-specificity" debate, elaborated in Chapter 17, "Implications for Research." To date, there is no clear evidence that problem-solving ability developed predominantly in one content domain is transferable to another. Further work on this question is in progress and is awaited with considerable interest.

Combined Quantitative and Qualitative Aspects

There are some areas of educational activity in which both quantitative and qualitative aspects of differentiation apply. A classic example is the clinical clerkship, but similar issues arise from the residency programs in family medicine or rotating internships where the trainee passes through an arbitrary sequence of specialty services. Let us examine the clinical clerkship in more detail.

From several clerkship studies, it is clear that learning experiences and assessment expectations differ markedly from one specialty setting to another (Bryne and Cohen, 1973; Patel, 1981) and considerable variation occurs from one institutional setting to another in the same specialty rotation. These qualitative differences are compounded by the rather arbitrary time sequences of the clerkship. Typically, students enter the clerkship with presumably similar levels of competence and are allocated to various sequences, either at random or by the students' choices. The result is that a particular student might begin with psychiatry and do the surgery rotation eight months later while a second student may do the reverse sequence. Does the clerkship sequence influence performance at graduation? Is it practical or desirable to adjust the teaching activities and assessment standards to the "stage of development" of students? Are there competencies which are independent of the content and clinical setting of a given rotation? Although there have been some attempts to look at these issues, much more work must be done.

We propose a basic approach to this dilemma of educational differentiation. Underlying this approach is the assumption that collaboration among specialty groups, programs, agencies, and institutions is desirable and potentially useful. The results of such collaboration would include increased understanding about activities, expectations, areas of interest and expertise, and improved efficiency by avoiding unnecessary overlap of activities.

The prototype for this approach might be a newly formed

clerkship committee in a medical school, consisting of the directors of each of the clinical clerkship rotations. Let us assume that each director is responsible for the clerkship for a given specialty in all participating institutions and settings. The task of this committee would be to plan a coordinated educational experience for students in the clerkship. Let us also assume that these directors had not worked together before but rather had run their own rotations independently.

The first step would be a display of the objectives, learning opportunities, and assessment methods for each rotation. These could then be compared. This comparative display might use, as a framework, a commonly agreed upon structure or categorization scheme (such as Table 15.1). This would make it possible to identify gaps in the clerkship or areas of unnecessary overlap. Some overlap may be desirable, but it should be justifiable and intentional. It may be possible to explore how and where certain unacceptable gaps could be handled.

A further stage might be the realization that there are some general goals which are relevant throughout the clerkship and which are independent of the content or clinical setting of a given rotation. Examples of such components are medical record keeping and systematic clinical problem solving, basic clinical skills and independent learning ability. Other objectives, while applicable across the clerkship, would logically be emphasized in a specific rotation. Some examples would be basic technical skills (suturing of cuts in the surgery rotation), mental status examination (emphasized in psychiatry), or use of community health resources (particularly relevant in the family medicine rotation). This activity could lead to the realization that a clerkship has both differentiated and undifferentiated features which would then allow for more rational decisions about the relative importance (or unimportance) of sequencing.

This approach could be used in other educational settings. For example, there may be some value in reviewing a postgraduate residency program to see if there are some objectives that are general rather than specialty-specific. An initial attempt at designing educational programs to meet general residency objectives is the Academic Studies program described by Sibley (1978). A similar application, although at a more general level, is evident when representatives of educational institutions, testing agencies, and professional organizations come together to discuss issues of licensure and certification.

Conclusion

To conclude, we have presented some general strategies designed to be useful to educators reading this book. The strategies were presented as possible solutions to problems identified in each of the three major sections of this book.

References

American Board of Medical Specialties: Report of conference on research in evaluation procedures. Chicago (1978).

Becker, H. S., et al.: Boys in white—student culture in medical school. Chicago: University of Chicago Press (1961).

Burg, F. D., et al.: A method for defining competency in pediatrics. J Med Educ 51, 824-828 (1976).

Byrne, N., Cohen, R.: Observational study of clinical clerkship activities. J Med Educ 48, 919-927 (1973).

Clemente, C., et al.: External examinations for the evaluation of medical education achievement and for licensure—a position paper. J Med Educ (suppl) 56, 933-962 (1981).

Corley, J.: Evaluation techniques in family practice residency training. Can Fam Phys 23, 202-204 (1977).

Diseker, R., Michielutte, R.: An analysis of empathy in medical students before and following clinical experience. J Med Educ 56, 1004-1010 (1981).

Gonnella, J. S., Storey, P. B.: Continuing medical education and clinical competence: a matrix approach to a complex problem. AMA Continuing Medical Education Newsletter 10, 3-15 (1981).

Harden, R., Gleeson, F.: Assessment of clinical competence using an objective structured clinical examination. Med Educ 13, 41 (1979).

Levitt, E.: Summary of Working Sessions on the Comprehensive Qualifying Evaluation Program, Annual Board Meeting, National Board of Medical Examiners, Philadelphia, Penn. (1979).

Maatsch, J. L.: Model for a criterion-referenced medical specialty test. Office of Medical Education Research and Development, Michigan State University in Collaboration with the American Board 1979 (1980).

Miller, G. E.: The orthopedic training study. JAMA 206, 601-606 (1968).

Newble, D. I., Elmslie, R. G., Baxter, A.: A problem-based criterion referenced examination of clinical competence. J Med Educ 53, 720-726 (1978).

Newble, D., et al.: The validity and reliability of a new examination of the clinical competence of medical students. Med Educ 15, 46-52 (1981).

Norman, G. R., et al.: Clinical experience and the structure of memory. Proceedings, 18th Annual Conference on Research in Medical Education, Washington, D.C. (1979).

Painvin, C., Neufeld, V., Norman, G., Walker, I., Whelan, G.: The triple jump exercise—a structured measure of problem-solving and self-directed learning. Proceedings, 18th Annual Conference on Research in Medical Education, Washington, D.C. (1979).

Patel, V.: The effects of a clinical clerkship program on the clinical competence of senior medical students. Unpublished thesis, McGill University (1981).

Powles, A. C. P., Wintrip, N., Neufeld, V. R., et al.: The triple jump exercise—Further studies of an evaluation technique. Ann Conf Res Med Educ 20, 74-79 (1981).

Sibley, J. C.: Postgraduate (residency) training at McMaster: A strategy for change. Med Educ 12, 76-81 (1978).

CHAPTER 16

Implications for Licensure and Certification

C. BARBER MUELLER

License and Licensure: The Privilege to Practice Medicine

Licensure is the process by which society, acting through a governmental agency or an agency authorized by government, grants permission to an individual to engage in a given occupation and use a particular title. After ascertaining that the applicant has met predetermined qualifications and obtained the minimal competence necessary to safeguard public health, safety, and welfare, the award of a medical license bestows the privilege to practice the art and science of medicine—in any or all of its branches (NBME, 1973, pp. 85-88).

The practice of medicine, however, does not lend itself to precise definition, either in terms of knowledge required, necessary skills, or procedures specific to it, and licensing bodies deal with a general concept of what constitutes the practice of medicine, a concept created by people who practice it and who have an intuitive knowledge of its domain (Derbyshire, 1969).

General statements about this domain have been written into provincial and state legislation to regulate human input into the profession in order to protect the public from incompetent and unethical practitioners. As these statutory mechanisms grant an unlimited scope of practice to the licensees, they also prohibit the practice of medicine by other individuals. Modern-day treatments, shaped by technologic advances unforeseen when most statutes were created, have made it impossible to apply vaguely worded laws to a definition of physician competence (Tancredi and Woods, 1972).

The most complete exposition of the principles embodied in these many statutes may be found in the *Essentials of a Modern Medical Practice Act* recently designed by a subcommittee of the Federation of State Medical Boards (1977).

This act states:

a. For the purposes of this act, a person is practicing medicine if he or she is authorized to practice medicine in this state.
b. Offers or undertakes to prescribe, give or administer any drug or medicine for the use of any other person.
c. Offers or undertakes to diagnose, correct and treat in any manner, or by any means, methods, devices or instrumentalities any disease, illness, pain, wound, fracture, infirmity, deformity, defect or abnormal physical or mental condition of any person.
d. Offers or undertakes to perform any surgical operation upon any person.
e. Uses, in the conduct of any occupation or profession pertaining to diagnosis or treatment of human disease or condition, the designation "Doctor," "Doctor of Medicine," "Doctor of Osteopathy," "D.O." or any combination thereof unless such a designation additionally contains the description of another branch of the healing arts for which a person has a license.

A concise statement representative of many statutes regarding the scope of medical practice is found in the California Statutes (1977):

The physician's and surgeon's certificate authorizes the holder to use drugs or what are known as medical preparations in or upon human beings and to sever or penetrate the tissues of human beings and to use any and all other methods in the treatment of diseases, injuries, deformities, or other physical or mental conditions.

The State Medical Board now feels this statute is no longer capable of meeting the needs of changing medical practice, and revisions are under consideration. Its vagueness has created problems as patients, practitioners, and government respond to technical innovations, the rise of unforeseen and unsettling ethical dilemmas, and the demand by patients for a more active role in their own health care (Wilkins, 1980).

A license to practice medicine grants the privilege to commit actions considered assault and battery or invasion of privacy when performed by an unlicensed individual. This license is the means whereby society recognizes treatment as a legitimate activity even though it may cause pain, suffering, bodily harm, or physical injury. When carried out without hostility and with the intent to cure, it permits wounding, assault, and even accidental homicide. The use of needles, knives, and other instruments to invade the body, the administration of anesthetic agents, narcotics, sedatives, or drugs prohibited to the rest of the people, and the invasion of another's privacy by examination of orifices and private parts are made legitimate by this license. With equal vigor it restricts these actions to situations specifically directed toward relief of pain and diagnosis or curing of disease. In criminal law, treatment is characterized as an application of force upon the body of another and its lawfulness for the physician derives not from the nature of the act, but from the rightfulness of someone to engage in it. Specific references in the Canadian Criminal Code permit surgical procedures by physicians while the Narcotics Control Act and the Food and Drugs Act deal with the dispensing of prescription drugs (Medical Treatment, 1980).

In return for the privilege to practice medicine and in acknowledgment of its obligations, the profession evolved codes of behavior which limit and govern professional conduct. Later it developed a scientific base for medical care. A close relationship developed between the educational systems which train the candidates and those bodies which examine and/or grant licenses. In viewing the educational process, the acquisition of technical knowledge and clinical skills seems to be given more formal emphasis than the acquisition of medical values.

The codes of proper physician behavior which reflect these medical values have been stated since antiquity. The earliest citations in the Smith papyrus were followed two thousand years later by the Oath of Hippocrates. Recent versions are seen in publications of all medical organizations, e.g., Canadian Medical Association, the American Medical Association, State and Provincial Medical Associations, the World Health Organization (Etziony, 1973). These authoritative restatements continue to reflect the issues of "confidentiality," "do no harm," "practice solely for the patient," "relate to colleagues," and "instruct the novices." Serving as behavioral constraints upon actions of the physician and the medical profession, social custom and the law reflect honor and respect for these traditional behaviors, and gross breaches of the code generally result in expulsion, i.e., loss of license.

Acquisition of this acceptable behavior, an understanding of its limitations, its obligations, and the responsibilities inherent in the profession occurs during medical school, residency training, and the early years of practice. Increasing conformity to this particular set of obligations and responsibilities constitutes a progressive professionalization for the physician role and has been the object of considerable study with regard to personal and social values, candidate selection, curriculum design, and medical school subcultures (Bloom, 1979). Suffice it to say that medical students gradually develop a professional self-image and begin to think of themselves in doctor-patient rather than student-teacher relationships. A sense of collegiality, secrecy, an ability to deal with uncertainty, and increasing confidence and competence in the activities of doctoring finally develop with increasing levels of training. Although the information explosion of the past half century has led to new knowledge and required new skills for the practice of medicine, these attitudes and behavior codes have not been altered significantly.

The practice of medicine is varied, its horizons are broad, and huge bodies of information have been developed which characterize each of perhaps 70 to 75 specialties. Attempts to define a core of required knowledge or skills have been productive only as they have evoked certain processes of thinking about education, even as they have been unable to define core knowledge common to all. Basic sciences such as Anatomy, Biochemistry, Physiology, and clinical sciences such as Surgery, Medicine, and Obstetrics are important disciplines in the basic medical educational process, but specific topics and specific information within this broad realm of basic and clinical disciplines is left to each of the medical schools and to the individuals who are studying therein (Derbyshire, 1969).

The licensing agencies of the 10 provinces and the 50 states use fairly similar licensing methods, with common techniques and reasonably similar standards. This process generally requires (1) minimum age, (2) graduation from an approved medical school, (3) internship in an approved program, (4) the meeting of implicit and unstated requirements for the "behavioral/professionalization" component, (5) testimony relating to moral and ethical standards, and (6) examination in a range of subjects related to the preparation for practice. Admission to the licensing process requires authorization from some accredited agency. In Canada a Provincial Medical Council awards the enabling certificate whereas in the United States the National Board of Medical

Examiners (NBME) and the State Medical Boards require a certificate from an accredited medical school. The medical school's involvement in both instances provides an assessment of the professional behavioral component included in elements (1)-(4) listed above. Admission may also occur by authorization of a Provincial Medical Council or State Medical Board after the survey of credentials of those applicants who apply from other than accredited schools—a process which again attempts to satisfy the "professional/behavior" component and the "moral standards component." In the GAP report of NBME this process is called "Internal A" (NBME, 1973).

In Canada, the Medical Council of Canada, established in 1912, under governmental auspices and representing schools and Provincial Councils, designs and administers an examination for licensing purposes. Subject to other supplementary requirements, candidates who pass are eligible for licensing by a Provincial Medical Council (Information Pamphlet, 1979). This examination attempts to assess a candidate's factual knowledge of clinical medicine and his ability to solve and treat clinical problems. Using six clinical discipline committees it draws material from the R. S. McLaughlin Center item pool to create a two-day examination composed of multiple-choice items, pictorial material, and patient management problems. Candidates are eligible to sit for the examination following receipt of an enabling certificate issued by a Provincial Medical Council. This certificate is normally issued during the final year in medical school. After achieving the M.D. degree, one year of postgraduate training is required before a candidate is enrolled on the Canadian Medical Register and eligible for license in a Province.

In the United States most candidates are now licensed by successful completion of an NBME examination. The National Board of Medical Examiners creates its three-part examination with material drawn from its own item pool. Part I consists of a two-day examination in seven preclinical disciplines (Anatomy, Physiology, Behavioral Sciences, Biochemistry, Microbiology, Pathology, and Pharmacology). Part II, composed of multiple-choice and pictorial material items, consists of a two-day examination in six clinical disciplines. Part III consists of a one-day examination using Patient Management Problems. Eligibility to sit for Part I or II is created by enrollment in an accredited medical school. Part III eligibility requires at least one year of postgraduate training. Successful completion of all three parts is acknowledged by a diploma granted by the NBME and recognized by 48 states in their licensing process (National Board of Medical Examiners, 1973; AMA, 1979).

The various U.S. State Medical Boards, working through the Federation of State Medical Boards (FSMB), combined with the NBME to create an alternative examination to be used for licensing. Items from the NBME item pool drawn by a committee of the FSMB are used to construct the examination known as the Federation Licensing Examination (FLEX). There is reasonable equivalence of content between it and the three parts of the NBME examination. Admission to the three days of FLEX is authorized by a State Medical Board after the candidate has satisfied other criteria for licensure in the state. Although the FLEX was designed to provide a national standard, particularly for the foreign medical graduate unable to sit for the three-part NBME examinations, it has become increasingly popular with U.S. medical graduates (National Board of Medical Examiners, 1973; Morton, 1977).

Both Canadian and U.S. testing agencies use short-answer, multiple-choice, computer-scorable test items and construct an examination whose scope is sufficiently broad and sufficiently difficult that no individual may achieve a correct answer on every item. The examinations also have items which are sufficiently easy that no individual fails every item. Reference groups, usually first-time candidates from Canadian and U.S. medical schools, are used to establish the norms against which all other are scored, and by this technique a standard set by the current output of U.S. and Canadian medical schools determines the pass/fail levels for the examination. Internal controls are used on a year-to-year basis to ensure that the examinations are consistent in complexity and difficulty and with changing medical information; both agencies attempt to keep their examinations current in depth and scope.

The licensing process, which includes the licensing examination, does not purport to measure clinical competence. Although the PMP component is an attractive test and attempts to measure some aspects of clinical reasoning and judgment, the mechanics of PMP design and scoring are difficult to validate against "on the scene" professional judgment and reasoning. Most of the reasoning in multiple-choice examination is internal to the exam and is related to item design, i.e., the A, C, or K item types. Hubbard and Schumacher (1971) in their book *Measuring Medical Education* document the current ability of multiple-choice examinations to measure medical educational achievement, not clinical competence. The licensing process thus documents an individual's achievement in educational, professional behavior, and moral and ethical terms, and, satisfied that an individual has achieved these ends, the agency awards those privileges which accompany the medical license.

Large numbers of applicants—2,500 per year in Canada via LMCC and approximately 27,000 per year in the United States by NBME and FLEX combined—have necessitated mass testing with machine scoring, large numbers of crisp items, and clear choices in the responses. This has accentuated the separation of the knowledge component from the behavior/performance component in the licensing process. There has been relatively little success in designing machine-scored examinations which incorporate questions to measure behavior and attitudes. These large-scale examinations are currently incapable of evaluating the use of data, clinical judgment, and clinical reasoning, even though the PMP makes such an attempt. The value of "cueing," so important in clinical medicine, is denied in multiple-choice examinations and those furtive observations and unique insights which are that part of the clinical setting which plays a role in clinical reasoning and problem solving or the method of arriving at unique and novel solutions do not lend themselves to mass testing.

Testing agencies have concentrated more on relative objectivity, reliability, validity, and security in numbers, leaving to the educational process the unwritten and imprecise obligation to instill that appropriate professional behavior—scientific, social, moral, and ethical—which marks the physician.

A Provincial Medical Council or State Medical Board after evaluating all facets of a candidate awards a license on the basis of presented data. Although objective data are present for cognitive aspects, there are little objective data for the behavior aspect. Consequently, as with the use of all subjective data, there is always an accompanying subjective decision about the awarding of a license. Changing social values, new ideas, and changing concepts enter the licensing system as the personnel who make subjective judgments are changed on a recurring and repetitive basis, and the licensing process thus continues to be modern and current.

In the United Kingdom the licensing process is even more closely tied to the educational process than in the systems described above. Acquisition of a medical degree is tantamount to a license to practice medicine, since the central licensing authority (General Medical Council) establishes national standards and imposes general conformity through accreditation of the educational system. It does not conduct an external evaluation of candidates.

Universities grant the degree of MB-ChB or MB-BS upon completion of the prescribed course, and final examinations held with external examiners from other universities set a common educational standard. The General Medical Council first issues a Provisional license which permits one year of practice under supervision in a hospital setting (i.e., internship). Following this year of approved training, the General Medical Council issues a full license to practice without statutory restrictions, and then after two or three years of further house officership a physician may enter the National Health System as a general practitioner. Specialist training is initiated by applying for ever more senior appointments made on a competitive basis at each level. After fulfilling the basic training requirements set by each of the several Royal Colleges, candidates sit for an examination which may serve as the admissions process into a College for further training, or in some Colleges constitutes admission to Fellowship and certification as a specialist. In either case, it signifies a serious intent on the part of the individual to pursue that specialty. With appointment to house officer posts of increasing responsibility, a candidate finally achieves sufficient experience to compete for a consultant post in the National Health Service. With physician mobility enhanced by entrance into the European Economic Community, Britain has developed some interest in a general licensing procedure not unlike that now used in Canada or the United States.

Certification—The Mark of Special Competence

Certification is the process by which a nongovernmental agency or association grants recognition to an individual who has met certain predetermined qualifications specified by that agency or association (NBME, 1973).

In the United Kingdom, starting in 1518, Colleges of Physicians, Surgeons, or Obstetricians chartered by the Crown were authorized to educate, train, and ultimately register individuals who would practice within limits defined in the charter. Thus was created a special relationship between a clinical educational process and subsequent certification of special competence. These Royal Colleges encompassed the broader areas of medicine, surgery, and midwifery and did not discriminate between the subspecialties or the subsubspecialties, as occurred on the North American continent.

In North America, medical schools chartered by local or regional authorities arose as agencies of religious organizations, sometimes of colleges or universities and frequently as proprietary schools operated by a group of interested physicians. By the mid 1880s, in response to frontier needs, both Canadian and U.S. medical schools produced individuals educated in the general principles of medicine, surgery, and midwifery—"general physician"—without a defined special interest, an educational thrust apparent in the early decades of the twentieth century which has continued to the present (Stevens, 1971).

In 1929 the Royal College of Physicians and Surgeons of Canada [RCPS(C)] was established as a nonteaching college that would confer higher degrees in medicine and surgery. It proposed to identify individuals "of high quality in one or more branches of medicine" and "encourage post-graduate education." After developing procedures to evaluate candidates applying for College Fellowship or certification as a specialist, it later began to review the programs that trained the candidates who applied for certification in its defined specialties. Canadian specialty organizations were influential in shaping committees, constructing examinations, and setting requirements for training (Graham, 1969). Thus were linked the educational processes and the examination processes in 36 specialties, wherein the examination component could reflect the educational effort just as the educational component was made responsive to standards established by the examination effort. In 1967, the examination arm of the RCPS(C) was greatly strengthened by the establishment of the R. S. McLaughlin Examination and Research Center, permitting the development of high-quality objective examinations of acceptable reliability and credibility, gradually replacing many, but not all, of the essay examinations used in the evaluation process. Now only those specialties that examine fewer than 50 candidates per year continue to use essay or short answer written examinations.

Growing emphasis on the attainment of competence rather than simply the fulfillment of required number of years of training led the RCPS(C) in 1973 to inaugurate the submission of final In-Training Evaluation Reports (ITERs) in order to acquire information about a candidate's attitudes, technical capabilities, skills, interpersonal relationships, and other elements related to clinical competence which are difficult to assess in a formal written or oral examination (Perey, 1977). The examination process now requires an ITER indicating that the program director believes the candidate has satisfied several attitude and skill requirements before being admitted to the examination process (Waugh, 1979). No Canadian-trained candidate is examined without such assurance. This is a counterpart to the "internal" assessment of acquisition of professional behavior during the medical school years. It is directed, however, more at the professional conduct of the budding technical specialist with regard to technical and specialist professional behavior than to the general attributes of becoming a physician.

Eligibility to enter the Royal College certification process varies from specialty to specialty. Usually a minimum number of years and frequently a period of subspecialty experience is required. Most specialties now require an acceptable ITER, followed by a written examination whose successful completion permits entry into a final oral examination in a three-step evaluation procedure (RCRS(C), 1980). Accreditation committees now require formal in-training evaluation procedures to document a candidate's progress through a residency training sequence, in the expectation that last minute adverse decisions may be eliminated and that only candidates ready for certification appear for examination. However, a comparison of ITER results to oral examination results in Internal Medicine showed no correlation, raising questions as to whether the ITER may possibly replace the oral examination (Skakun et al., 1975).

In the United States, the late 1800s and early 1900s saw the creation of societies and colleges formed by individuals with similar professional interests in order to serve educational, social, and other supportive functions. Admission to these bodies usually required an application, the self-profession of special interest, and approval by recognized peers. Membership in such a society indicated an interest in the defined specialty area and generally carried some recognition of special competence, without the requirement of a formal examination or predetermined qualification other than a restricted practice. By the 1920s individuals in many of these professional societies believed that special competence could be defined and should be insisted upon, and that the public would expect it and would be well served if standards of excellence were established in each special field (Stevens, 1971). Definitions of each specialty area, with educational or other requirements leading to specialty certification, were developed by these societies. The first nationally recognized Medical Specialty Board—Ophthalmology—was established in 1917, and certification of special competence has now become the chief mission of 22 autonomous specialty boards and has remained separate and very distinct from the issues of licensure. The American Specialty Boards remain outside federal or state jurisdiction with regard to the content of their special domain, even though all are incorporated in some state for administrative, fiscal, and legal purposes (Holden, 1979).

Although the primary function of the Boards has been to evaluate individual candidates who appear voluntarily for examination, the Boards are also interested in improving the quality of medical education and medical care, particularly in the post-medical school period. Accreditation programs in each specialty are carried out by Residency Review Committees generally composed of members drawn from the appropriate Board, the Council on Medical Education of the AMA, and in some cases from a related specialty society.

There are now 22 formally recognized American Specialty Boards plus two areas in which primary Boards have established an additional certificate of special competence. In 1970 the several American Boards, by reorganizing the Advisory Board of Medical Specialties, created the American Board of Medical Specialties (ABMS) to coordinate many of their activities and deal with matters common to all Boards.

Eligibility to enter the certification process varies from board to board, but in general, all require a minimum number of years in an accredited residency program or a cluster of years in several programs (AMA, 1979). There may or may not be a requirement for graded experience, and frequently time to be spent in one or more prescribed subspecialty areas is specified. Upon completion of the required clinical work, a candidate is admitted to a written examination which, if successfully completed, is followed by an oral examination. Only a few Boards require testament to the candidate's readiness for the examination, capability as a resident, or honesty and ethical behavior.

In-training assessment by either observation, anecdotes, or formal examinations is being increasingly introduced into the educational process in many of the specialties. In 1972 the American Board of Internal Medicine discarded the oral examination and substituted a Program Director's Evaluation which testifies to several facets of the resident's behavior, attitudes, and skills. From information gleaned by observing the candidate during his daily work and compiled by the training faculty, the program director acknowledges the candidate's competence in interviewing and examining patients, keeping adequate medical records, and planning patient management (Ebert, 1971; Petersdorf and Beck, 1972). Following such testimony, the written examination serves as the certifying examination.

Certification as a specialist carries little legal acknowledgment except in the federal service. Both the U.S. military services and Veteran's Administration organizations give pay and advancement advantages to Board certified specialists. This certificate of special competence has not yet been related to the issues of license. It is a record of personal achievement awarded to an individual subsequent to performance in a residency program (internal), followed by the successful completion of a written and oral examination (external). The individual may use the certificate any way he sees fit, and this use frequently depends upon the specialty in which he has been certified and the institutional or hospital connections which are desired. A Board certificate is indeed a mark of special competence, and its usefulness to the individual is visible when the specialist applies for institutional privileges or other special arrangements.

Problems with Validation

The evaluation process leading to a license requires documentation of appropriate professional behavior (internal) and knowledge acquisition (external) and testifies to a special medical educational achievement. Validation of the process (its internal as well as its external components) would be possible only if performance, as scores generated in the licensing process, could be related to either grades or rank in medical school, performance as an intern, or performance in later years as a physician. The licensing process, however, uses minimum pass criteria with no ranking or grading except at the pass/fail point, and it is impossible to validate licensing as a discrimination process, even against medical school educational achievement. The North Carolina study by Peterson (1956) showed that better grades in medical school were not reflected in better performance as a physician, but this type of study does not satisfy validation criteria for the awarding of a license, since performance as a physician by those individuals who fail the licensing examination cannot be tested—they are not permitted to perform. Validation of the licensing examination is currently impossible against subsequent physician performance, and the licensing process should only be regarded as an assessment of educational achievement.

Residency training which leads to specialty certification

begins to inculcate professional technical competence. Each candidate creates a record of performance as a physician, as a resident trainee, as a budding specialist—and it might be possible to review the performance of a resident in his chosen specialty, for while practicing under supervision he nevertheless demonstrates some degree of professional competence. It might be possible to examine a training record and compare it to a record developed in the certification process. This could be done in order to validate the certification examination or to increase the efficiency of the examination process. In either case it requires precise and standardized measurements of candidate performance during residency years, to which a rank in the examination process may be compared. But the RCPS(C) and most boards report only in pass/fail terms and the candidates are not ranked in the formal examination process. A most difficult alternative would be to assess a candidate's record in the certification process against subsequent performance as a specialist.

In 1971, the American Board of Anesthesia used the written examination for an objective reference standard against which its oral examination procedures were analyzed. The authors found a variation in grading standards used by the oral examiners and felt that "the rate of disagreement among examiners evaluating identical content and performance is considerably higher than would be tolerated in the scoring of an objective examination." It was concluded that correlations between the oral and written examinations were positive, even though moderate (Kelley et al., 1971). The American Board of Internal Medicine attempted to validate its written examination by comparing the test performance of first- and third-year trainees. Finding the differences to be statistically significant, it was concluded that the examination was a valid measure of achievement. Notable, however, was the observation that the largest differences between the two resident groups were in those sections of the test that required the examinee to arrive at a correct diagnosis or prescribe appropriate treatment, rather than in the section dealing with factual information (Schumacher, 1973).

In two studies of the In-Training Evaluation Report (ITER) Skakun et al. (1975) found that the ITER did not measure the same elements of performance measured in either the written or oral examinations. They also found that some exceptional students performed well on all three components—the ITER, the written, and the oral—but that some who did well on the ITER did not necessarily do so on either the written or oral examinations (Skakun et al., 1977).

Describing those actions which comprise the function of a physician in the practice of medicine is difficult, and a ranking according to degrees of competence in these actions is currently impossible. Without ability in this sphere it probably is impossible for the licensing process to separate bad from good applicants and the certification process to select the specially competent from the mediocre. Both processes therefore assess achievement in a special educational setting and those cognitive features which are easy to assess have become an overt and visible means of measuring this achievement. Those more subtle features of attitude, skills, interpersonal relationships, critical thinking, and continuous learning remain anecdotal, and their measurement depends upon subjective observations made during the educational period. These features, which are so essential to performance as a competent physician, seem unlikely to be measured in a quantitative fashion in the near future, and validation of either the licensing process or the certification process against practicing physician performance seems impossible with our current techniques. This issue is at the crux of the relicensure/recertification debate.

Relicensure and Recertification

The expansion of knowledge accompanied by changes in our social structure has brought a reevaluation of professional status with suggestions that lifetime medical licensure may not be in the best interest of society and periodic reassessment should be required. This concept has introduced difficulties into a licensing system which has generally dealt with educational achievement and not with clinical competence at the time of licensure, for most applicants for a medical license—recent medical school graduates— have not yet demonstrated clinical competence; they have merely demonstrated ability to achieve an education in an accredited educational setting. In 1971, the New Mexico legislature took an action which linked continuing medical education (CME) to reregistration of a license to practice in that state. Since then 26 states have opted to require voluntary continuing medical education as a prerequisite for the annual reregistration of license that heretofore required only the payment of a fee. With this CME requirement, problems have arisen regarding accreditation of the educational offering. Who does it? Where is the ultimate accreditation authority? By which state is it recognized? Beyond which state boundaries is CME permissible and what constitutes national (interstate) CME? The American Medical Association instituted an accreditation system in 1964 using several medical agencies, chiefly the state medical societies, and acknowledged physician participation in these accredited sessions by a Physician's Recognition Award initiated in 1968 and awarded after 150 hours of CME. AMA authority in the area has recently been challenged by the Coordinating Council on Medical Education, and universal CME accreditation processes are currently unsettled. No province in Canada has yet made CME mandatory and accreditation difficulties have not arisen.

The major professional societies have accepted the obligation to provide continuing education of their members since the world of clinical medical practice has no formally defined agency. Most continuing medical education uses traditional education methods wherein the students are passive observers while a teacher demonstrates either wisdom, an art, or a technique, usually of overriding interest to the teacher. The extent of student-physician participation is frequently only that action taken to enroll in or reject the course. The teaching faculty is usually medical school faculty personnel, and the educational offerings are random, voluntary, and almost always in traditional, simple pedagogical modes. Little change in CME methodology has occurred in the past 50 years.

Education of the physician practitioner is an individual function neither institutionally ordained nor discipline defined. There is no formal faculty, no observation of the trainee (physician-student), and no counterpart of that "internal" component which was so important in both initial licensing and subsequent certification. There is nothing forseeable in the field of medical practice that can or will evaluate physicians on their professional skill and professional behavior. Peer observation of professional behavior is generally infrequent and usually uncritical, and formal peer review does not always clearly identify professional performance as distinct from personal likes and dislikes. Assessment of adequate professional behavior cannot be measured by continued membership in medical professional societies for there is no means by which professional societies create institutional judgments or shape professional behavior in ways similar to that which either undergraduate medical school or residency training programs are privileged to do. Attempts to view the "internal" component for relicensure have utilized HMOs, PSROs, and Quality Assurance Programs but have not satisfactorily dealt with that component of professional behavior which separates the quality physician from the incompetent or unethical.

It is possible to assess cognitive achievements of the practicing physician by using a formal examination which deals with up-to-date biomedical knowledge, but it may not necessarily be related to those patient-care problems seen by the individual practitioner. If cognitive assessment is to be included in future relicensure actions, it must be related to an individual's practice profile or it will be seen as irrelevant and arbitrary.

The causes of physician obsolescence are more likely to be found in nonprofessional behavior—drug addiction, mental incompetence, fraud, alcohol abuse, and other social and lifestyle problems—than in problems created by obsolescence of biomedical knowledge (Derbyshire, 1969). The educational schema of CME, even though random, voluntary, and disorganized, may perhaps provide the optimum means whereby a physician may pick and choose his desired relevant information. For the immediate future, it appears that relicensure will likely be closely related and increasingly linked to continuing medical education, with some refinement occurring as specifications are tightened. Hopefully, this will be accompanied by major changes in the form and methodology of continuing medical education; changing it from a passive exercise in which the physician/student watches the experts to an active exercise in which the physician/student is a leader in designing his own education, for his own needs, for his own patient problems.

Recertification as a specialist is an issue formally approved by each of the 22 American Specialty Boards, but not yet dealt with on the Canadian scene. It seems likely that those states which wish to move beyond an educational requirement for relicensure may ultimately accept specialty board recertification as an acceptable demonstration of continuing competence. If so, the several specialty boards will be placed in a position vis-à-vis formal civil licensure which is new to them, bringing with it quite different responsibilities from their current status as certifiers of individual competence. If so, there may be civil scrutiny in regard to methods and standards before they are permitted by state licensing agencies to act in lieu of state authority. Recertification by the specialty boards, accepted in principle, has now been implemented by five boards, and several boards are still considering their position relative to the recertification issue.

Simple cognitive testing within the domain of a specialty seems to have little or no relevance to competent performance and up-to-dateness of the individual specialist. Each specialty board may define cognitive features which cover an entire specialty area, but each board seems to recognize that not all, if any, of its certificants practice in such broad domains, and no board has yet been able to relate selected cognitive aspects of its examination to an individual's practice profile.

Many specialty societies have developed voluntary self-assessment examinations which carry a large educational return to those individuals undertaking the exercise (Directory of Self-Assessment, 1977). The American Boards of Internal Medicine and Surgery have elected to relate their recertification efforts to the self-assessment programs of the related specialty society, and the exact format or relationship between the two has begun to be worked out in some detail. In the initial certification process the specialty boards focused chiefly on testing cognitive aspects of the special discipline, for this area of "external" assessment is their overt function. The American Board of Internal Medicine (ABIM) instituted its voluntary recertification process in 1974 and repeated it in 1977, based upon the general format of its initial certifying examination. By using material covered in the self-assessment program (MKSAP)—with multiple-choice items and PMPs—the ABIM provided elective as well as mandatory sections in its test.

Specialty board influence wielded through the accreditation process by the Residency Review Committees has been significant in upgrading training programs, but is noticeably absent in efforts to upgrade CME activities. In general, the boards have been interested in residency education and have left education of the practicing physician to the specialty societies. Only recently have they begun to create a tenuous link between the educational effort of the specialty society and the assessment effort of the comparable specialty board.

References

American Medical Association: 1979-1980 Directory of residency training programs accredited by the Liaison Committee on Graduate Medical Education. Chicago (1979).

Bloom, S. R.: Socialization for the physician's role. In: E. C. Shapiro and L. M. Lowenstein (Eds.), Becoming a physician. Cambridge, Mass.: Ballinger (1979).

Bulletin of information and description of National Board Examinations. Philadelphia: National Board of Medical Examiners (1973).

California Statutes: Business and professions code, Section 21377 (1977).

Deming, L. H.: Personal communication (1980).

Derbyshire, R. C.: Medical licensure and discipline in the United States. Baltimore: John Hopkins Press (1969).

Directory of self-assessment programs for physicians. Chicago: American Medical Association (1977).

Ebert, R. V.: Further changes in the requirements and procedures of the American Board of Internal Medicine. Ann Intern Med 75, 121-123 (1971).

Etziony, M. B.: The physician's creed. Springfield, Ill.: Charles C. Thomas (1973).

The Federation of State Medical Boards of the United States: A guide to the essentials of a modern medical practice act (1977).

Graham, J. H.: Relations with Canadian medical organizations. Royal College of Physicians and Surgeons of Canada 50th Anniversary Publication (1969).

Holden, W. D.: The American specialty boards. In: T. Samph and B. Templeton (Eds.), Evaluation in medical education: Past present and future. Cambridge, Mass.: Ballinger (1979).

Hubbard, J. R., Schumacher, C. F.: Measuring medical education. Philadelphia: Lea & Febiger (1971).

Information pamphlet. Ottawa: Medical Council of Canada (1979).

Kelley, P. P., Matthews, J. H., Schumacher, C. F.: Analysis of the oral examination of the American Board of Anesthesiology. J Med Educ 46, 982-988 (1971).

Medical treatment and criminal law. Working Paper 26, Law Reform Commission of Canada, Ottawa (1980).

Morton, J. H.: Licensure and certification in the United States; present development and future plans. JAMA 237, 47-49 (1977).

National Board of Medical Examiners: Evaluation in the continuum of medical education. Philadelphia (1973).

National Board of Medical Examiners: Annual report. Philadelphia (1980).

Perey, B.: The measurement of professional competence in specialty certification. Ann R Coll Phys Surg (Can) 10, 270-273 (1977).

Petersdorf, R. G., Beck, J. C.: The new procedure for evaluating clinical competence of candidates to be certified by the American Board of Internal Medicine. Ann Intern Med 76, 491-496 (1972).

Peterson, O.: An analytical study of North Carolina general practice. J Med Educ 31, 1-65 (1956).

Royal College of Physicians and Surgeons of Canada: General information and regulations on training requirements and examinations. Ottawa (1980).

Schumacher, C. F.: Validation of the American Board of Internal Medicine written examination. Ann Intern Med 78, 131-135 (1973).

Skakun, E. N., Wilson, D. R., Taylor, W. C., Langley, S. R.: A preliminary examination of the intraining evaluation report. J Med Educ 50, 817-819 (1975).

Skakun, E. N., Wilson, D. R., Taylor, W. C.: A comparison of performance on multiple choice tests, oral examinations and intraining evaluation reports. Ann R Coll Phys Surg (Can) 10, 284-285 (1977).

Stevens, R.: American medicine and the public interest. New Haven and London: Yale University Press (1971).

Tancredi, R., Woods, J.: The social control of medical practice. Milbank Mem Fund Q 1, 99-122 (1972).

Waugh, S.: The certification procedure: how the system works. Ann R Coll Phys Surg (Can) (1979).

Wilkins, H. E.: Personal communication (1980).

CHAPTER 17

Implications
for Research

GEOFFREY R. NORMAN

The reader of the past several chapters, seeking some solutions to the challenge of assessing clinical competence, may be experiencing a certain discomfort. When subject to critical review, many of our measures of clinical competence are found wanting. Despite the best of intentions, and substantial investment of energies and resources, many of the innovations over the past two decades have followed a similar historical course.

1. Identification of a clear need for evaluation methods in a particular domain.
2. Initial development of a new approach.
3. Early studies, using methods of marginal rigor and yielding positive results.
4. Widespread adoption and enthusiasm.
5. Later studies, using more rigorous methods, casting some doubt on the initial findings.
6. Some disenchantment and a search for new methods.

As a general observation, this discouraging sequence of events points out a need for rigorous research before, rather than after, widespread adoption. Nearly every method reviewed has possessed face validity, that is to say, it appeared capable of assessing what was intended. And virtually every study of acceptability has reported enthusiastic response from all participants (and a certain lack of awareness of the Hawthorne effect by the investigators). Furthermore, it has been relatively easy to show that, whatever the attribute being assessed, senior students have more of it than junior students, although it has been somewhat more difficult to demonstrate a similar gradient in postgraduate training and practice. But when subjected to more rigorous analysis of test-retest reliability or concurrent validity, the results of most studies usually fall in the range from equivocal to clearly discouraging.

The cause of this unhappy state of affairs is not easy to pinpoint. There is no shortage of rigorous research methods in behavioral and clinical science, many of which have direct application to the investigation of evaluation methods. Nor, when we examine the funds which have been invested by funding agencies and licensing bodies in the development of such methods as computer simulation, can we conclude that research is hampered by a shortage of funds. Yet when the accomplishments and efforts of the last two decades are viewed in a critical light, we appear to have made little progress toward the precise definition and valid assessment of clinical competence. Perhaps the blame rests mainly on those doing evaluation research. We who are active in the development of methods appear to fit Whitehead's characterization of "the narrowness of men with a good methodology." Our simplistic questions are frequently confused, rather than clarified, by weak experimental designs followed by impressive and incomprehensible statistical analysis.

In the present chapter, I hope to outline strategies which may redress the balance to some degree. I intend to point out some fundamental questions which must be addressed by empirical research in order to achieve an understanding of the important dimensions of clinical competence. And I will critique the methods we have used in the past to evaluate the usefulness of various evaluation methods, and suggest better experimental strategies.

Basic Research Questions

The early postwar years saw a proliferation of objective methods of testing knowledge, paralleling the development of computer hardware capable of automatically scoring such tests. The adoption of such methods, however, apparently succeeded in reducing the assessment of competence to a series of pencil marks in boxes, which sowed the seeds of a debate still raging in the literature (Ebel and Senior, 1976; Newble, 1979) regarding the role of multiple-choice tests. In part, this debate led to concerted efforts to define other components of competence which could not be assessed by objective test items (American Institutes for Research, 1960) and the development of a number of measures of such general skills as "problem-solving," "interpersonal skills," and "self-assessment ability." Unhappily, although objective measures of these skills can be shown to have high internal consistency, the reliability of such measures across different problems (McGuire and Babbott, 1967) is low to moderate at best, and validity is usually limited to a demonstration of positive change with education. Basic research has begun to define the components of problem solving (Barrows et al., 1978; Elstein et al., 1978), but little is known about the determinants of successful problem solving. Specific research questions which require further elaboration include:

1. What are the important and relevant variables to be measured in the clinical encounter?
2. How are the dimensions of clinical performance related to outcomes, e.g., quality of care?
3. What are the important predictors or determinants of clinical performance?
4. What is the relationship between various instructional methods (e.g., problem-based learning) and clinical competence?

The Measurement of Clinical Performance

At present, there exists no consensus about precisely what is clinical competence or clinical problem solving. The discussion of Chapter 2 illustrated the variety of approaches which have been used to define the components of competence. But the situation is further complicated when one proceeds from definition to measurement. Precisely what variable or combination of variables should one measure in assessing "diagnostic thinking," "clinical judgment," or "problem-solving ability"? As we indicated, basic research has begun to provide some direction, at least in terms of describing the complexity of the measurement problem. Elstein et al. (1978) measured 12 variables thought to be related to problem-solving ability. Barrows et al. (1978) assessed 21 variables in each encounter. None of the variables assessed in either study was found to be a general measure of competence to the extent that it was highly correlated across encounters.

It is probably the case that not all these variables are necessary to describe the cognitive aspects of clinical problem solving in a single encounter. Yet the possibility remains that these investigators may have omitted or inappropriately characterized some critical variables. For example, subjective probability has been a fruitful source of investigation in a variety of professional domains (Beach, 1975) yet was not characterized in either study. Decision analysis, described briefly in Chapter 2, uses two parameters—the probability and utility of various end points—to define optimal choice under uncertainty, yet little is known about how or whether physicians use such parameters in their decisions. Interpersonal skills have been assessed using a number of theoretical foundations, but there is very little research relating the interpersonal and cognitive features of clinical competence.

Research into the components of clinical competence is of more than academic interest. As Elstein et al. (1978) have indicated, if, for example, problem solving is content specific, then an assurance of competence may require evaluation of the physician's approach on each class of problem he is likely to encounter in practice. Yet the apparent low reliability across problems may be a consequence of the instability of the variables used to define problem solving, and a more judicious choice of variables may reveal consistency of performance across problems.

Such research also has implications for teaching and learning. In the past decade, several new medical schools have opted for a problem-based curriculum. The rationale for the approach is the goal of providing a different type of physician, who might be characterized by greater problem-solving, self-learning, and self-assessment skills. At the present time, follow-up studies of McMaster graduates using, among others, the measure of performance on licensing examinations has revealed only that graduates of new schools are no worse than graduates of more conventional approaches. A sensitive evaluation of this curriculum approach must be preceded by basic research to better understand, and measure, the characteristics which are thought to be enhanced by these programs.

Relationship Between Clinical Competence and Other Measures

Construct validity is a notion which has proven useful in psychological research for many years, finding application both in validation of an instrument and in achieving a better understanding of the underlying features assessed by the instrument. It is an indirect test of validity used in circumstances where no criterion or concurrent measure exists. The investigator begins with a study hypothesis, and the study of validity tests both the validity of the measure and the coherence of the theory relating the measure to other variables.

Construct validity, relating measures of competence to other aspects of education and health care, could be a sensitive tool to explore the dimensions of competence. Unfortunately, the approach has been subject to abuse by educational researchers. By far the most common construct is that, whatever the trait being assessed, senior students have more of it than junior students. Unfortunately, senior students have more of many things than junior students—knowledge, clinical skills, gray hairs, wrinkles, and debts, and the only theory being tested by this construct is that people change as a result of education and/or getting older. Although a few cynics may doubt the former, the latter theory is unassailable.

Although this section, in part, addresses methodological weaknesses, it is intended to point out a lost opportunity. Construct validity may, as a general technique, have great utility in advancing the state of the art in evaluation of competence. A major problem facing anyone intending to assess competence is the overwhelming diversity of knowledge, attitudes, and skills subsumed under the term. The task might be eased if we had greater awareness of which aspects of competence are important in effecting particular changes in patients' health, and conversely which components may be quite irrelevant to the actual delivery of health care. An example of the former is the relationship between certain aspects of interpersonal skills and compliance as outlined in Chapter 12; an example of the latter is the lack of relationship between compliance with antihypertensive medication and patient education (Sackett et al., 1976). Similarly, although thoroughness of data gathering is a virtue prized by generations of physicians (or their supervisors), evidence is beginning to accumulate that it is unrelated to diagnosis and management (Barrows et al., 1978) and inversely related to experience (Marshall, 1977). Careful study of the construct validity of measures of the process dimensions of competence, relating these measures to defined outcomes of health care, may yield important insights into the weighting to be placed on various dimensions of competence, in both learning and evaluation.

The Determinants of Clinical Competence

We know very little about the attributes of a competent physician. Up to perhaps two decades ago, competence was treated as a synonym for knowledge—given sufficient knowledge, competence would automatically follow. Educational programs were geared to inculcation of this body of knowledge, and admissions procedures were based on selection of students with appropriate prior knowledge as evidenced by high marks on undergraduate prerequisites and high MCAT scores. Unfortunately, the accumulated findings of two decades of research on the predictive power of undergraduate grades and the lack of relationship between tests of knowledge and other measures leads to the inevitable conclusion that although knowledge may be a necessary aspect of competence, it is far from sufficient. As a result, we have cast a broad net in searching for other dimensions which may assist us in selecting and training future physicians. We seek "personal qualities" at the time of admissions; we teach and nurture "problem-solving skills," "interpersonal skills," and "technical skills" in our curricula. The basic research to clarify the meaning of these terms, however, has not been done. We do not know whether problem solving is general or content specific, and we do not know whether problem solvers are born or made; should we be selecting students on the basis of performance on a general problem-solving test, or should we attempt to teach it? Very little research exists linking performance on clinical problems to the mastery of formal knowledge relevant to the solution of the problem. As a result, the finding of a low relationship between tests of knowledge and tests of problem solving may simply be a result of little overlap in the required knowledge to solve the problem and knowledge assessed on the parallel test.

A general practitioner spends about 50 percent of his training in a clinical setting; for a subspecialist, this figure is closer to 80 percent. The role of this clinical experience in the attainment of competence is not clear. At the one extreme it may simply be an opportunity to practice and apply knowledge acquired in the preclinical phases and acquire technical skills; conversely, the clinical experience may have a direct educational role in implanting a broad series of patient-based experiences in memory—patient prototypes whose recall may be a major determinant of diagnostic ability (Norman et al., 1979).

Basic research is needed to clarify the role of these and other predictors of clinical competence—research which may have broad implications ranging from medical school admissions to specialty certification.

A Critique of Methodology

Winifred Castle, a British statistician, recently wrote a handbook attempting to explain statistical concepts to nonstatisticians, in which she wrote that "We doctors seem to use statistics like drunken men a lamppost—for support rather than illumination" (Castle, 1979, p. 4). A brief perusal of the proceedings of the American Conference on Research in Medical Education (RIME) over the past few years may lead the reader to conclude that researchers in medical education are the down-and-out winos of the research enterprise.

Our collective strength is our analytical tools; our weakness is our limited ability to ask appropriately circumscribed questions and implement rigorous experimental designs to test these questions. A randomized trial, the hallmark of clinical research, is conspicuous by its absence in the literature on medical education, and most studies are based on what Campbell and Stanley (1966) label a "pre-experimental design"—the one group, before–after study—or on retrospective regression or factor analysis of convenient data sets. When we do bring up the statistical heavy artillery, it is often used inappropriately. For example, a rule of thumb in factor analysis is that the ratio of the number of subjects to the number of variables should be at least 10 to 1. A study in a recent RIME proceedings reported a factor analysis (varimax rotated, of course) involving 11 variables and 27 subjects—a ratio of 2.4 to one. The author had no qualms in interpreting all 5 factors which emerged from the analysis.

A critique of research on clinical competence assessment reveals a number of weaknesses and some clear directions for change.

Inappropriate Questions

It is an unfortunate truism that most research is done by researchers; and a corollary in medical education is that most researchers were trained to do educational research. The majority of faculty and staff in offices of medical education (in North America) are not physicians and have no clinical training. We tend to view the world through the eyes of our own discipline of education or psychology. While many of the research paradigms of our training are highly appropriate for research in medical education, all too often the questions which come to our minds are not equally appropriate. To return to a favorite example, the term *problem solving* has become commonplace in both public school and medical education. However, the similarity may end with the term. A public school student's ability to "problem solve" may be assessed by arithmetic or logical problems; by contrast, a medical student's problem-solving ability is interpreted as his ability to gather data from a patient and integrate the data into an appropriate diagnosis and management plan. There may be little or no similarity between these two cognitive skills, and the questions and methods applicable to the former may be nonsensical when applied to the latter. If we, as educational researchers, are to develop the facility to ask appropriate research questions which get to the heart of the matter, we must be prepared to establish working relationships with clinicians and basic scientists, patiently nurture these relationships, and learn from the anecdotal observations of these individuals. All too frequently we presume to the role of teacher, rather than learner, and view our job as training clinicians to understand our jargon and adopt our world view. A little humility would be a welcome advance.

One other piece of evidence regarding the communication gap between clinicians and "magicians" is the use of jargon by educational researchers. When a paper is presented which speaks of an experimental trial of "census and force field analysis," a jargon term for solving medical problems in a small group, and follows up with an "orthogonal varimax rotated factor analysis," the glazed look in the eyes of the practitioners should be no surprise.

Inappropriate Experimental Designs

Although educational researchers lack the relevant background or firsthand experience to ask appropriate questions, they do have a valid contribution to make in terms of their knowledge of appropriate experimental methods and approaches to statistical analysis. It is nearly impossible to acquire a graduate degree in education or psychology without formal training in research methods, a training which emphasizes the essential role of random sampling and random allocation in making causal inference. We are repeatedly trained in the potential bias which may result from comparing nonequivalent groups, or from generalizing the results of surveys where there were a significant number of nonrespondents.

In light of the admonitions of our teachers, it is disheartening to examine the approaches we use as professionals. I recently reviewed eight months of the *Journal of Medical Education* and found 44 papers which presented research findings with statistical analysis. Of the 44 papers, 26 (59 percent) were based on survey data, or analysis of a single group of subjects; 14 (32 percent) used some form of pre-experimental design such as pre- and post-test of a single group, or comparison with a nonequivalent control group; and only 4 (9 percent) used a true experimental design. Although many of the surveys had adequate response rates, one study reported results based on a response rate of 17 percent.

I am not suggesting that all our research in clinical competence should be based on randomized trials. A randomized trial is a useful design for decision making, since it minimizes bias and maximizes the likelihood of an appropriate decision, but it is not appropriate for research designed to reveal association between variables. An appropriate random sampling procedure from a defined population, however, rather than the present overuse of volunteer samples, is a minimum prerequisite to ensure a generalizable result.

Inadequate Measures Development

In addition to improving our experimental designs, we might consider applying more stringent measurement criteria—reliability and validity—to our instruments prior to their dissemination.

Reliability is a deceptively simple concept which in practice can become exceedingly complex. The reliability of a test cannot be adequately reduced to a single number. If we consider a test such as a PMP or an observed student-simulated patient encounter which attempts to measure a general competence based on the solution of a single problem, we must ask about the reliability of the test for different observers, repeated administrations of the same problem, different problems, different specialties, and so on. Too frequently the reliability of an objective test is calculated from even- versus odd-numbered responses, and the reliability of subjective ratings is based on two observations of the same performance. In both cases, the calculated reliability is an upper limit of what might be obtained if other sources of variation were included.

Another feature of test reliability which is usually ignored is that it is based on the ratio of the "true" variance between subjects to the total variance in observations. It is therefore intimately linked to the heterogeneity of the sample on which it is based, and a test which is useful in distinguishing first-year from final-year students may be hopelessly unreliable when used to discriminate among clinical clerks or residents. Some time ago, Cronbach et al. (1972) reformulated the concept of reliability, suggesting that it be expressed in terms of "generalizability"—the degree to which a test result can be generalized to different situations in which one or more factors influencing the test differ. It is time to incorporate these notions into analysis of tests of clinical competence.

Validity remains a difficult concept in evaluation of competence. Unlike clinical medicine, we have no educational pathologists to establish, by autopsy or biopsy of the mind, the accuracy of our measurements. As a result, a multitude of indirect measures of validity, described briefly in Chapter 3, have evolved. Some are more sensitive or powerful than others, and unfortunately, it is the weakest among these which have found the most widespread application. Face (or faith) validity is rarely tested empirically, and few tests have failed to meet this requirement, since all that is required is to assemble a small group of friends and ask them whether your new test looks reasonable as a measure of whatever. Content validity can be approached rigorously by prior definition of all the relevant content and random sampling from this "population," but usually it is used as a synonym for, or variation on, face validity.

I have already alluded to the difficulty with construct validity as it is applied in educational measurement. The finding that senior students perform better than junior students on a test says virtually nothing about the specific traits or skills assessed by the test. The approach may be useful if constructs are developed which yield specific insights into the skills being assessed, but as it is presently applied, construct validity is of limited value.

Concurrent validity requires the existence of some other instrument which approximates a "gold standard." Although we frequently despair of identifying such a standard, we should not lose sight of the fact that the final test of clinical competence is performance with patients in a clinical setting. In validating a simulation test, it may not be unreasonable to compare performance with actual clinical performance as Goran et al. did (1973). Quality-of-care approaches provide some methods to assess performance in real settings.

Appropriate Statistical Analysis

In contrast to our research questions and experimental designs, our data analyses suffer from an abundance of riches. We have little hesitation in conducting our factor analyses and, when they yield nothing more than one general factor, then examining the reliability of the data. We too often confound statistical with clinical significance, the former a prerequisite to an inference of clinical or meaningful differences, but of itself revealing nothing about the strength of the relationship. Statistical significance depends on three factors—the magnitude of the relationship, the variability of the sample, and the sample size; and as someone said, "Too small a sample, and you can prove nothing—too large a sample and you can prove anything." As researchers, we owe it to our readers to convey sufficient information about the properties of our data—means and standard deviations—so that statistically significant differences can be examined in the light of the data, rather than considered an end unto themselves. The communication of basic statistical data serves two ends; it is a prerequisite for scientific credibility, and it enhances communication with those of our audience who are not as facile at interpreting a multiple regression coefficient or an eigenvalue as we are. The statistical heavy artillery has a role to play in rigorous testing of research hypotheses, but it should supplement, rather than replace, more basic descriptions of the data.

Summary and Conclusions

The development of measures of clinical competence has too frequently seen the supplanting of scientific rigor by general enthusiasm and the natural tendency to fill the gap. Unfortunately, viewed in the harsh light of retrospection, many of these efforts have not resulted in progress toward the goal. If we are to make solid gains in this difficult area, we must be prepared to work cooperatively with those who have the greatest experience in the multiple dimensions of competence, the clinicians, and combine their insights with our research tools in the development and rigorous testing of new approaches. We must be prepared to not accept terms such as "problem solving" or "interpersonal skills" at face value, but must conduct basic research to achieve an empirical understanding of the terms. Finally, the testing of new evaluation methods must be conducted using the most rigorous methods available, and results should be communicated in such a manner that the analyses clarify, rather than obscure, the relationships.

References

American Institutes for Research: The definition of clinical competence in medicine. Palo Alto: Author (1960).

Barrows, H. S., Norman, G. R., Feightner, J. W., Neufeld, V. R.: Analysis of the clinical methods of medical students and physicians. Toronto: Ontario Ministry of Health (1978).

Beach, B. H.: Expert judgment about uncertainty: Bayesian decision-making in realistic settings. Org Behav Hum Perf 14, 10-59 (1975).

Campbell, D.T., Stanley, J. C.: Experimental and quasi-experimental designs for research. Chicago: Rand-McNally (1966).

Castle, W.: Statistics in operation. Edinburgh: Churchill Livingstone (1979).

Cronbach, L. J., et al.: The dependability of behavioral measurements: theory of generalizability for scores and profiles. New York: Wiley (1972).

Ebel, R. L., Senior, J. R.: Toward the measurement of competence in medicine. Philadelphia: American Board of Internal Medicine (1976).

Elstein, A. S., Shulman, L. S., Spraffa, S. A.: Medical problem solving: an analysis of clinical reasoning. Cambridge: Harvard University Press (1978).

Goran, M. J., Williamson, J. W., Gonnella, J. S.: The validity of patient management problems. J Med Educ 48, 171-177 (1973).

Marshall, J.: Assessment of problem solving ability. Med Educ 11, 329-334 (1977).

McGuire, C. H., Babbott, D.: Simulation technique in the measurement of problem-solving skills. J Educ Measurement 4, 1-10 (1967).

Newble, D. L.: A comparison of multiple-choice tests and free response tests in examinations of clinical competence. Med Educ 13, 263-268 (1979).

Norman, G. R., Feightner, J. W., Jacoby, L. L.: Clinical experience and the structure of memory. Proceedings, 18th Annual Conference on Research in Medical Education, Washington, D.C. (1979).

Sackett, D. L., Haynes, R. B., Gibson, E. S., et al.: Improvement of medication compliance in uncontrolled hypertension. Lancet 1, 1265-1268 (1976).

CHAPTER 18

Implications for Health Care

J. FRASER MUSTARD

The main focus of this book has been the competence of an individual physician working with an individual patient. Such a focus is practical since it has provided a framework for a realistic review of how we have attempted to define and measure clinical competence and how new knowledge about clinical competence has been applied in various settings. In this chapter we wish to broaden this perspective by examining the role of the physician as seen by society more generally. Specifically, the perspective will be that of population health and the role of health care planning. We will begin by considering the role of health care in our society and then proceed, in the light of the role of physicians in health care, to suggest some expectations which society should have of the competent physician.

In order to understand the role of the physician in contributing to the health of an individual patient, it is useful to review some of the considerations concerning the determinants of human health and the role of health care. From a variety of recent studies and considerations, three key points stand out in relation to the role of health professionals such as physicians. These points have direct relevance on a society's expectations for the role and quality of work provided by physicians, and are as follows:

1. The major determinants of human health are where we live and how we live.
2. The main contribution of health care and the profes-

sionals who promote care is on the quality of life of individuals who are ill or think they are ill.

3. Individual physicians have a major impact on the effectiveness and efficiency with which health care interventions are used to affect the quality of life.

Let us examine the basis for these assertions.

Determinants of Health

It has been widely assumed by many social scientists and economists that health care is an important determinant of health. As an example, this assumption was part of the basis of the British National Health Service, introduced by Lord Beveridge (Banham, 1977; Eltis and Bacon, 1978). When he recommended the public funding of health care, he argued that removing financial barriers to health care would provide universal access to the benefits, reduce the burden of ill-health, and eventually reduce the needs for health care. His assumption that health care is a major determinant of human health is still a cherished concept. The Ontario Economic Council's "Statement of Issues for 1979," for example, includes these sentences:

> Moreover a consensus is emerging that our current outlays [on health care] should, and could be bringing higher levels of health for our population or, conversely, that existing levels of health could be achieved with lower resource commitments. We are coming to realize that health status can be influenced at the margin only to a limited extent by the current health care delivery system [Ontario Economic Council, 1979, p. 3].

The idea that health care should be a major determinant of health also underlies recent concern about the fact that increased expenditure on health care does not have a proportional impact on life expectancy. Gori and Richter (1978) point out, for example, that in the United States, between 1940 and 1975, the average life span for individuals increased 15 percent while per capita expenditures on health care (in constant 1967 dollars) increased by 314 percent.

One of the most important contributions to our understanding of the determinants of human health has come from McKeown, a British physician interested in social medicine, who has analyzed the factors that contributed to changing life expectancy in Britain over the past century (1976). He estimated that improved nutrition accounted for more than 70 percent of the gain in life expentancy; that the improvement of the physical environment (housing, improved water systems and sanitation) accounted for an additional 20 percent; and that the contribution of the health care system, mainly through immunization, was about 5 percent. McKeown summarizes his conclusions in this way:

> Medical science and services are misdirected and society's investment in health is not well used, because they rest on an erroneous assumption about the basis of human health. It is assumed that the body can be regarded as a machine whose protection from disease and its effects depends primarily on internal intervention. The approach has led to indifference to the external influence and personal behavior which are the predominant determinants of health.

It is too easy to dismiss this by assuming that it may have been true in the past, but that surely at the present time health care has a significant impact on health. Such major recent advances as antibiotics, the treatment of hypertension, intensive care units, and surgery must contribute to a gain in life expectancy. But the facts do not fully support this expectation. The major causes of death in Canada are:

Cardiovascular and renal disease	51%
Cancer	18%
Accidents	6%
Diseases of the respiratory system	5%
Diabetes	2%

Since many of these conditions contribute to death before a normal life expectancy is achieved, control of these conditions should lead to further improvement in life expectancy in developed countries. Will the reduction in premature mortality from these disorders come from health care interventions or from changes in the effect of environment or lifestyle? It has recently been estimated that the bulk of human internal cancers are the product of either lifestyle or our environment. Doll and Peto (1981) conclude that 30 percent of these cancers can be attributed to smoking, 35 percent to diet, 7 percent to social behavior and 4 percent to place of work. In the case of coronary artery disease, two of the key risk factors are smoking and diets rich in saturated fat and cholesterol. The reduction in deaths from ischemic heart disease in the age-groups 35 to 45, 45 to 55, and 55 to

65 since 1964 in the United States has been associated with a reduction in cigarette smoking and dietary saturated fat, and an increase in the proportion of dietary polyunsaturated fat. Although it is still uncertain whether these changes in risk factors are important in the reduced incidence of deaths from ischemic heart disease, the evidence is compatible with the hypothesis that reduction in the risk factors will reduce the incidence of ischemic heart disease. Moderation in the use of alcohol could also significantly reduce premature deaths from accidents.

In an insightful recent analysis, Fries (1980) has stated that improvement in life expectancy for developed countries could be as much as 12 years if the right steps were taken. By adopting a better lifestyle and adjusting environmental hazards to health, Fries believes that mean life expectancy could reach 85 years. This figure, on the basis of present evidence, appears to be the biological limit to maximum human life expectancy.

While these estimates by Fries apply to the so-called developed countries of the world, it is likely that the same story is true in the developing countries. This perspective has recently been described by Evans and his colleagues of the World Bank (Evans et al., 1981).

To summarize this first consideration; the available evidence indicates that the major determinants of health, as measured by improved life expectancy, have been achieved primarily by improved nutrition, improvements in the physical environment and changes in behavior—and not by the existing health care system. The majority of the estimates indicate that continuing improvement in the life expectations of our population will be primarily determined by changes in our way of life and the environment in which we live and work. If health care is not a major determinant of health, what then is its role? This is our next consideration.

The Role of Health Care

We have seen in the previous section that health, at least as indicated by life expectancy, is determined mainly by factors outside of the so-called health care delivery system. The major contribution of health care is in the improvement and/or sustaining of the quality of life by providing appropriate care for acute and chronic illness and by relieving illness-related anxiety.

Typically health care workers, and physicians in particular, are concerned with the question: "Does this individual have a disease or not?" On the other hand, patients are individuals who either are ill or think they are ill. These two perspectives can be brought together (as shown in Figure 18.1). Four classes of individuals are thus defined, all of which can be viewed as being legitimate concerns of health care workers. The first category includes those individuals who have a disease and are ill. Second, there are those who think they are ill but have no demonstrable disease. There is another class of individuals who have a disease but who do not know it and who do not feel "ill" or deny that they are ill. Finally, there is the group who have no disease and are not ill. This classification can assist us in examining the spectrum of interventions available in the health care system and the health care objectives to which they may be applied.

Let us remind ourselves about the possible outcomes of ill-health and disease: they are recovery (with or without any intervention from the health care system); partial recovery with some residual disability; and death. It must be remembered that death is a normal outcome for all of us. With this in mind, what are the goals of health care? They include the following:

1. Assist to prevent disease and to minimize or delay the effects of disease.
2. Cure: To effect complete recovery from a disease as a direct result of an intervention. An example might be the use of antibiotics in bacterial meningitis, or appendectomy of a gangrenous appendix.
3. Stabilization and rehabilitation: Cure of a disorder is not possible, and efforts are directed toward stabilizing the disease and helping the individual within his or her capabilities to the best possible emotional function.
4. Support: Relief from pain and suffering, provisions of effective strategies for the management of a patient's problem, taking into account therapeutic limitations; reassurance and explanation in order to minimize anxiety and facilitate personal planning. It includes providing access to appropriate allied health professionals and agencies so as to provide optimum support for the affected individual. This important contribution is frequently neglected in training and devalued in practice. It is particularly important for those individuals who have acute or chronic disorders for which there is no effective therapy and for those who think they are ill, but who do not have detectable disease.

FIGURE 18.1.
A Perspective on Illness and Disease

		HAVE DISEASE	
		YES	NO
ARE ILL	YES	"Cure" Rehabilitation Support	Support
	NO	"Cure" Prevention Support	(Prevention)

Terms in cells are goals of health care interventions.

The Role of the Individual Physician

In most cultures there is a segment of society that is concerned with illness, life, and death. In Western societies, the physician is the individual who is given the official responsibility to determine the presence or absence of illness. The manner in which this responsibility is used not only determines the quality of health care, but has wider effects in a society of a social and economic nature. For example, if an individual feels ill and would like to stay away from work, it is the physician who has the power to confirm illness and allow the individual to stay home. In another situation, if a person's behavior is thought by colleagues or family to deviate from normal, it is the physician that has the mandate to label this behavior pattern as an illness or disease and designate the degree of disability and appropriate institutional care.

Because of the considerable responsibility delegated by society to the physician, certain tensions develop. Concerns are expressed about the power of the physician and strong criticisms are raised from time to time. George Bernard Shaw's *Doctor's Dilemma* (Shaw, 1946), is in this vein. Ivan Illich's *Limits to Medicine* (1976) is a more recent treatment of the same subject. Among the concerns expressed are the following: first, how does a society ensure that physicians use their power appropriately and do not abuse their privilege? Second, how can a society ensure that physicians apply their skill and knowledge to the management of patients' problems at the highest possible level of performance? And third, how can a society ensure that physicians fulfill their total responsibility to patients, including prevention, support, and reassurance? These considerations, which involve honesty, integrity, effectiveness, sensitivity, and a broad range of responsibility, relate directly to considerations of clinical competence.

The safeguards that have been developed to assure quality and competence are largely those of self-governance, with only limited appeal by the patient in circumstances where physician self-governance seems to have failed. Theoretically, hospital boards, through their medical advisory committees, should be able to exercise some discipline on the standards of care and physician performance in an institution. But the hosptial boards tend to delegate most of this responsibility to the professional staff in the institution and only rarely become directly involved. The Colleges or Boards that are established to grant licenses for the practice of medicine also exercise a watchdog role; they can receive complaints and, if appropriate, discipline physicians. Finally, individuals can resort to the courts if they are dissatisfied with the quality of care delivered by a group of physicians or and institution.

Given these concerns and the limited arrangements which a society has to ensure that responsibilities granted to physicians are fulfilled, what specific expectations should society have of a competent physician? These will be considered in the next section.

Expectations by Society of the
Competent Physician

Many writers, both within the medical profession and in society more widely, have described expectations of the competent physician. These descriptions usually include such characteristics as technical competence, humanity (the ability to care and listen), efficiency in the provision of health care, and the ability to recognize personal strengths and limitations. The following examples illustrate some of the expectations which society can place on a physician:

A specialist physician sees a patient referred by a family physician in a small community. The physician is technically competent and does an excellent job of determining the patient's problem and recommending an appropriate course of action. However, the specialist does not describe his opinion and conclusions to the patient in an understandable manner. Furthermore, he fails to communicate this information to the family physician. As a result, both the patient and the referring physician are dissatisfied and angry. Here the expectation is for the physician to communicate in an effective manner with the referring physician as well as with the patient.

A patient who feels ill is seen by a physician but the physician, in reviewing the case, concludes that the patient does not have any disease which would explain the symptoms of the patient. He tells the patient that there is nothing wrong with him and implies that he is a hypochondriac. This patient, dissatisfied with this statement, goes to another physician who recognizes the nature of the patient's problem and helps the patient develop some insight into why he feels ill even though there is no underlying disease. The expectation here is for the physician to be interested in and competent to handle illness regardless of whether it is associated with disease.

An individual with chest pain is referred to a cardiologist. With the aid of modern technology (in this case, coronary arteriography), the cardiologist determines that the pain is ischemic in origin and that the patient has major arteriosclerotic disease in two of his coronary arteries, but the myocardium is still healthy. He advises the patient to undergo coronary bypass surgery to "improve" the blood flow to the myocardium. The patient asks whether a trial of medical management would be as effective, and what the benefits and risks are. The cardiologist replies that although the evidence from randomized trials does not clearly favor a surgical approach, in his professional judgment, bypass surgery is appropriate for this individual, and he believes the benefits outweigh the risks. Here the expectation is that the physician will know which therapeutic interventions are effective.

A group of physicians is advising a Workman's Compensation Board. They are given the records of patients with asbestosis who have had exposure to asbestos in the work place and are asked to evaluate the degree of disability. The purpose of their assessment is to determine the degree of disability the individual should be given by the Workman's Compensation Board. The workers are generally aware of the evidence that asbestos in lungs produces progressive changes (asbestosis) leading to a shortened life span. Based on a physical examination, chest X-rays, and pulmonary function tests, they estimate that a given worker's disability should be 25 percent. Here the expectation is that the physican can accurately predict disability from laboratory tests (including X-rays) and that the judgment is fair.

What expectations should our society have of the physicians in these stories? They can be summarized as follows:

1. A physician should be both technically competent (in in terms of knowledge and skills) and competent in his ability to communicate clearly with patients and other health professionals.
2. A physician should understand and contribute to all goals of health care: prevention, cure, rehabilitation, and supportive care. He should recognize that his main contribution is to enhance the quality of life of his patients.
3. A physician should be informed about scientifically validated knowledge of the effectiveness of new thera-

pies or diagnostic tests and use only therapeutic and diagnostic procedures that have been shown to be effective in appropriate clinical situations.

4. Where information required for clinical decisions is incomplete, the physician should recognize this and contribute to the development of new knowledge.

Conclusion

The performance of physicians must be understood within the context of health and health care. There is considerable evidence that health care per se is only a small contributor to health, as measured by life expectancy. Much stronger determinants of health are nutrition, the physical environment, socio-economic factors, and human behavior. The role of health care is primarily directed toward improving the quality of life for individuals who are ill. The goals of prevention, cure, rehabilitation, and support must be directed appropriately to various categories of individuals, based on whether they have or do not have disease and whether they are ill. Increasingly, health care will be applied at the extremes of the life cycle, in particular to the aging population.

A physician has a special, powerful role in society. He can label individuals as having a disease or not. His decisions have not only medical but social and economic consequences. A society is rightly concerned about ensuring that its physicians are sensitive to the range of responsibilities they have been given, that they are technically competent, that they are informed about scientifically validated evidence of new investigations and therapies and use this new knowledge appropriately, and that they are good listeners and communicators.

These are the elements of physician competence that will contribute to an excellent health care system.

References

Banham, J.: Report to the Royal Commission on the National Health Service: London, England. McKinsey and Associates (1977).

Doll, R., Peto, R.: The causes of cancer: Quantitative estimates of avoidable risks of cancer in the United States today. Oxford: Oxford University Press (1981).

Eltis, W., Bacon, R.: Britain's economic problem: too few producers. London: Macmillan (1978).

Evans, J. R., Hall, K. L., Warford, J.: Shattuck Lecture—Health care in the developing world: problems of scarcity and choice. N Engl J Med 305, 1117 (1981).

Fries, J. F.: Aging, natural death and the compression of morbidity. N Engl J Med 303, 130 (1981).

Gori, G. B., Richter, B. J.: Macroeconomics of disease prevention in the United States. Science 200, 1124 (1978).

Illich, I.: Limits to medicine: Medical nemesis—the expropriation of health. London: Marium Boyars (1976).

McClure, W.: Health Care Cost Commission—Choice for medical care. Minn Med 61, 261 (1978).

McKeown, T.: The role of medicine: Dream, mirage, or nemesis (2nd ed.). Princeton, N. J.: Princeton University Press (1976).

Ontario Economic Council: "Statement of Issues for 1979." Government of Ontario (1979).

Shaw, G. B.: The doctor's dilemma. Hammondsworth: Penguin Books (1946).

Index

Abrahamson, S., 73-74, 88, 201, 207, 208, 212, 214
Adler, L., 238, 239, 244
Affective Sensitivity Scale, 238
Allport, G. W., 135
American Board of Anesthesia, 323
American Board of Emergency Medicine, 104
American Board of Family Practice (ABFP), 148, 154, 174
American Board of Internal Medicine (ABIM), 16, 20, 72, 204, 208, 261, 277-279, 281-282, 289, 321, 323, 327
diagnostic competence defined by, 278-279 (table)
American Board of Medical Specialties (ABMS), 6, 16, 307, 321, 326
American Board of Obstetrics and Gynecology, 148, 174
American Board of Orthopedic Surgery, 21, 72, 302
American Board of Pediatrics, 20, 277, 299
American College of Anesthesiologists, 106
American College of Emergency Physicians, 260-261
American College of Physicians, 108, 279-282
American Conference on Research in Medical Education, 336

American Heart Association, 270
American Medical Association, 5, 325
American Specialty Boards, 321
Anderson, J., 83, 103, 238
Andrew, B. J., 17, 19, 20, 261, 265
Animal models in technical skills assessment, 262-263, 267-272
Assessment methods, selection of, 297, 301-305. See also Measurement properties
Association of American Medical Colleges (AAMC), 298, 306
Audience effect on direct observation, 56, 57-58
Audit, chart, see Medical record review

Bales, R. F. 239, 243
Barnes, E. J., 74, 83
Barrows, H. S., 27, 111, 112, 332
Bayesian diagnosis, 17, 28-29, 201, 214
Behavior Test of Interpersonal Skills for Health Professionals, 239, 245
Bendig, A. W., 130
Bentsen, B. G., 144, 146, 152, 153
Berner, E. S., 113
Best, A., 238
Bligh, T. J., 193
Bloom, B. S., 100

Board certification, *see* Certification

Board of Censors of the Royal College of General Practitioners, 113

Branching PMPs, *see* Patient management problems

Brigham, C. R., 205

British National Health Service, 343

Brockway, B., 238

Brockway Medical Interview Checklist, 238

Brody, D. S., 253

Brook, R. H., 31, 144, 146, 149, 159-160, 173

Brown, C. R., 171

Brumback, G. B., 125, 134

Bull, G. M., 72, 75, 81, 83, 84, 97

Campbell, R., 238

Campbell, D. T., 336

Canada
    certification in, 319-320
    licensing in, 314-315, 317

Canadian Council of Hospital Accreditation, 171

Carkhuff, R. R., 235, 238, 242, 243

Carkhuff Rating Scale for Empathy, 238, 242, 243

Carter, H. D., 75, 83

CASE system, 204, 206, 208, 210, 212. *See also* Computer simulations

Castle, W., 336

Categorization of clinical competence, 32, 297, 298-301

CBX project, 204, 206, 207, 208, 210. *See also* Computer simulations

Ceiling effect, 130

Center for the Study of Medical Education, 72

Certification, 5-6, 11, 302, 318-324
    re-, 6, 11, 148, 154, 174, 324-327
    validation problems, 322-324

Chart audit, *see* Medical record review

Clemente, C., 298, 306

Clute, K. F., 23-24, 30, 96, 144, 146, 157, 159

CME, 170-171, 324-326

Codes of physician behavior, 313-314

College of Family Physicians of Canada, 6, 20, 21, 62, 108, 226, 261, 302

Collopy, B. T., 157

Colton, T., 77, 83, 84, 88

Competence, clinical
    assessment methods, selection of, 297, 301-305
    categorization of, 32, 297, 298-301
    defining, *see* Defining clinical competence
    historical perspective on, *see* Historical perspective on clinical competence
    research needs, see Research needs
    variation in range of, 144-147
    see also Measurement properties

Comprehensiveness, 42, 43
    direct observation, 54-55
    essay examinations, 96, 114
    MCQ, 100-102, 110, 114
    medical record review, 152
    MEQ, 112, 114
    PMPs, 185-186
    simulated patients, 222
    technical skills assessment methods, 262-263
    written examinations, 96, 100-102, 112, 114

Comprehensive qualifying evaluation (CQE), 299

Computer-aided diagnosis, 202-203

Computer-aided instruction (CAI), 202-203

Computer simulations, 201-216, 304
    for assessment of technical skills, 267-272
    vs. CAI, 202
    vs. computer-aided diagnosis, 202-203
    credibility, 206-207, 209
    educational considerations, 206-207, 214-215

feasibility, 206-207, 212-214
measurement properties, 205-
215
vs. other forms of simulation,
advantages of, 203-205
precision, 206-207, 209-210
validity, 206-207, 210-212
Concurrent Quality Assurance
(CQA), 162-163, 166
Concurrent validity, 42, 45-46
direct observation, 63
MCQ, 103-105
medical record review, 155-164
MEQ, 113
PMPs, 189-192
written examinations, 103-105,
113
see also Validity
Construct validity, 42, 47
direct observation, 63
MCQ, 105-107
medical record review, 164-165
MEQ, 112-113
PMPs, 187-189
research needs, 333-334, 339
written examinations, 105-
107, 112-113
see also Validity
Consumer opinion definition of
competence, 17, 29-30
Content validity, *see* Comprehen-
siveness
Continuing medical education
(CME), 170-171, 324-326
Coordination Council on Medical
Education, 325
Corley, J. B., 60, 62
Corley, K. F., 194
Cost, *see* Feasibility
Cost containment policies, 8
Cowles, J. T., 21, 97-98, 121, 125,
129, 131
Cox, K., 77, 107
CPMP, 207. *See also* Computer
simulations
Credibility, 41, 42
computer simulations, 206-
207, 209
direct observation, 53-54

essay examinations, 95, 114
MCQ, 98-100, 110, 114
medical record review, 149-151
MEQ, 112, 114
oral examinations, 73-74
PMPs, 185
simulated patients, 221-222
technical skills assessment methods, 262-263
written examinations, 95, 98-
100, 110, 112, 114
CRISYS, 207. *See also* Computer
simulations
"Critical incident" approach to competence, 20-22
Cronbach, L. J., 339
Curriculum, 7
"informal," 7-8

Data collection in medical record
review, 144-145
Data interpretation in medical
record review, 144-145
David, F. B., 41, 49
Dawes, K. S., 158
Death, major causes of, 344-345
Decision analysis approach to competence, 26, 28-29
de Dombal, F. T., 167, 206, 209,
211, 214-215
Defining clinical competence, 3
categorization, 32, 297, 298-
301
descriptive studies, 17, 23-25
dimensions of competence, 15-
16
epidemiologic and quality-of-
care approaches, 17-18,
30-31
methods of defining physician
activity (overview), 16-18
patient and consumer opinion,
17, 29-30
reflective/philosophic approach,
17, 18-19
studies of diagnostic thinking,
17, 26-29
task analysis approaches, 17,
19-22

Delaney, P. V., 261, 265
DeNio, J. N., 86, 126
Derbyshire, R. C., 5
Dershewitz, R. A., 153
Descriptive studies of competence,
    17, 23-25
Diagnostic management problem
    (DMP), 184, 196, 197-
    198. *See also* Patient
    management problems
Diagnostic tests, 275-292
    accuracy in, 283
    bias in, 283
    concepts essential to effective
        ordering and interpretation
        of, 283-287
    current teaching and learning
        concepts essential to effec-
        tive use of, 287-288
    definition of competence in use
        of, 277-282
    excessive use of, 275-277
    future teaching and evaluation
        of use of, 289-291
    and medical record review, 144-
        145
    observer variation in, 283
    and PMPs, 185
    precision in, 283
    predictive value in, 283-286
    range of normal of, 286-287
    sensitivity in, 283-286
    specificity in, 283-286
Diagnostic thinking, studies of,
    17, 26-29
Diamond, H. S., 207, 213
Dickie, G. L., 144, 146, 164, 170
Dickinson, C. J., 206
Diederich, 121
Dielman T. E., 132, 134
DiMatteo, R., 240
Dinsdale, S. M., 173
Direct observation, 17, 23-24, 51-
    67, 304
    audience effect in, 56, 57-58
    comprehensiveness, 54-55
    credibility, 53-54
    definition of term, 52
    educational effect, 66-67

expectation bias in, 55-56
feasibility, 64-65
historical perspectives on, 51-
    52
interaction between observa-
    tional task and observer,
    59-60
measurement properties, 53-67
precision, 55-62
reactivity of process, 56, 58-62
realism of, 54-55
sources of bias in, 56
technical skills assessment, 262-
    263, 264-267
traits/training of observer, 61-
    62
uses and rationale, 52-53
validity, 62-63
Dixon, R. H., 144, 146, 170, 276
Doctor-patient relationship, 233-
    254
assessment methods, 236-252
assessment of the information
    base regarding skills for ef-
    fective, 241-243
comparison of discrimination,
    formulation, and perfor-
    mance tests on selected test
    characteristics, 238-239
    (table)
and consumer movement, 234
defining, 235
deterioration in, 234
discrimination tests, 241-242
formulation tests, 242-243
history of, 233-234
information provided by patient,
    246-250
measurement of physician/stu-
    dent attitudes and attri-
    butes, 237-240
measures of doctor-patient
    agreement on, 250-252
measures of physician/student
    behavior with patients,
    243-246
patient-based information re-
    garding, 246-252
Doll, R., 344

Donabedian, A., 52
Donnelly, M. B., 123, 127, 188, 189, 191, 193
Dowaliby, F. J., 127
Doyle, B. J., 249
Doyle, M., 78

Ebel, R. L., 96, 98, 138
Education, implications for, of competence assessment, 297-309
   categorization, problem of, 297, 298-301
   educational differentiation, problem of, 297-298, 305-308
   selecting assessment tools, problem of, 297, 301-305
Educational considerations, 43, 48-49
   computer simulations, 206-207, 214-215
   direct observation, 66-67
   essay examinations, 97, 114
   MCQ, 108-109, 110, 114
   medical record review, 167-175
   MEQ, 113, 114
   oral examinations, 88
   simulated patients, 224-225
   written examinations, 97, 108-109, 114
Edwards Personal Preference Schedule (EPPS), 237
Ekwo, E. E., 54, 64, 66
Elements of Effective Communication, 238, 244
Ellis, J., 89
Elstein, A. S., 26, 27, 54, 112, 333
Emergency care and medical records review, 146-147
Engel, G. L., 65
Epidemiologic definitions of competence, 17-18, 30-31
Epidemiologic studies of competence, 17, 24-25, 30-31
Erviti, V., 125, 129, 131
Essay examinations, 94, 95-97, 114
   comprehensiveness, 96

credibility, 95
educational considerations, 97
feasibility, 97
precision, 96
validity, 96-97
   see also Written examinations
Essentials of a Modern Medical Practice Act, 312
Evans, J. R., 345
Evans, L., 76, 78, 83, 84
Examinations, *see* Oral examinations; Written examinations
Expectation effect in direct observation, 55-56
Experts, consensus of, approach to competence, 19-20

Face validity, *see* Credibility
Family Medicine Residency Programs (Canada), 62, 63
Feasibility, 43, 47-48
   computer simulations, 206-207, 212-214
   direct observation, 64-65
   essay examinations, 97, 114
   MCQ, 108, 110, 114
   medical record review, 165-167
   MEQ, 113, 114
   oral examinations, 87
   technical skills assessment methods, 262-263
   written examinations, 97, 108, 110, 113, 114
Federation Licensing Examination (FLEX), 316, 317
Federation of State Medical Boards (FSMB), 312, 316
Feedback
   direct observation, 66
   global rating scales, 123-124
Feightner, J. W., 212
Feinstein, A. R., 215
Feletti, G. I., 112
Fessel, W. J., 150-151, 160
Fiel, N. J., 266
Finchman, S. M., 209
Fletcher, R. H., 166

Foreign medical students, assessing,
148
FORTRAN, 213
Freeman, J., 113
Free-response tests, 111
Friedman, R. B., 207, 208, 209,
210, 211, 212, 213, 222
Fries, J. F., 345
Funkenstein, D., 9
Futcher, P. H., 72

Gallagher, R., 123
Gardner, B., 127, 133
Geertsma, R. H., 129
General Medical Council (U.K.),
317-318
Gerrard, B., 239, 245, 246
Global rating scales, 101, 104, 119-
138, 304
advantages of, 122-124
anchoring, 131, 136
checklists, use of, 136
history of, 121
items of, as source of imprecision, 128-132
limitations of, 135-136
measurement properties, 124-
128
number of points, 137
pooling ratings, 137-138
precision, 124-125
raters, as source of imprecision,
133-135
raters, training of, 137
recommendations on, 135-138
scale, as source of imprecision,
132-133
validity, 125-128
Goetz, A. A., 164
Goldstein, A., 77
Gonnella, J., 151
Goran, M. J., 31, 45, 190, 339
Gori, G. B., 343
Gorry, G. A., 207
Gough, H. G., 126, 134
Governmental influence on clinical
competence, 8
Graded problem-oriented record
(GPOR), 155

Grayson, M., 238
Green, E., 78-79
Greenfield, S., 151, 158, 160
Grimm, R. H., 167
Griner, P. F., 277
Guildford, J. P., 130

Halio, J. L., 88
Halo effect, 75, 135, 136, 137
Hammett, W. H., 144, 146, 155
Hammond, K. R., 125, 134
Harden, R. M., 64, 266-267, 271,
303
Harless, W. G., 201, 206, 208
Harper, A. C., 226
HARVEY, 272
Hastings, G. E., 144, 146, 154, 163
Hawthorne effect, 330
Health, determinants of, 343-345
Health care, implications for, of com-
petence assessment, 342-
351
Health care research, 10-12
Helfer, R. E., 197, 239
Hermann, N., 154
Hess, J., 235, 239
Hippocrates, 18
Historical perspectives on clinical
competence, 4-11
force fields, convergence of,
10-12
profession, influence of, 4-8
research and development, in-
fluence of, 9-10
society, influence of, 8-9
History taking
computerized, 201
direct observation assessment
of, 53, 54-55, 61, 66
and medical record review, 144-
145
and PMPs, 185
Hodgkin, K., 110
Hollifield, G., 239
Holloway, C. D., 166
Holloway, P. J., 76, 78, 79, 83
Holt, R. R., 135
Hopkins Interpersonal Skills Assessment, 238

Hubbard, J. P., 71, 72, 75, 94, 187, 193, 206, 316
Hulka, B. S., 30, 249-252
Hutter, M., 239
Huxham, G. J., 97

Illich, I., 348
INDEX, 206, 210. *See also* Computer simulations
Index of Communication, 238
Index of Facilitative Discrimination, 238
Information-processing approaches to competence, 26-28
Insurance
    malpractice, 8
    medical, 8
Interaction Process Analysis (IPA), 239, 243-244
Internal consistency, 44
Interpersonal Relationship Rating Scale, 239
Interpersonal-relationship skills
    direct observation assessment of, 54-55, 61, 66, 67
    and global rating scales, 122-123
    oral examination assessment of, 73
Interview Evaluation Scale, 238
Interviewing skills
    direct observation assessment of, 53, 54-55, 61
    oral examination assessment of, 73
In-training evaluation reports (ITERs), 86, 101, 104, 120, 319-320, 323

Jackson, D. N., 129
Jarrett, F., 239
Johnson, P. E., 207
Joint Commission on the Accreditation of Hospitals, 171, 174
Jordan, A., 241
Jungfer, C. C., 157

Kagan, N., 238, 244
Kane, R. L., 144, 146, 160, 164

Kegel-Flom, P., 126, 133
Kent, R. N., 53, 57, 61
Kessner, D. M., 144, 146
Kleinmuntz, B., 27
Kling, S., 100-101
Knox, J. D. E., 111, 112
Korsch, B. M., 29, 247
Kroeger, H. H., 157-158, 166

Laboratory tests, *see* Diagnostic tests
Lamont, C. T., 226
Landy, F. J., 132, 133
Leeper, D. J., 206, 211
Lembcke, P. A., 156
Levine, H. G., 72, 80-81, 83, 84-85, 87, 131, 186, 188
Lewy, A., 186
Licensing agencies, 314-315
Licensure, 5-6, 311-318
    re-, 6, 11, 324-327
Life expectancy, 343-345
Likert, R. A., 121
Lindsay, M. I., 145, 147, 161
Linear PMPs, *see* Patient management problems
Linn, L., 131
Lipscomb, P. R., 73
Lipton, A., 240
Lipworth, L., 31
Littlefield, J. H., 83, 88
Liu, P., 265
Lloyd, G., 145, 147
Logs, procedural approach to competence, 22
Ludbrook, J. H., 76, 83, 85
Lyons, T. F., 152, 159

Maatsch, J. L., 75, 82, 83, 85, 87, 104, 106, 219
MACMAN, 206. *See also* Computer simulations
MACPEE, 206
MACPUFF, 206
Maguire, G. P., 66
Malpractice, 8-9
Management skills
    direct observation assessment of, 54-55, 61

Management skills (*continued*)
  and medical record review, 146-
    147
  and PMPs, 185
Margolis, C. Z., 145, 147, 155, 159
Marshall, J., 193-194
Marshall, V. R., 76, 83
Martin, A. R., 169-170
Martin, I. C., 196
Mash, E. J., 61
Mathews, B., 238, 242
MATRIX, 207. *See also* Computer
    simulations
McCarthy, W. H., 191
McGuire, C. H., 77, 80-81, 84-85,
    100, 106-107, 185, 186,
    188, 189, 190, 191, 192
McKeown, T., 343-344
McLeskey, C. H., 106
McMaster University, 88, 220, 248,
    303
MCQ, *see* Multiple-choice questions
McSherry, C. K., 166
Measurement, definition of, 39-40
Measurement properties, 3, 40-49
  comprehensiveness, 42, 43-44.
    See also Comprehensiveness
  of computer simulations, 205-
    215
  credibility, 41, 42. *See also*
    Credibility
  of direct observation, 53-67
  educational considerations, 43,
    48-49. *See also* Educational
    considerations
  feasibility, 43, 47-48. *See also*
    Feasibility
  of global rating scales, 124-128
  of medical record review, 149-
    175
  of oral examinations, 73-88
  outline of, 42-43 (table)
  of patient management prob-
    lems, 184-192
  precision, 42, 44-45. *See also*
    Precision
  of simulated patients, 221-225
  of technical skills assessment
    methods, 262-263

  validity, 42, 45-47. *See also*
    Validity
Mechanical simulations for technical
    skills assessment, 267-272
Medical Council of Canada, 43-44,
    101, 315
Medical education, *see* Education
Medical Interview Satisfaction Scale
    (MISS), 247-248
Medical Knowledge Self-Assessment
    Program (MKSAP), 108,
    279-282, 306, 327
Medical record review, 48, 63, 142-
    176, 304
  completeness of recording,
    155-159
  comprehensiveness, 152
  concurrent validity, 155-164
  construct validity, 164-165
  credibility, 149-151
  educational considerations, 167-
    175
  feasibility, 165-167
  formative applications, 168-
    173
  format of records, 148-149
  vs. PMPs, 190-191
  precision, 152-155
  predictive validity, 165
  relationship to patient out-
    comes, 155, 159-163
  relationship to physician judg-
    ments, 155, 163-164
  strengths of, 175
  in undergraduate education,
    142-143
  validity, 155-165
  variation in the range of compo-
    nents in clinical competence
    in different studies, 144-
    147 (table)
  weaknesses of, 175-176
Medical schools
  assessment of, 5
  training programs, quality of,
    6-8
MEQ, *see* Modified essay questions
MERIT, 207. *See also* Computer
    simulations

Merrill, J. A., 145, 147
Meskauskas, M. S., 76, 83
Michigan State University Office of
    Medical Education, 205
Miller, G., 47, 84-85, 87
MKSAP (MKSAP-V), 108, 279-
    282, 306, 327
Modified essay questions (MEQ),
    94, 110-111
    measurement properties, 112-
        113, 114
    see also Written examinations
Morehead, M. A., 153, 173
Moses, L. E., 30
Mueller, C. B., 260
Multiple-choice questions (MCQ),
    11, 41, 43, 45, 94, 97-
    110, 114, 123
    comprehensiveness, 100-102,
        110, 114
    concurrent validity, 103-105
    construct validity, 105-107
    credibility, 98-100, 110, 114
    educational considerations,
        108-109, 110, 114
    feasibility, 108, 110, 114
    vs. oral examinations, 81-85
    vs. PMPs, 189
    precision, 44, 102-103, 110,
        114
    predictive validity, 105
    validity, 103-107, 110, 114
    see also Written examinations
Murphy, J., 286
Murray, H. A., 237
Murray, T. S., 113

Naeraa, N., 95
Naftulin, D. H., 225
National Board of Medical Examiners
    (NBME), 20-21, 71-72,
    127, 183, 186, 193, 196,
    204, 208, 299, 314-316
National Library of Medicine, 205
National Self-Evaluation Program of
    College of Family Physi-
    cians of Canada, 108
Nelson, A. R., 145, 147, 168
Nerenberg, R. L., 192

Neufeld, V. R., 145, 147, 170
Newble, D. I., 61
Nobrega, F. T., 150-151, 161
Norman G. R., 157, 159, 191, 221,
    223
Nunnally, J. C., 130
Nurse practitioners, assessing compe-
    tence of, 148

Objective Structured Clinical Exam-
    ination (OSCE), 303
Objectivity, 44-45. *See also* Preci-
    sion
Observation, *see* Direct observation
O'Donohue, W. J., 76, 81, 83, 86
ODSAL, 206. *See also* Computer
    simulations
Ontario Economic Council, 343
Open-ended questions, 111. *See
    also* Modified essay ques-
    tions
Oral examinations, 44, 46, 71-90,
    304
    credibility, 73-74
    current and historical impor-
        tance of, 71-73
    educational considerations, 88
    feasibility, 87
    level of training and perform-
        ance on, 87
    vs. MCQ, 81-85
    measurement properties, 73-88
    vs. other measures of clinical
        competence, 81-86
    precision, 74-81
    triple jump exercise, 88, 303
    validity, 81-87
    variation in, due to candidates,
        77-79
    variation in, due to examiners,
        74-77
    variation in, due to oral type and
        content, 80-81
    and written examinations, cor-
        relation between, 81-86
Osborne, C. E., 152
Osler, W., 18
Ostrow, D. N., 222
Owen, A., 226

Page, G. G., 192
Palva, I. P., 188
Paper-and-pencil tests, *see* Written
    examinations
Paper simulations, 94
Parker, S., 237
Parlow, J., 237
Pascoe, L., 237, 238, 242
Paterson, D. G., 121
Patient card decks, 184, 196-197.
    See also Patient manage-
    ment problems
Patient definitions of competence,
    17, 29-30
Patient education, 9
Patient feedback form (PFF), 248
Patient management problems
    (PMPs), 24-25, 44, 45-46,
    47-48, 63, 72, 104, 111,
    123, 127, 183-198, 304,
    316, 317
  branching, 186, 188-189
  comprehensiveness, 185-186
  computerized, 204, 209, 211.
    See also Computer simula-
    tions
  concerns regarding, 195
  concurrent validity, 189-192
  construct validity, 187-189
  credibility, 185
  educational effect, 194
  educational perspective, poten-
    tial from, 184
  evaluation perspective, potential
    from, 184
  history of use, 183-184
  linear, 186, 187
  measurement criteria, 184-192
  other written simulations, 196-
    198
  precision, 186
  predictive validity, 192
  scoring, 193-194
  strengths of, 195
  validity, 187-192
Patient record review, *see* Medical
    record review
Patient satisfaction questionnaire
    (PSQ), 249-250

Pawluk, W., 192
Payne, B. C., 145, 147, 154, 162,
    165-166
Payne Process Audit, 174
Peer Scientific Review Organization,
    171
Penta, F. B., 271
Performance
  vs. competence, 15
  definition of, 39-40
Personality characteristics and oral
    examination performance,
    79
Personality Research Form (PRF),
    237
Personal Orientation Inventory
    (POI), 237, 240, 242
Peterson, O. L., 23, 30, 157, 159,
    322
P4 Deck, 196-197. *See also* Patient
    management problems
Physical examination
  direct observation assessment of,
    53, 54-55, 61, 66
  and medical record review, 144-
    145
  and PMPs, 185
Physician(s)
  expectations by society of the
    competent, 349-351
  role of the individual, 347-348
Physician assistants, assessing compe-
    tence of, 148
Physician-patient relationship, *see*
    Doctor-patient relationship
Physician-Patient Situation Test,
    238, 241
Physician Performance Index (PPI),
    154, 162, 174
Physician's Recognition Award, 325
Pickering, E., 11
Pickering, G., 98
Pierleoni, R. G., 127
Plato, 18
PMPs, *see* Patient management
    problems
Pokorny, A. D., 77, 78, 83, 84
POMR (POR), *see* Problem Oriented
    Medical Record

Portable patient problem pack, 184, 196-197. *See also* Patient management problems
PPI, 154, 162, 174
Practice activities, studies of, 25
Precision, 42, 44-45
    computer simulations, 206-207, 209-210
    diagnostic tests, 283
    direct observation, 55-62
    essay examinations, 96, 114
    global rating scales, 124-125
    MCQ, 102-103, 110, 114
    medical record review, 152-155
    MEQ, 112, 114
    oral examinations, 74-81
    PMPs, 186
    research needs, 338-339
    simulated patients, 222-223
    technical skills assessment methods, 262-263
    written examinations, 96, 102-103, 110, 112, 114
Predictive criterion validity, 46. *See also* Predictive validity
Predictive validity, 42, 46
    diagnostic tests, 283-286
    direct observation, 62
    MCQ, 105, 114
    medical record review, 165
    MEQ, 113
    PMPs, 189-192
    written examinations, 105, 113
    see also Validity
Pressey, S. L., 74
Printen, K. J., 125
Problem box, 111
Problem formulation, 144-145
Problem identification, 144-145
Problem Oriented Medical Record (POMR. POR), 148, 155, 156, 166, 168-173, 176. *See also* Medical record review
Problem-solving skills
    direct observation assessment of, 54-55, 61, 67
    oral examination assessment of, 73

Procedural logs approach to competence, 22
Process Check Sheet, 239
Professional Standards Review Organizations (PSRO), 5, 8, 162
Profile of Non-Verbal Sensitivity (PONS), 238, 240
Prognostic accuracy, 46. *See also* Predictive validity
Programmed patients, *see* Simulated patients
Provincial Medical Council (Canada), 314-315, 317
Pseudopatients, *see* Simulated patients
Psychotherapy Interaction Scale (PIA), 239, 244

Quality assurance, 5, 8, 12, 30-31, 325
Queen's University Interviewer Rating Scale, 239

Rakel, R. E., 145, 147
Rasche, L., 238, 241
Recertification, 6, 11, 148, 154, 174, 324-327
Record review, *see* Medical record review
Reed, D. E., 145, 147, 171
Reflective/philosophical definitions of competence, 17, 18-19
Reid, J. B., 59
Reliability, *see* Precision
Relicensure, 6, 11, 324-327
Renaud, M., 226
Repeatability, *see* Precision
Research and development influence on competence, 9-10, 10-12
Research needs, 330-341
    appropriate statistical analysis, 340
    basic questions, 331-335
    critique of methodology, 336-340
    determinants of clinical competence, 335

Research needs (*continued*)
   inadequate measures develop-
     ment, problem of, 338-339
   inappropriate experimental de-
     sign, problem of, 337-338
   inappropriate question, problem
     of, 336-337
   measurement of clinical per-
     formance, 332-333
   relationship between clinical
     competence and other meas-
     ures, 333-334
Residency Review Committees, 321
Response-to-Patient Inventory, 238,
   242
Resusci-Ann, 270
Rimoldi, H. J. A., 183
Rimoldi card deck, 183, 196, 197.
   See also Patient manage-
   ment problems
Robbins, A. S., 237, 244
Robinson, S. A., 198
Role-playing oral, 85
Romm, F. J., 162
Rosenthal, R., 238, 240
Rosinski, E. F., 88
Rothman, A. I., 103-104
Royal College of General Prac-
   tice of Australia, 194
Royal College of General practi-
   tioners, 110
Royal College of Physicians and
   Surgeons of Canada, 6, 47,
   319, 323
Royal Free Hospital, London, 174
R. S. McLaughlin Examination and
   Research Center, 315,
   319
Rugg, H., 134
Ryden, M., 239

Sackett, D. L., 286
Samph, T., 4
Sanazaro, P. J., 21, 145, 147, 148,
   150, 162, 167, 168
Sandler, G., 281
Sanson-Fisher, R. W., 223
Saywell, R. M., 145, 147, 153
Schneiderman, H., 203, 206

Schumacher, C. F., 109, 187, 207,
   210, 211
Scope and style of review, 12-14
Scott, H. M., 145, 147, 164
Self-assessment and medical record
   review, 146-147
Senior, J. R., 15, 204, 206, 210, 213
Sensitivity of diagnostic tests, 283-
   286
Sequential management problem
   (SMP), 184, 196. *See also*
   Patient management prob-
   lems
Shaw, G. B., 348
Short-answer tests, 111. *See also*
   Modified essay questions
Sibley, J. C., 104-105, 145, 147,
   150, 151, 153, 308
SIM-1 project, 201, 204, 207, 208,
   214, 272. *See also* Computer simulations
Simborg, D. W., 172
Simulated clinical encounters (SCE),
   104
Simulated Patient Encounter (SPE),
   219
Simulated patients, 219-227
   advantages of technique, 220
   applications of, 225-226
   comprehensiveness, 222
   credibility, 221-222
   educational effect, 224-225
   measurement criteria, 221-225
   precision, 222-223
   for technical skills assessment,
     267-272
   training of, 220-221
   validity, 223-224
Simulated recall and direct observation, 54, 64, 66
Simulations, *see* Computer simulations; Patient management
   problems; Simulated patients
Sixteen Personality Factor Test
   (16PF), 240
Skakun, E., 86, 104, 211, 323
Skendzel, L. P., 283
Smith, P. C., 132